CHILDREN
OF
PSYCHIATRISTS

and other
psychotherapists

THOMAS
MAEDER

PERENNIAL LIBRARY

HARPER & ROW, PUBLISHERS, New York

Grand Rapids, Philadelphia, St. Louis, San Francisco
London, Singapore, Sydney, Tokyo, Toronto

A hardcover edition of this book was published in 1989 by Harper & Row, Publishers.

First PERENNIAL LIBRARY edition published 1990.

Designed by Karen Savary

The Library of Congress has cataloged the hardcover edition as follows:

Maeder, Thomas.
   Children of psychiatrists and other psychotherapists.
   Bibliography: p.
   Includes index.
   1. Children of psychotherapists—Mental health. I. Title. [DNLM: 1. Child Psychology.   2. Parent–Child Relations.   3. Psychotherapy. WS 105.5.F2 M184c]
RJ507.P84M34   1989   155.4   88-45524
ISBN 0-06-016064-0

ISBN 0-06-091663-x (pbk.)
90 91 92 93 94   FG   10 9 8 7 6 5 4 3 2 1

To
Shawn
Morgan
Sara
and
Max

Contents

Si notre vie manque de soufre,
c'est-à-dire d'une constante magie,
c'est qu'il nous plaît de regarder
nos actes et de nous perdre en
considérations sur les formes
rêvées de nos actes, au lieu
d'être poussés par eux.

——ANTONIN ARTAUD

Introduction

"Shrinks' kids are nuts."

The saying is frequently heard, and it is widely, cheerfully, often seriously believed. Anyone identified as the child of a psychiatrist or psychoanalyst is suddenly viewed in a new light: "Oh, so that's why you're crazy?" or "Well, why *aren't* you crazy, then? They all are, you know." Nothing comparable afflicts the children of plumbers, dermatologists, businessmen, or painters: no one asks "Does your sink drip?" or "How come your complexion's so clear?"

Psychoanalysis, psychiatry, and other forms of psychotherapy were devised to help people resolve personal difficulties and grow to lead free and satisfying lives. This is part of a parent's role as well. Unlike lay parents, psychotherapists are trained to observe and understand, to deal with life's crises, to know when to intervene and when to let things follow their natural course. Assuming that more knowledge is better than less, that understanding and experience are useful things to have, then—other things being equal—therapists *ought* to have a slight edge over the ordinary, amateur parent who just muddles along with common sense and Dr. Spock. Certainly they should not do worse. Yet psychotherapists are reputed to fail at child rearing on a spectacular and grotesquely comical scale. Is this indeed true? And why? Or why not?

The simple and rather unexciting answer is that some "shrinks' " kids are "crazy" and most of them are not, much the same as everyone else. The more interesting question, to my mind, is a less trivial one: whether those therapists' kids who are emotionally troubled, as well as those who are sane, brilliant, foolish, fascinating, charming, obnoxious, boring, or anything else, are so in ways discernibly different from their peers and directly attributable to their parents. Are there common features to be found among the children of psychotherapists, ones more subtle than mere demographic and economic similarities, that stem from different manners of behaving and of understanding behavior? It appears that there are.

3

If psychotherapist parents do have significant effects upon their children, does it result from their training alone, from their personalities, or from both? What, if any, advantages do their education and experience give them in helping their children through developmental and practical crises? Can techniques originally devised for the cure of existing problems be profitably used in a prophylactic or pedagogical manner? Do therapists analyze their children? (always the first question everyone asks). Are they better at understanding their children's behavior, and if so, are the consequences beneficial or harmful? To what extent do the children absorb therapeutic or analytic knowledge and techniques, and does it affect their manner of viewing themselves and of interacting with others?

My own interest in this topic stems from a very simple origin: my father was a psychoanalyst and my mother a clinical social worker. Psychoanalysis formed a large part of my family's identity, just as, with the first floor of our house entirely occupied by offices and my parents working long hours each day, six or seven days a week, it dictated much of the household's daily routine. I heard about psychoanalysis, read about it, took pride in it, and held beliefs my friends did not share about what people are like and why they act as they do. I sometimes felt that I was different from other children, as most children do, though I, unlike them, was offered the chance to attribute part of this real or imagined difference to a convenient external factor—my parents' profession.

I was not alone in these sentiments. A good friend of mine in high school was also the child of a psychiatrist and a psychoanalyst. We found that we shared certain somewhat uncommon intellectual, literary, and artistic interests. We prided ourselves on being slightly bizarre, and we occasionally, though usually in jest, exchanged speculations on how much of this might be attributable to our parents' professions and how much credit we deserved ourselves. At one point he and his sister and I toyed with the thought of a "Shrunken Kids Party" for the children of psychiatrists, most appropriately held, someone suggested, in a Hall of Mirrors.

Years later, when I began looking into the subject more seriously, in part at the urging of a friend and editor who, it turned out, had been my parents' patient, I found that it intrigued far more people than I suspected, both professional and lay. The American Psychiatric Association had hosted sessions on "Children and Psychiatrist Parents" at its 1979 and 1980 annual meetings. Various regional psychiatric organizations had held panel discussions. These sessions always drew unusually large audiences and tended to be remembered years afterward, but somehow discussions never progressed very far, as though it were uncomfortable to delve too deeply. David Reiser, an analytically trained psychiatrist and the son of a psychoanalyst, presented a paper entitled "The Sorcerer and the Mirror—Psychiatrists and Their Children" at a 1980 meeting of the Colorado Child and Adolescent Society. It is a very thoughtful and serious paper, and he was consequently surprised to learn that the first announcements mailed out about his presentation billed it as "My Father the Shrink, by David E. Reiser," something he found offensively flippant and felt betrayed a certain amount of anxiety over admitting that it was a truly significant topic. At his insistence, new flyers were issued.[1]

As part of my research I wrote to the presidents of all the regional psychoanalytic and psychiatric associations in the United States to ask whether the topic had been discussed by their members and to solicit their personal views. I anticipated a cool reception, since psychiatrists and psychoanalysts take considerable abuse under the best of circumstances, and might understandably look askance at someone doing research on whether or not they damage their children. On the contrary, they were very interested and encouraging. Some, of course, thought there could be nothing to the myth that psychotherapists' children are unusual, and predicted that my conclusions would boil down to a disappointingly brief disclaimer; yet they were willing to keep an open mind and to provide whatever help I might need. Of more than 110 letters sent out, well over half elicited replies, of which only 2 were genuinely hostile.

In light of the interest in the topic, it is surprising to learn how little has been written. There are six pages on analysts' children in one of psychoanalyst Heinz Kohut's impenetrable theoretical works, and brief sections in German analyst Alice Miller's various books on child rearing and emotional child abuse. Several general articles in the professional literature on the emotional problems of psychotherapists or the emotional burdens of practicing therapy mention repercussions in the family. The most specific piece on psychiatrists' children was a 1977 article by Ross Wetzsteon in the *Village Voice*.[2] A number of psychiatrists told me they had thought of writing something on the subject, but when they searched the literature and found that nothing had been written before, they decided, with that incomprehensible logic peculiar to certain academics, that they therefore could not write about it either. Any number of the therapists' children I interviewed had dreamed about writing something on the subject, and virtually without exception they welcomed my research.

The conclusions in this book are based on interviews with more than two hundred children of psychotherapists—mostly psychoanalysts and psychiatrists, fewer clinical psychologists and social workers. On average the interviews lasted an hour: the shortest were just under half an hour, the longest was more than twenty hours spread out over six sessions. I also interviewed about fifty psychotherapists who are not also the children of therapists, either in their capacity as parents or because they specialized in child and adolescent psychiatry or had treated numerous therapists' children. In addition, I have carried on an extensive correspondence. At one point I attempted to use a questionnaire to obtain large amounts of information from more people than could be individually interviewed, but the response rate to the lengthy questionnaire was so poor, and the results generally so much more superficial than what could be learned in even brief interviews, that this attempt was abandoned.

Locating psychotherapists' children was something of a problem.* There is no easy way to find them in large numbers: for obvious reasons professional directories give little personal information about therapists. Many were found through friends and acquaintances, and, by word of mouth, through their friends and acquaintances. Therapists and several professional organizations supplied the names of children of colleagues and members. My doctor's receptionist, a publicist at Harper & Row, a co-speaker at a Book and Author luncheon, a librarian helping out with a reference, and many other such miscellaneous folk supplied names of friends, acquaintances, or people they had heard of or read about who were psychotherapists' children. I asked each person I interviewed for the names of others.

An "Author's Query" in the *New York Times Book Review* yielded several dozen responses that ranged geographically from one mile from my house to Alaska, arrived between one week and two years after the query ran, and varied in tone from a twenty-page autobiographical sketch to an offer from a literary agent to handle the book, a note from a woman I had never met saying she had introduced my parents to each other (apparently true), and the following intriguing anonymous note from New York:

---

* "Children" is something of a misnomer, since my interview subjects are nearly all adults, several of them in their seventies and eighties, but I will call them this nonetheless, since their importance in this project is due solely to their relationship with their parents, no matter how long ago it may have been.

Dear Mr. Maeder,

With regard to your book—I do hope you explore what *others* think of the children of psychiatrists and therapists.

There is a general consensus of parents here in NY, that the most disturbed (mostly meaning neurotic) children are (in order)

1st—children when both parents are psychotherapists

2nd—children whose mother is a psychotherapist

3rd—father is psychotherapist

4th—both parents are psychiatrists

5th—mother is psychiatrist

6th—father is psychiatrist

This general consensus or informal poll has been taken at sandboxes and "the best" private schools in Manhattan.

I am not qualified to speculate why the above breakdown occurs but, trust me, it does. Psychiatrists and therapists make lousy parents!!!

My haphazard manner of locating interview subjects, though slow and unpredictable, had the unforeseen advantage of effectively randomizing my population. Aside from a slightly disproportionate concentration of people from New York, Philadelphia, Boston, and Washington, and a correspondingly slight underrepresentation of Californians and midwesterners, there is no unduly heavy swing in any identifiable direction. Some subjects were suggested as unusually healthy, and some as particularly bizarre. On the whole I believe that a balanced representation was offered, which was what I had sought.

Lawrence Hartmann, a psychiatrist at Harvard and the son of famed analyst Heinz Hartmann, cautioned, "In general I find myself hoping that you will be patient with the drab and the ordinary. I think it is so tempting to take the picturesque, the kinds of things one could write a novel about, or the kinds of things one would make a *New Yorker* cartoon about, as typical. I am always wary of the picturesque getting dramatically more attention than it deserves. I think there is a lot of ordinariness about psychiatrists and psychoanalysts as parents."[3] It is true that there is some risk of making something from nothing, of distorting such a subjective picture, of creating a self-fulfilling prophecy. Moreover, people who have a complaint may rather blame their parents than themselves. Asked to assign a cause for something, particularly when society offers a ready-made explanatory myth, and even more particularly when a writer comes and asks what they blame on being a psychiatrist's child, they may reach for the obvious explanation, and in their eagerness to be helpful may reach unreasonably far. Clearly, some of their attributions will be incorrect, and some of the similarities that appear may be due to other factors or to pure coincidence, and should be regarded at first with skepticism. But eventually, after the same themes recur in one interview after another and emerge as long-standing preoccupations of the children themselves, one must conclude that they mean something.

This book does, admittedly, concentrate on the unfavorable effects that psychotherapists have on their children. It is therefore a somewhat lopsided account in its overall message. I do not claim that most therapists harm their children more than other people do, nor that therapists mostly do harm to their children, neither of which I believe. Most therapists, most of the time, act like anyone else, for better or for worse. But the therapeutic population includes a sizable minority of people who have problems and who create or encourage certain very distinctive problems in their children. As Freud commented, "pathology, by making things larger and coarser, can draw our attention to normal conditions which might otherwise have escaped us."[4] By observing how things can go wrong, we are better equipped to perceive how they might go right, not only among psychotherapists, but for any parent.

It is harder to be a good parent than to be a good therapist. The good effects that therapist parents have on their children are predominantly the result of their personalities and affection, not the consequence of theoretical training. To be a genuinely good parent one must be a good human being, whereas a great deal of help has been rendered to patients by therapists who are personally miserable, self-centered, and even vicious, but who could introduce a little knowledge and objectivity into what had been a totally subjective mess. Conversely, the bad effects of therapist parents are predominantly the result of flaws that afflict them as people rather than by-products of their training, but here the flaws are often much the same ones that led them to become therapists and which encourage them to use therapeutic concepts and techniques in inappropriate ways. "My job hasn't affected me a bit," many therapists have told me. "I came out of my training the same person I was when I went in." Sometimes that is a shame.

Hundreds of people helped with this project, and regrettably the need to protect their and their parents' anonymity prevents me from thanking them publicly. Rather than arbitrarily mentioning the few names that I can, I shall therefore thank none individually, with the exception of David E. Reiser, who not only offered his experience and wisdom, but read a draft of my manuscript and contributed many valuable comments.

As few details as possible have been changed in the quotes and case histories, but whenever a choice had to be made, I chose to protect rather than expose. Alterations have been limited to changes in names, locations, and occasional slight shifts in profession.

Note: In the absence of a gender-neutral third-person-singular pronoun, *he* has been used at various points in this book when speaking of a nameless, faceless, hypothetical individual. This grammatical usage is not intended to imply any assumption about the sex of therapists, children, or patients.

1

The Myth
About
Psychotherapists' Kids

> Of course we're crazy. But unlike most crazy people, we're proud of it.
>
> —A PSYCHIATRIST'S SON

As the curtain goes up in *The Impossible Years*,[1] a successful 1965 Broadway play, Dr. Jack Kingsley, a psychiatrist ("as well adjusted as a psychiatrist can be," the stage directions say), is dictating material for a chapter in a book on raising teenagers. "If I've given you the impression so far that the teen-age girl of today is a trifle sloppy, a trifle wanton, and considerably inconsiderate, don't give up hope. In future chapters I will outline the methods of coping with the typical adolescent girl. As a psychiatrist and a parent I have applied these methods, and as a result I am able to point to my teen-ager and say proudly, 'There is *my* daughter.'" Absolutely no one is surprised when his daughter enters a few moments later, the picture of sloppiness, wantonness, and disrespect. In fact, Dr. Kingsley fares rather well, since the general expectation of psychiatrists' children is far worse.

For most people, the belief that psychiatrists' children are crazy is the logical sequel to a conviction that psychiatrists themselves are nuts. Crazy people have crazy kids. Others suppose that the children's alleged lunacy is the product of the parents' arcane techniques—they are little monsters created by Dr. Sigmund Frankensteins who analyzed and manipulated their children's behavior in strange, unnatural ways. Their methods may or may not be effective in helping adults with existing problems, but they are utterly inappropriate for raising little children. Still others believe that psychiatrists are merely variants on the caricatured absent-minded professor, ineffectual bumblers so lost in abstract theories of behavior and grand images of themselves that they never perceive the real world around them.

The children themselves are divided in their opinions: of those whom I asked why the myth should exist, 47 percent replied "basis in fact," while the rest laid the blame on a gullible world. The parents don't know, either: most of them can think of good reasons why therapists' kids *ought* to have problems and will cheerfully relate horror stories about families they know, yet, not very surprisingly, they assert that their own children are healthy, charming, mature, and that they all get along most wondrously well. They generally suggest that the reputed craziness of therapists' kids is no more than a maliciously witty fictitious belief. But why should such a belief exist?

The notion that psychiatrists are crazy is certainly nothing new to our time. In the late-nineteenth century, when mental health care was almost exclusively institutional, the humor centered around the arbitrary dividing line between eccentricity and insanity. Patients were depicted as quick-witted, lighthearted, fun-loving eccentrics ill tolerated by a sour and pedestrian society. Psychiatrists were venal and foolish at best, vicious and stupid at worst. Possibly the best series of humor books on this theme, beginning with *The Lunatic at Large*, was written by Scottish author and historian J. Storer Clouston, the son of an eminent Edinburgh psychiatrist.[2]

In the 1930s psychiatrists outstripped ministers and general practitioners as preferred butts of social humor, an accurate measure of their growing significance. By the 1950s, between 1 and 2 percent of all cartoons in the *Saturday Evening Post* and *The New Yorker* concerned psychiatrists and their patients[3] and in a randomly chosen 1968 issue of *Medical Economics*, a trade journal for doctors, more than 17 percent of the 110 cartoons dealt with psychiatric topics, though at the time psychiatrists constituted less than 6 percent of the actual medical population, and considerably less of its economics.[4]

In recent years the number of psychiatrist jokes has slightly declined, along, perhaps, with the practice of traditional psychiatry and psychoanalysis themselves. Yet scarcely a week goes by without at least one psychiatrist joke in the newspaper, the subject generally identified by the now largely anachronistic cigar, beard, and Viennese accent. Psychiatrists and analysts are shown as obsessed with sex, interested in nothing but their hourly fees, eager to see problems where none exists, and most often, of course, as crazy.

These jokes and beliefs exist in part because people wish to believe them. Psychiatrists make people uneasy. They represent authority and judgment, much as priests do. They are often suspected of having powers to discern people's deep, dark secrets during casual conversations. One need only watch people's response when they learn that a person they have met is a psychiatrist to know that it is a powerful bit of information, not at all like "I am a lawyer," or "I'm a developer," or "I am a gastroenterologist." Some suddenly look uncomfortable and slip quickly away. Others begin to talk surprisingly intimately about their own problems or personal therapy. As a result, many psychiatrists try to avoid revealing their profession to strangers. They hedge and say "I'm a physician," or "I'm in the mental health field," or else they lie outright. One psychoanalyst told people he was an undertaker, which generally veered the conversation away from the topic of work. Another said whatever came to mind at the time, until the day on the golf course when he said he was a barber and then couldn't find anything to talk to his partners about for the rest of the afternoon.

People ridicule things that make them uncomfortable. How better can one ridicule psychiatrists than to say that they are crazy and that, far from being frighteningly adept at understanding other people, they can't even raise their own kids. Once such a jocular stereotype takes hold, it perpetuates itself and grows. The recollection of a friend of a sister's college roommate who was a shrink's kid and once acted rather strange will fasten the stereotype firmly in place while a dozen humdrum psychiatrists' children, and a hundred troubled cardiologists', schoolteachers', bankers', and shopkeepers' kids slip unobtrusively from memory.

Psychiatrists, moreover, very conveniently fill the role of a stock character needed in social commentaries. To the extent that J. Storer Clouston's novels criticize society's intolerance of individuals who are different, the psychiatrist is merely a handy plenipotentiary representing social stodginess and repression in a highly polished form. Dr. Kingsley of *The Impossible Years* is ultimately little more than any other pompous, self-righteous parent who flounders along trying to raise his children and to persuade himself that he is doing a good job. Being a psychiatrist merely accentuates the large gap between what he thinks and says he does and what he does in fact.

Psychiatrists have grown weary of psychiatrist jokes, though some still collect the cartoons in scrapbooks for their waiting rooms. Many like to believe that such psychological explanations as those mentioned above entirely account for the myth about them. "Psychiatrists aren't crazy," they say smugly, exhibiting one of the dialectical gambits people most often object to in them, "People just need to think that they are." Or, in other words, "It's not me, it's *you*."

These explanations are, indeed, plausible and account for a great deal, yet myths do not spring out of nothing. They may depend heavily upon the projected needs of the believer, but there must be a kernel of truth to begin them and to guide their growth and development. Some psychiatrists are obsessed with sex, some are more interested in money than in cures, and some can scarcely refrain from seeing everything in abstract, psychodynamic terms. And though I will not say something so silly as that psychiatrists and their children are crazy, it is even sillier to deny outright and without reflection that there is anything at all to the notion. Perhaps much of what laymen say in jest has a basis in fact—less grotesque, extreme, and comical, to be sure, and certainly by no means ubiquitous, but nonetheless there.

Many psychotherapists believe that their profession has little or no discernible effect on their children. One psychoanalyst listened indulgently as I outlined my topic, then said that he thought I was wasting my time. The premise was misguided and absurd—the sort of thing laymen like to believe. Psychiatry and psychoanalysis are jobs like any other. One leaves them at the office. One's children are not one's patients. So on and so on—a litany of claims I would come to recognize as clichés of the profession. He went on to say he made sure his profession did not affect his family life, a suspicious statement in itself. When I suggested that a therapist, if faced with a crisis, might resort to his learning rather than his heart, he dismissed the notion. "Personally, when I am faced with a potentially emotionally charged situation at home I stop and think: first, how would a normal parent act under these circumstances? Second, how would a psychiatrist behave? And third, how should I, as a psychiatrist not acting like a psychiatrist, act?" He followed this lunatic and, one hopes, exaggerated statement with the complacent observation that his professional and personal lives were so separate that his children scarcely knew what he did for a living. His college-age daughter, interviewed several days later, said, "I always tell people that I've been in analysis since the day I was born."

Another man, a child psychiatrist who is himself the son of a psychiatrist, while denying that psychiatrists have adverse effects on their children, was much less sanguine about psychoanalysts. "I think that, as a group, *those* people are not well grounded in reality. They think in terms of projection and displacement. They think of relationships in terms of *transference*, not as something that is happening between two human beings here and now on planet Earth. I can see where this tendency toward detachment, intellectualization, and all of these splitting and defense mechanisms might interfere with one's dealing with life. I don't do that myself. I'm a family therapist, and I don't think in terms of that bullshit. At home, if my son is good, I just reinforce the hell out of him." The jarring use of the word "reinforce" did not even register in his mind as something that conflicted with his boast.

The truth of the matter is that psychotherapy is not just a job. Whereas the education of a surgeon, dentist, mathematician, or engineer equips him with a set of intellectual working tools, just as a craftman's training teaches him to work with the tools of his trade, the psychiatrist's education is designed to change the way that he thinks about his own and other people's behavior. As with the two men described above, elements of their learning remain a constantly active concern in their minds as they conduct their daily lives, and their learning is precisely related to what takes place between people in daily life. This in itself sets them apart from most other workers. The extent to which one can relate to people and conduct one's affairs in terms of surgery, teeth, mathematics, or mechanical structures is, after all, severely limited.

In a 1968 paper, researchers who studied the therapeutic training process stated that one of the most difficult obstacles to the mastery of psychiatric skills is that the psychiatrist must " 'unlearn' the major sorts of interpersonal orientations which he acquired as a 'normal member of society.' "[5] He replaces them with strange new attitudes and skills. The psychiatrist must, for example, learn to maintain an unusual degree of objectivity and poise in the face of emotional crises, to elicit deep confessions from relatively casual acquaintances, to refrain from standard socially dictated responses, to visualize people in terms of their family histories and unconscious motivations, to discern the importance of seemingly insignificant verbal or postural clues, and to scrutinize his own feelings while dealing with patients and, perhaps, with everyone else. Psychiatry is far more than an intellectual utensil that can be picked up, applied, and returned to its place; the psychiatrist ascribes to a philosophy that permeates every part of his life and tinges his sense of values. It would be surprising if psychiatrists did *not* exert an unusual influence on their children, whether beneficial or not.

A more interesting comment on the possible effects of psychotherapists on their children is that though there may be differences, they might not be of real interest. Everett Dulit, director of Child and Adolescent Psychiatry at Montefiore Medical Center in New York, was once asked to address a Long Island group of psychotherapists on the subject. He gave the topic considerable thought and spoke with some dozen of his colleagues, and he reached the conclusion that there was no distinctive psychopathology among therapists' children, and that any differences one might find would most likely be artifacts or stylistic variations without any profound significance. Dulit likened psychotherapy to other intensely absorbing occupations that pervade the family life:

People who go into music think a lot about music, people who go into athletics are very absorbed in the use of the body, and people who become executives are interested in the uses of power in this world. Likewise people who go into psychological work end up making that a central theme in their lives. They talk about it and think about it and they are aware of it all the time, and their children grow up in an environment where psychological-mindedness is front stage center from beginning to end. It is a presence in the children's lives, and they may take to it or they may recoil from it, but they cannot simply ignore it. But the differences in someone who is psychological-minded are stylistic, not better or worse, healthy or unhealthy. *When* things go wrong they may go wrong in certain ways, but I'm not sure that they go wrong any more often than with anyone else. It's not easy to put together a good, effective, well-balanced life, and most people do it to a reasonable degree with some flaws. But whether you do it in French or you do it in English, you do it hysterical or you do it obsessional, you do it psychological-mindedly or you do it non-psychological-mindedly, those are just stylistic variants.[6]

This is a valid point to keep in mind, and it pinpoints influences that can at times obscure the issues. One does not want to confuse, for instance, differences in vocabulary for actual differences in meaning. When a therapist's child sitting at the dinner table asks her father why he is angry, and the father denies it, saying "I'm not angry, you're projecting," does it have special meaning or not? Does it have a unique effect on the relationship, or is it simply a question of style? Arguably this is a merely an odd way of saying "No, I'm not," and nothing more. Conceivably, the child even understands it that way, performing a simultaneous translation of the father's jargon-infested conversation. But in fact, and one supposes not purely by coincidence, four different therapists' children described this identical incident to me, and not one of them regarded "You're projecting" as mere idiosyncratic word choice. "You're projecting" does not mean "I'm not," it means "*I* am not even involved here, the problem is in your *own* mind." It makes a very significant difference in terms of the way that parent and child get along with each other and resolve disputes that arise between them.

The most common objection I have heard in the course of research for this book, one raised in the first few sentences of virtually every interview, is that it is impossible to distinguish what was the effect of one's father or mother being a psychotherapist and what was simply his or her natural personality. One never had any other parents, nor the same parents in the same circumstances but practicing a different profession. There is no control group, and the issues are hopelessly confused.

This is true, yet in an important sense it does not matter. Much of what gives psychotherapy its particular complexion is the set of personalities of the people drawn into it. Few people are dropped into a profession by sheer happenstance. Though there are undeniable constraints upon one's choice—economic, social, geographical, familial, ethical, and physical—there remains enough leeway within those limits, and even within a given profession, that one can generally end up in a field that somehow resonates with aspects of one's personal interests, ambitions, or needs. A person chooses a profession because of what he thinks it will do for him, whether his anticipated gratification is measured in money, prestige, power, or some other more subtle emotional coin.

It may, then, be the similarities in personality types as much as or more than the similarity of what therapists do for a living that makes it interesting and worthwhile to discuss the effects that they have upon their children. In that sense it might be more accurate to say that I have studied, not the children of psychotherapists, but the children of people who have become psychotherapists. If therapists are unusual, it is not because otherwise undistinguished individuals were abruptly transformed by therapeutic training into monsters, like werewolves under a rising full moon, but because psychotherapy lures certain people in the first place, then makes them even more similar through the practice of a common profession.*

If one could conduct a strange magical experiment in which one abducted a hundred random passers-by from the street, and with the wave of a wand magically converted them into psychotherapists, they would bear many similarities to those people who became psychotherapists through more arduous and orthodox means. They would have similar work schedules and environments, similar patients and colleagues, similar incomes and expenses. They would go to the same conferences, hold many of the same philosophical beliefs, use some of the same jargon, and be viewed similarly askance by the general public. To the extent that professions define one's associates and friends, the two groups might send their children to the same schools and engage in many of the same cultural and recreational activities, such as all migrating to Truro in August. They would both doubtless show many of the purely stylistic consequences of practicing psychotherapy that Dulit describes. But there would also be important differences related to the personal motivations that had led one group and had not led the other group to the profession: the lacks they had felt within their lives, the ambitions they had, the gratifications they sought to derive. These differences would determine the more profound significance that psychotherapy has in their respective lives, and the degree to which it affects their families.†

* Along similar lines, Jay Rohrlich, a New York psychiatrist who specializes in treating Wall Street businessmen, says that a frequent problem among his patients is that they treat their personal lives much as they conduct their professional lives. *Quantities* of things matter: how well their sons do in sports, what grades their daughters get on their tests, how often they have sex with their wives or lovers, how big a house they have or how many cars. The very quantification and lust for more that drives them to excel at work causes problems at home. Yet Rohrlich points out that these were not utterly nonmaterialistic people who, for reasons beyond their control, went into finance, where an acquisitive, competitive outlook was thrust upon them. They began with materialistic strivings, and then sought to satisfy them. The profession served as a magnet for such people, brought many of them together, and created a subculture in which quantification and acquisitiveness were the norm and permitted them to deviate yet further from the rest of the world.[7]

† Curiously enough, such a control group may exist, though it was not magic that transformed them, but war. Early in my research, psychiatrist Howard Page Wood[8] suggested that I might find a difference between psychiatrists who had entered the profession during World War II and those who did so before or after. During the war, the armed forces recruited many general practitioners and undifferentiated residents into psychiatry to meet the tremendous wartime need for psychiatric care—one of thirteen soldiers had at least one neuropsychiatric admission.[9] As opposed to prewar and postwar psychiatrists who had chosen the field of their own free will and perhaps to satisfy certain needs in themselves, these wartime psychiatrists were not "psychiatrist types," yet many of them liked the work, found that they were good at it, and when the war was over they found themselves in a specialty that was growing in popularity and prestige more rapidly than any other. It is my impression, based on informal observations, that

It is widely believed that many people who become psychotherapists have had significant emotional problems or came from families where there were severe emotional problems. This is a delicate topic to raise with the therapists themselves. One man I spoke to, the president of a regional psychoanalytic society, flew into a rage when I suggested that troubled people go into psychotherapy: "*I* didn't become a psychoanalyst because I had problems," he shrieked, "I became a psychoanalyst because my *mother* had problems." Twenty minutes after our telephone conversation ended he called me back to further rebut what he perceived as a slanderous accusation against his profession. Yet it is hard to avoid the issue of childhood emotional turmoil. In conversations, it is truly astounding how many children of psychotherapists spontaneously bring up the subject of their therapist parent's horrendous early life and subsequent difficulties in coping with the family, something they credit with being the critical determinant in their parent's choice of profession.

The fact that psychotherapists may have been troubled people need not be a drawback in their professional lives. Many resolve their problems in the course of training and personal therapy, and end up stronger and more compassionate as a result. Certainly one would rather seek help from a therapist who had successfully dealt with his own personal misery than from one who had led a life of unrelenting bliss and whose knowledge of unhappiness came exclusively from textbooks.

There are those, however, who deal with their problems incompletely or not at all. Studies examining various measures of maladjustment such as suicide and alcohol abuse indicate, though not conclusively, that psychotherapists remain discernibly troubled as compared to their social, economic, and ethnic peers. Anecdotal studies reach even less cheerful conclusions about the total life patterns of psychotherapists. Though this does not of necessity prevent them from effectively helping their patients, it leaves a definite stamp on the field as a whole, as well as upon the therapists' children. A

---

the wartime psychiatrists tend to be very competent in a pedestrian sort of way compared to their prewar and postwar brethren, who include more of the greatest and the worst, the most exalted and brilliant, and the most severely troubled. A number of psychiatrists and psychoanalysts to whom I have mentioned this observation said, after a moment's reflection, that their own experience would support it.

Not coincidentally, the wartime psychiatrists also have a less distinctive effect on their children. In a majority of cases where children I interviewed said that their father's profession had had a negligible impact on family life, and where they even seemed puzzled by my study and not especially interested in it, the father had been recruited into psychiatry during World War II.

more insidious and interesting factor, which will be discussed in detail later on, is the fact that many therapists discover, in the course of their training, a convenient way to *avoid* dealing with problems. They acquire authority, methods of justifying themselves and deflecting criticism, and an arsenal of defensive techniques and rationalizations that insulate and protect them so well that they no longer feel compelled to resolve the underlying problems. This combination of resolved problems, persistent problems, and encapsulated problems is responsible for much of the profession's amalgamated personality and underlies many of its strengths and its weaknesses.

The extent to which all these personal and professional considerations exist and affect psychotherapists' children is a complicated question with no simple or single answer. Psychotherapists are not a distinct breed of creature walled off from the rest of humanity, and their problems and those of their children are simply a somewhat definable slice taken from a continuous spectrum of human concerns. Therapists' children are not crazy in the sense of being psychotic, mentally ill, or insane. Effects are often absent, and when present are subtle and widely varied. The psychological inheritance of therapists' children does not set them conspicuously and constantly apart in the way that, for example, rich kids' wealth affects every part their lives: their clothing, their houses, their hobbies, their vacations, the schools they attend, and the social world they inhabit.

There have been a few previous studies on the specific effects that psychiatrists and psychoanalysts have on their children. An excellent 1977 article by Ross Wetzsteon in the *Village Voice* with the somewhat sensational title "Do Psychiatrists Drive Their Children Crazy?" concentrated on the effects when psychiatrists become too caught up in their theories to deal adequately with reality, and with the problems that result when they consciously or unconsciously use their training as an offensive and defensive weapon.[10] The only two serious theoretical treatments that have been published within the profession are short fragments in books on other topics, Heinz Kohut's *The Restoration of the Self* and Alice Miller's *The Drama of the Gifted Child*.

The late Heinz Kohut painted a rather depressing portrait of psychoanalysts' children based on observations of several he had in analysis.[11] They complained of a sense of unreality and an inability to experience emotions. They tended to be walled off and secretive, and had an intense though ambivalent need to attach themselves to powerful people in order to feel meaning and vitality in their lives. They applied themselves amiably and unquestioningly to the therapeutic task, but without making significant progress, owing to a curious reluctance to reveal themselves and participate without reservation.

Kohut's explanation of the problems of these children was that the analyst parents had been overly intrusive into their children's minds, with damaging consequences. According to a fairly standard theory of early childhood development, all infants at first recognize no distinction between themselves and the world around them: various pleasures and discomforts ebb and flow, and the infant has virtually no control over this seemingly random succession of states. It is up to the parents to more or less correctly anticipate, divine, and satisfy the baby's limited needs for food, comfort, and stimulation. As the infant grows, its needs become more numerous and complex, and the parents' capacity to comprehend and satisfy the full range of its secret yearnings is proportionately diminished. At this stage the infant begins to perceive the limitations of its parents, or more accurately, to perceive the boundaries between parents and self, between self and other. In an embryonic way, it realizes that if you want something done in this world, you must do it yourself. The infant's self emerges as that volume of its life that parents do not automatically understand, and its sense of vitality and personal power stems from an increasing ability to manipulate the connections between its self and the other.

In Kohut's theory, the analysts' children diverged from their peers because their parents had a qualitatively different, almost preternatural empathic ability to understand what was going on in their children's minds, and they often told their children of their insights. Long past the point that is healthy or normal, back where other parents' empathy is left in the dust, analysts continue to attempt and often succeed in understanding their children's thoughts, wishes, and feelings without, however, grasping the more general developmental need of the child to be treated as a whole and allowed to grow. The result is a diminution in the child's sense of self, because more space is ceded to the parents' apprehension, and the lines of misunderstanding delimiting the boundaries between self and other become diffuse and unreliable. The child does not question the parents' intrusion (as he does not later question the intrusions of psychotherapy), since it is simply the way that life is, and not something intended or perceived as an assault. Nonetheless the children react against this insidious invasion with an ongoing tendency toward secrecy and obscurity through which they try to protect some small coherent sense of self.

One shies away from generalizing Kohut's description in its extravagant original form, which is due, perhaps, to the fact that his observations were based on analysts' children who not only were analytic patients and thus ipso facto unusually disturbed, but were all analytic patients who had been through a first failed analysis before coming to him. Kohut never states or implies that the situation he describes is true of all analysts' children. He uses it to illustrate a point at which his theory of "self psychology" diverges from classical psychoanalysis and triumphs over it, not because analysts' children held intrinsic interest for him.

Moreover, few people, even analysts themselves, seriously believe that psychoanalysts' empathic abilities are so preternaturally acute and qualitatively different from those of lay parents that this fact alone would account for such dramatic harm to the child. While analysts may have penetrating insights in the controlled, dispassionate circumstances of their practice, amidst the give and take of daily life at home they can be as baffled as anyone else. Instead, what may be more significant than real empathic intrusion is that there is a faith in the powers of intellectual analysis, a belief in the appropriateness of entering into another's emotional life, and an attitude of presumed understanding that is as harmful to the child as correct empathic perceptions would be. I believe this to be the case—but it arises in large part from a very different quarter: from the pathological intent of the parent rather than from pathogenic aspects of benignly intended technique.

German psychoanalyst Alice Miller has described a population of children similar to Kohut's, but from a slightly different angle. The patients she describes were very gifted. They had been precocious and unusually responsible as children; they were their parents' pride. Their adult lives, too, are admirable and enviable, yet despite their success in most endeavors, they feel empty and dissatisfied, and are plagued by depression, guilt, and anxiety whenever they feel they have failed at something.

In the very first interview they will let the listener know that they have had understanding parents, or at least one such, and if they ever lacked understanding, they felt that the fault lay with them and with their inability to express themselves appropriately. They recount their earliest memories without any sympathy for the child they once were, and this is the more striking since these patients not only have a pronounced introspective ability, but are also able to empathize well with other people. Their relationship to their own childhood's emotional world, however, is characterized by lack of respect, compulsion to control, manipulation, and a demand for achievement. Very often they show disdain and irony, even derision and cynicism. In general, there is a complete absence of real emotional under-

standing or serious appreciation of their own childhood vicissitudes, and no conception of their true needs—beyond the need
for achievement.[12]

The people Miller is discussing are the children of narcissistically
impaired parents. Such parents, unable to experience the full vitality
of their own lives, seek to fill some of their own emotional vacancy
vicariously through those around them. The parents, when children
themselves, had been deprived of the unquestioning love and admiration that ennoble the child's sense of self. They had learned to
manage and conceal their distress, but in certain ways, and particularly when they had their own children, they sought to exact from
others the lost love and admiration they needed to repair themselves.
Their children are raised—quite innocently but no less harmfully—so
that much of their sense of worth comes from divining and gratifying
the parents' expectations, while they themselves, though they tend to
be talented, sensitive, and appealing, end up with a fundamental void
at their core that prevents them from experiencing the full vitality of
their own lives. They, too, are narcissistically impaired, and unless
something intervenes to break the chain, their children may be as well.

According to Miller, narcissistically impaired people are often
drawn to psychoanalysis. They tend to be good at it because of the
skills they unconsciously cultivated in their relationships with their
parents, and it gratifies certain needs that they have: "our own mother
seldom or never listened to us with such rapt attention as our patients
usually do, and she never revealed her inner world to us so clearly
and honestly as our patients do at times."[13] In contrast to Kohut,
Miller attributes a set of emotional characteristics often found among
analysts' children not to the intrusive techniques of the parents'
profession but to the parents' personality.

The two viewpoints are easily combined, and correspond closely to
what I have found in the course of my research. The effect upon the
children is not, however, simply that of having a parent who is emotionally impaired in some way, like the child of an alcoholic or of a
schizophrenic, nor of having a parent in a psychologically potent
profession, such as a famous actor or significant thinker. The children
of therapists have parents whose pathology has found a home in a
profession that is equipped with its own redeeming philosophy, whom
society has chosen to respect in part *because of* their emotional oddity,
rather like shamans and visionaries of old, and, one might add, like
some clergymen of today. It is interesting, for that matter, to note that
the clergy is the only professional group whose children have their own

initials: "PKs," for preachers' kids. With some reluctance, but urged on by a desire for simplicity in the pages to come, I have taken the liberty of coining a parallel term, "PsyKs" (pronounced SIGH-kays), for psychiatrists', psychoanalysts', and other psychotherapists' kids.

Before examining the specific subpopulation of therapists in question and the effects that they have on their children, it is worth reviewing the overall profession of psychotherapy, its social and demographic characteristics, its aims and its philosophy.

What and
Who Are
Psychotherapists?

At that time it took a certain lack of balance to be interested in Freud's work at all, for psychoanalysis was a deviant activity.

—PAUL ROAZEN

The history of psychotherapy is very different from the history of psychiatry. Psychiatry and its medical antecedents were concerned for most of their existence with the treatment of neurologically damaged patients, and of psychotics and severe neurotics whose behavior was so grossly disordered that they were disruptive to society or were clearly unable to function on their own. The precise definition of these severe forms of mental illness may change significantly from one time or culture to another, but in any context there eventually comes a point where an inability to function and to participate in society becomes an incontrovertible fact.

Until the late eighteenth and early nineteenth centuries insanity was considered to be largely incurable and therefore more of a custodial problem than a subject of interest to the medical profession. This was just as well for the insane. To combat the black bile and overheated blood presumed to be responsible for their afflictions, centuries of unfortunate lunatics were given hellebore purges or bled. Erasmus Darwin, the grandfather of Charles, developed a gyrating chair that spun the patient into unconsciousness, thus redistributing errant blood, and the kindly Benjamin Rush devised the "tranquillizer," a chair to which the patient was tightly strapped, thus stopping all muscular activity and permitting the blood to slow its frenzied rush through the brain.

In 1815, Dr. Thomas Monro, one of an unbroken series of Monros, fathers and sons, who served as resident physicians at Bethlehem Royal Hospital, or Bedlam, from 1728 to 1891, told a parliamentary committee: "Patients are ordered to be bled about the latter end of May, or the beginning of June, according to the weather, and after they have been bled, they take vomits once a week for a certain number of weeks; after that, we purge the patients. That has been the practice invariably for years, long before my time; it was handed down to me by my father, and I do not know any better practice."[1]

Other physicians believed in breaking the patient's will, as though the insane mind were one whose parts had aggregated into a crazy form and must be shattered and allowed to coalesce again normally. Or, if the madman had strayed from the memory of the real world, the vision of death might recall him to more tangible pursuits. Lunatics were dropped suddenly into freezing baths, or chained to the bottom of a well that was slowly filled with water. A Massachusetts physician devised a perforated coffinlike box in which madmen were locked and then lowered underwater until the bubbles ceased to rise, then raised and sometimes revived. Beating was also a popular remedy, whose rationale derived from the view that a wandering mind was like a recalcitrant child that just needed a little discipline.

These brutal and dangerous treatments were reserved for the well-to-do. King George III of England was purged, leeched, and flogged assiduously during his recurring bouts of insanity. Other lunatics did not receive so much attention, and were simply confined in almshouses, workhouses, bridewells, prisons, and the few public insane asylums. Such treatment as there was in asylums, both public and private, was atrocious. English parliamentary investigating committees who visited asylums in the early nineteenth century scrupulously mentioned in their official reports that they vomited at what they saw. They found emaciated wrecks who were filthy, louse-ridden, and sometimes broken and scarred from repeated beatings. They were packed into tiny, unventilated dungeons whose floors were of straw, saturated with urine and excrement. There were lunatics in private asylums whose feet were amputated when mortification set in from the constriction of their chains, and rats sometimes gnawed at the flesh of madmen in close restraint. Some were beaten to death or suffocated. Many buildings were unheated throughout the winter to cut costs. There was a convenient theory that madmen did not feel cold. Some of the inmates froze to death, disproving the theory, but cutting costs even further.

In the late eighteenth century, enlightened groups in France,

England, and Italy experimented with nonrestraint methods of care. The most famous of the new lunatic asylums was the Retreat, in York, England, founded by a group of Quakers to provide an alternative to the York Asylum, which was one of the largest and worst of the county facilities. The notion of "moral management" or "moral treatment," as it came to be known, was to remove patients from their habitual environment and place them in an asylum somewhere in the country, where they could be surrounded by beauty and calm. To soothe a troubled mind and body there would be light, well-ventilated buildings, a regular schedule, and nourishing, easily digestible food. Exercise, reading, music, conversation, and the arts were encouraged, while potentially disturbing visits from family and friends were limited to certain times. Fears and anger were to be assuaged rather than opposed, and though physicians and keepers held absolute authority, they were to exercise it without force and to treat their patients with the honor and dignity that humans deserve. Asylums run according to these moral principles made a very favorable impression on observers. The occupants looked better and saner than the wretches in the county asylums. Since the hospitals were more humanely run, they could appeal to the families of less desperately ill patients, with the result that cure rates went up.

Asylums increasingly came under the jurisdiction of medical men who, for the first time, had the opportunity to observe many cases at close quarters over extended periods of time. Following the passion for classification characteristic of the time, as manifested by Linnaeus in biology and Lavoisier in chemistry, alienists attempted to divide mental illness into its various classes and subclasses, each precisely described by a constellation of behavioral and physiological symptoms. Pinel, Esquirol, Haslam, Bucknill, and others performed autopsies on hundreds of lunatics and were unable to discern any distinctive pattern of cerebral lesions, which reinforced the gradually dawning suspicion that insanity was not always organic, but often a psychic maladjustment and hence susceptible to cure. The previous medical sense of fatalism gave way to unbridled optimism over the asylum's potential, and medical superintendents and alienists fought battles of statistics proving their triumph over madness. In the United States, the Hartford Retreat boasted a 55 percent overall cure rate and an 82 percent rate for recent patients who had not already suffered from inappropriate care elsewhere. The Worcester Hospital boasted a 90 percent cure rate; and in 1842 and 1843, hospital directors in Virginia and Ohio claimed 100 percent recovery of recently admitted patients. True, these figures were often spuriously computed by selecting particularly favorable sample groups, or by tallying admissions in terms of numbers of patients, and releases in terms of number of times released. One woman was "cured" at the Bloomingdale Asylum in New York six times in one year, and forty-six times before she finally died in an asylum.[2] Still, the figures were very impressive and, armed with them, hospital superintendents propounded the notion that insanity was a curable ailment rather than a shameful and permanent affliction, and that lunatics would stand a far better chance of recovery if they were sent to an asylum promptly rather than cared for at home until they grew unmanageable.

This changing tradition that became institutional psychiatry touched upon the issues of psychotherapy at many points, but never led directly to its development. Conversely, most of the ambulatory patients who see psychotherapists would have been crazy to subject themselves to early alienists, or even to later institutional psychiatrists, whose insulin shock, electroshock, and psychosurgery were unpleasant treatments with little more real scientific basis than the brutal Victorian therapies. With the exception of various narcotics, no psychologically useful pharmaceuticals were available until the 1950s, at which point organic psychiatrists began to develop effective treatments for some hitherto intractable cases. Psychiatry has only very recently ceased to be predominantly custodial in nature.

The emotional complaints that afflict psychotherapeutic patients are much more elusive in nature than those that lead to institutional care. These people are in touch with reality, function more or less normally, and can be very successful in most aspects of life. They may suffer tremendously themselves and cause grief to those around them, yet their problems are fundamentally private, not social concerns. It is difficult to say at what point life's inevitable worries, fears, catastrophes, eccentricities, and bouts of ill temper verge into something qualifiable as needing professional help. Depending upon one's particular notions of who needs therapy for what, the group of patients requiring psychotherapy is arbitrarily large or small.

Traditionally, when people had problems in personal relationships, with their work and ambitions, and in their more ultimate and abstract relations with the world in general and with life itself, they kept them to themselves or discussed them with family, friends, or some trusted member of their community. The only institutionalized form of guidance to be found was in the church. Clergymen were, after all, among the best educated people in most communities, and had experience with the human condition of a breadth and intensity far greater than that of the ordinary citizen. Moreover, the clergyman supposedly partook of the deity's wisdom and impartiality and was bound to keep secret his parishioners' confidences. On the other hand, the clergy was usually judgmental: there was a right and a wrong. Though the clergyman might be compassionate and forgiving, his ultimate purpose was to guide the errant congregant back toward a preordained moral path, not to help him find his own independent way through the world, as many modern psychotherapists claim to do.

Before the mid-1890s, the only organized secular source of more or less therapeutic advice came from the marginal fields of mesmerism, phrenology, and various other specialties classifiable as faith healing. These would-be sciences attracted many of the same sorts of patients as modern therapy—people uncomfortable with themselves and searching for solutions, liberal agnostics and atheists in search of a higher but not theological morality, and the intellectual well-to-do, with both the curiosity and the cash to pursue nonessential efforts toward self-improvement.

Mesmerism, named after its founder, Franz Anton Mesmer, a theatrical healer who flourished in the late eighteenth and early nineteenth centuries, involved the use of "magnetized" materials to reshape the pathological distribution of magnetic forces around the patient and thereby cure him of various physical and psychological ills. It achieved great popularity in certain circles, though numerous scientific committees failed to detect the existence of Mesmer's mysterious universal fluids—not to be confused with ordinary magnetism—and labeled the technique either self-delusion or overt fraud. Nonetheless, mesmerists offered treatment, sometimes successful, to neurotics, hysterics, and psychosomatics, and their work led to significant understanding of hypnosis, the power of suggestion, and the nature of the therapist-patient relationship.[3] Phrenology further brought consideration of the internal architecture of the human mind into the realm of popular thought.

In the late nineteenth century there was a brief medical fad for "rest cures" in response to the neurological concept of neurasthenia—a vague notion that most unspecified cases of depression, frustration, and general ennui were attributable to nervous exhaustion resulting from the toll that modern industrial life takes on man's biologically unaccustomed nervous system. Rest cures worked sometimes, of course, and they were a fine source of income for certain psychiatrists, but little real treatment or theory was involved. Ultimately, it was the work of neurologists, who study the functioning and anatomy of the nervous system and the classification of disorders, that led to the development of modern psychotherapy: investigators such as Janet and Charcot, studying the etiology of hysteria, and Freud, whose work led to the founding of psychoanalysis.

The beginning of psychoanalysis marks the true beginning of psychotherapy, in large measure because it legitimized the concept of conducting treatment based entirely upon talk, in which the elicitation and discussion of the patient's memories and attitudes, rather than the administration of physical or pharmacological agents, was the operative part of the treatment. Arguably, the greatest of Freud's contributions was not the theoretical framework of psychoanalysis itself, much of which was radically altered or replaced, often by Freud himself, but the establishment of a system of thought or paradigm within which all aspects of normal and abnormal human behavior could be considered. The system began not at the levels of inorganic chemicals, biological cells, or medical tissues and organs, but at the level of human experience, and was expressed in terms that, however objectionable they may at times have been, were fully comprehensible to the educated public. Though it was a "talking cure," it was different from simple advice in that there was a structure to the relationship, and a formalization of the role of the therapist, who was supposed to facilitate and elicit rather than teach or direct.

Once the basic paradigm of psychotherapy had been established, various factors contributed to its spread. Clifford Beers' Mental Hygiene movement and the increased sympathetic awareness of mental illness that followed both world wars greatly encouraged government and community support for the creation of psychological services outside of the traditional institutional context. The popularity of psychoanalysis in intellectual circles and its resulting percolation down through the popular press led to universal familiarity with basic analytic concepts. By the 1960s, psychotherapy had not only become an accepted American solution to personal problems, but a commonplace one.

Though psychotherapy has grown quite familiar, it remains surrounded by a great deal of confusion, including justifiable uncertainty as to exactly who psychotherapists are. The term can apply to psychiatrists; medical and nonmedical psychoanalysts; psychologists; social workers; marriage, family, or pastoral counselors; and a host of other advisers, aides, and support personnel. An official of the National Association of Social Workers asked me, "When you say 'psychotherapists,' are you also going to include beauticians and hairdressers? Today even they are given some rudimentary training in recognizing mental illness and in certain psychotherapeutic methods."[4] One investigator, seeking to define individual psycho-therapy, ended with the frustrated conclusion that "currently, pro-fessional psychotherapy is defined by the context and agreements which bind the two people together. If they call it psychotherapy, then, in today's confusing world of hundreds of forms of psychother-apy, who is to deny that it is?"[5]

In the present context, "psychotherapist" will be used in a some-what more restrictive sense to include members of one of four pro-fessions: psychiatry, psychoanalysis, clinical psychology, and clinical social work. Though the formation and credentials of these various practitioners are very different, the work that they do may often be quite similar, and the general public, to the therapists' exasperation, has tremendous difficulty telling them apart.

The Psychiatrist

Psychiatry, alone among the four professions, is a medical specialty,* like pediatrics or cardiology. Following four years of med-ical school an aspiring psychiatrist generally spends four years in a psychiatric residency program before being eligible to take certifying board examinations. Whereas the most widespread image of the psy-chiatrist is of a private practitioner treating individual suburban neu-rotics through essentially psychoanalytic techniques, many take more biochemical, psychopharmacological, genetic, or epidemiological ap-proaches to mental illness, conceiving of the mind according to a physicalist medical model rather than as a distinct psychological en-tity. On the whole, 57.7 percent of psychiatrists list their primary work setting as private practice; 27.1 percent as private or govern-ment hospitals, clinics, or mental health centers; and 12.3 percent as medical schools.[6]

In 1946 there were about four thousand psychiatrists in the United States. In 1963 the number was 16,049, and by 1981 it had increased by 77.7 percent, to 28,524,[7] a large but not disproportionate growth, given that during the same period the total physician population grew from 276,475 to 485,123, an increase of 75.5 percent. The proportion of women in the profession had risen to 17.3 percent by 1982—a higher percentage than in any other medical specialty.[9] The densest

* A recent paper on the economics of psychiatric practice bemoans the fact that many customers cannot distinguish between psychiatrists and other psychotherapists or counselors, and suggests that psychiatrists should take advantage of their unique training: "To maintain their market share, psychiatrists will have to emphasize their medical diagnostic skills and their expertise in psychopharmacology."[8]

populations of psychiatrists are in the District of Columbia, Massa-chusetts, New York, and Connecticut, and the lowest are in Idaho, Wyoming, and Mississippi. This national distribution is probably roughly comparable for the other psychotherapeutic specialties.

The most recent figures on psychiatric fees, from a 1982 survey conducted by the American Psychiatric Association (APA),[10] give a nationwide mean fee for a 45-to-50-minute individual psychothera-peutic session with a psychiatrist as $69.54, with variations in state averages ranging from a low of $49 in Massachusetts to a high of $86 in Minnesota.* Since patients tend to see psychiatrists on a regular, ongoing basis, and not just for the emergencies or annual or biannual checkups typical with other medical specialists, psychiatric psycho-therapy tends to be expensive. A weekly session at the average rate would come to a total of $3,500 per year, and insurers have tradition-ally been reluctant to cover psychotherapy, so that a larger portion of this cost devolves upon the patient than for most other medical treatments.

Because psychiatric psychotherapy is so expensive, people think of psychiatrists as fabulously wealthy, which, coupled with the fact that they appear to do so little, exacerbates the already low esteem in which psychiatrists stand. In reality, the situation is quite different. According to the *Socioeconomic Characteristics of Medical Practice in 1983*, compiled by the American Medical Association, psychiatrists earned more than 23 percent less than the national average income of all physicians. The average doctor's net income from medical practice for 1982 was $99,500. The highest-paying specialties were radiology ($136,800), anesthesiology ($131,400), and surgery ($130,500). Until 1975 psychiatry was the lowest-paid medical specialty, without ex-ception. Since then the income from psychiatry has risen, or the income from pediatrics and general and family practice has fallen, so that psychiatry is merely the third lowest, paying a mean net income of $76,500, according to the American Medical Association, or a mean

---

* Comparable figures for the various types of psychotherapists are notoriously untrustworthy, since different surveys use different criteria and look at different populations. Among psychi-atrists alone the figures are hard to reconcile. A 1973 study of psychiatrists said the typical fee for a 45-to-60-minute visit was $36.73. A 1978 survey conducted for the journal *Medical Economics* found that the median fee for individual psychotherapy by psychiatrists was $51. A 1980 study gave an average charge per visit to office-based psychiatrists of $37.70, yet this study excluded visits for which there had been no charge and did not distinguish between 20-, 30-, and 50-minute visits. The figures given in the 1982 APA study cited above were subjected to cost-of-living adjustments on a state-by-state basis, which makes it impossible to compare them to anything else.[11]

gross of $82,180 according to a study by the American Psychiatric Association.*[12]

The relatively low earnings of psychiatrists are readily understandable if one considers the fact that other physicians, though they may earn less per visit, also spend less time on each visit. The average physician sees 131.8 patients per week. General and family practitioners see 160.6.[13] Psychiatrists see a mere 39.2 individual patients, and an additional 3.4 in groups.[14] Moreover, whereas many other specialists can delegate routine portions of examinations and treatments to nurses or technicians, psychiatrists are generally obliged, due to the very nature of the work, to conduct all of the treatment themselves.† They must do an hour's work for an hour's pay. They do not even have a set of short, lucrative special procedures, such as cataract surgery for ophthalmologists, to supplement their income from office visits, and if they increased their hourly office rate they could easily price themselves out of a practice.

The patient base of psychiatrists also tends to be more sensitive than that of other physicians. Since psychiatric patients return frequently, conceivably the forty patients who come one week are the same forty who come the next and the week after—the loss of a single patient would eliminate one hour of work from each week, and 2.5 percent of the psychiatrist's income. Other physicians draw their 130 weekly patients from a much larger total pool, any one of whom comes rarely and whose loss would be of little importance. It has, moreover, been argued that psychiatric services, being both more costly to each patient and more discretionary in nature, are more readily dispensed with in times of hardship than other physicians' services.

Another reason for the lower income of psychiatrists is that, contrary to the protestations of the psychiatrists themselves, who would have one believe that no one works harder than they, according to the American Medical Association they spend fewer hours per week in patient care than any medical specialist except pathologists (who do not really attend to patients at all), and fewer hours in overall professional activities than any specialist. Another study arrived at the

---

* The small difference between these two numbers is attributable to the fact that the professional expenses of psychiatrists are less than half the average for all physicians; only pathologists spend less. They spend less on payroll, medical equipment, and liability insurance than anyone else, and only anesthesiologists spend less on offices and supplies.

† There are exceptions. I did interview one psychiatrist *during* a group therapy session. He simply left the group alone to conduct itself and, when the session was over, to let itself out. Of course, as it turned out, three-fourths of the people in the group were psychiatrists themselves.

corollary fact that psychiatrists spend more hours per day engaged in personal, nonprofessional activities than any specialist except dermatologists. [15]

The Psychoanalyst

A psychoanalyst is someone who has completed training at a psychoanalytic institute and who has been psychoanalyzed; they are the only psychotherapists for whom personal therapy is an absolute requirement. Psychoanalysts may or may not be physicians. The early members of Freud's pioneer group came from a variety of disciplines, one of the factors that contributed such a vast and eclectic scope of interests to analysis and led analysts to venture into such diverse topics as the arts, literature, anthropology, and religion. Freud himself, though he was a medical doctor, opposed the restriction of analytic training to physicians. In the United States, however, the American Psychoanalytic Association chose to limit normal membership to licensed physicians, and though there are institutes unaffiliated with the American Psychoanalytic Association that do not have this requirement, the orthodox analytic establishment in this country, represented by the approximately three thousand members of the association, is predominantly composed of psychiatrists who have gone on to analytic training.

American psychoanalysts are about the most extensively educated people in the world. An analyst who follows a typical American Psychoanalytic Association program will generally have completed at least his first year of psychiatric residency before entering the analytic institute, meaning that he is already in his late twenties. Personal analysis usually begins before course work, as a way to ensure that the particular candidate is appropriate for analytic training. Course work lasts for four or, in some programs, five years. By the second year of courses the candidate can begin supervised analyses, of which there must be three, each supervised by a different analyst, none of whom is the candidate's personal analyst. There is generally a requirement that at least one, and perhaps two, of the supervised analyses must be in or approaching termination before the candidate can graduate, and since the successful completion of an analysis is not entirely within the analyst's control, this can be a frustrating and elusive requirement to satisfy. All told, a fairly typical analytic training lasts eight years, and very often much longer. Psychoanalysts tend to be forty before their education is complete and they emerge into full professional life, though of course they will already have been working as practicing psychiatrists for nearly a decade.

Psychoanalysis is very expensive for the patient. In 1976, the most recent year for which a nationwide survey is available, the average fee per session for analytic patients was $42, and the typical number of sessions in treatment was 848, spread over a period of three-and-three-quarters to four-and-a-half years, for a total cost of nearly $36,000, or about $10,000 per year. The cost has no doubt risen considerably in the dozen years since, but surprisingly, the American Psychoanalytic Association has no figures on this. Analysts treated other patients with nonanalytic psychotherapy—71 percent were not deemed appropriate for analysis, and the remaining 29 percent could not afford it—and these treatments were shorter and less costly, though they were billed at a higher rate per session. The total number of American Psychoanalytic Association members has remained quite steady over the past decade, while the number of analytic patients has declined. In 1976, the average analyst had about five patients in analytic treatment (though the figure was higher for training analysts and lower for the rest), an overall decline of 9 percent from the preceding decade. A 1984 study of the Boston Psychoanalytic Society and Institute found that the average analyst had a mere three analytic patients for a total of 11 hours per week, but when one excluded the training analysts, who are largely devoted to perpetuating the profession and have some analytic candidates as patients, and looked only at nontraining analysts, who are solely engaged in treating other patients, the numbers dropped to two-and-a-half patients and 9.4 hours per week.[16] A considerable number of older analysts have commented to me that they cannot imagine who is going into analysis now or why they are doing so, since classical analysis is clearly a dying profession.

The Social Worker

Social work was originally entirely associated with public assistance and child welfare agencies, the courts, schools, and various other community groups. Before the mental hygiene movement, the emphasis was on direct aid and relief rather than on the type of social casework that later became its domain. Having started with real, material problems, social work has throughout maintained a more pragmatic approach than the other psychotherapies, paying attention to people within the context of their real material and social circumstances instead of viewing them as isolated psychological entities.

In the United States it was recognized fairly early that there would be value in familiarizing social workers with basic psychoanalytic concepts and, by the thirties and forties, analysts were regularly teaching courses in schools of social work. It is surprising and fortuitous that analysts should have been willing to lend themselves to such programs given that, if any objection might be leveled against analysts it is that they concentrate on mental phenomena at the expense of practical reality, just the opposite of the social worker's plight. Partly owing to this new training, social workers began to emerge from the role of pure caseworkers and ancillary therapeutic support personnel to become primary independent therapists.

Private practice by social workers began early in the century, but according to one survey did not increase rapidly—something of an understatement, given the dutifully reported estimate that by 1940 there were, nationwide, only 4 full-time and 36 part-time private practitioners. In the psychological-minded sixties, social workers acting as private psychotherapists, first called psychiatric social workers, then clinical social workers, proliferated. By 1976 there were an estimated 2,189 social workers in private practice, 1,270 of them full time. Of these, 77 percent had been through personal therapy, two-thirds of them with a psychoanalyst. According to estimates by the National Association of Social Workers, by 1982 about 17,800 social workers, or roughly 20 percent of the organization's membership, were practicing psychotherapy in one setting or another as their primary employment. Licensing requirements vary more widely than those for physicians. In most states, a clinical social worker must have a master's degree in social work, followed by two years of supervised clinical experience, and meet continuing education requirements for license renewal.[17]

A 1985 survey found that nearly 60 percent of clinical social workers charged $50 to $60 per individual session, which usually meant a fifty-minute "hour." The average net income of social workers who considered themselves to be in full-time private practice was $36,864. The study did not give a separate figure for social workers, but found that among psychologists, social workers, and marriage and family therapists combined, the average number of patient hours per week was 28.7.[18]

The Psychologist

Psychology began as a purely academic offshoot of natural philosophy, but in the late nineteenth and early twentieth centuries it grew to include what are now physiological psychology; behavioral psychology; educational and vocational testing; certain industrial human factors studies; and aspects of child study, ethology, anthropology, and linguistics. In recent decades, an increasing number of people have used a background in psychology as the starting point for a career in individual or group psychotherapy. Most of the nonmedical psychoanalysts in the United States have a background in psychology.

To be licensed as a clinical psychologist, one must have a Ph.D. in psychology, perform three years of supervised clinical work, and pass a state licensing examination. The numbers of psychologists who practice individual therapy are virtually impossible to determine, but the proportion appears to be high. Of the 2,204 people who received doctorates in psychology in 1983, 61 percent had specialized in clinical psychology, counseling, community, or school work as opposed to research, industrial, or educational psychology.[19]

In 1985, the median fee per individual therapy session charged by psychologists was $70, and those in full-time private practice earned an average of $50,371, significantly more than social workers or marriage and family therapists, though much less than psychiatrists and medical psychoanalysts.[20]

The Psychotherapist

A psychotherapist is simply anyone who practices psychotherapy. The term is descriptive rather than the title of someone with specific professional training. Anyone in the above four professions who deals with troubled people, either singly or in groups, and whose primary mode of treatment is through conversation or acting rather than by pharmaceutical or physical means, can be termed a psychotherapist. People in the professions often limit the term to those who are not psychiatrists or medical analysts, in order to differentiate them from doctors and relegate them to an inferior position.

Despite the vast differences among the types of psychotherapists, however, all four subgroups—or those of them who engage in office-based individual psychotherapy of an essentially analytic nature—are linked by common types of practices, common sorts of patients, and a more or less common view of the world. A book by Henry, Sims, and Spray entitled *The Fifth Profession* is a study of the tremendous similarities among the analysts, psychiatrists, psychologists, and social workers who, viewed as an amalgamated "fifth profession" of psychotherapists, transcend the differences in their formation.[21]

This extensive 1971 study of 3,990 psychotherapists found that, demographically, they were largely upwardly mobile urban Jews, the children of Eastern European immigrants who had rejected their parents' political and religious beliefs in favor of more liberal views. There were, of course, tremendous variations within this gross picture: Catholics, who make up only 9.7 percent of psychotherapists, are overrepresented among social workers and greatly underrepresented among analysts, which fits well with the cultural background of the two specialties and with the ethical inclinations of the religious denominations.* On the other hand, more than 50 percent of psychiatrists and 62 percent of psychoanalysts are Jewish, which has added a unique blend of cultural and intellectual traditions to the fields, as well as brought about many of the most conspicuous stereotypes. The general population at the time of this study was estimated to be 25 percent Catholic and 3 percent Jewish.[22]

In terms of what the four professional groups of psychotherapists actually do, Henry, Sims, and Spray go so far as to say that:

> . . . it is important to query the social utility of having four highly organized, well-equipped, self-sufficient training pathways, each of which produces psychotherapists. Of course, these separate pathways produce other professionals who are not psychotherapists, but the point here is that the kinds of people progressively drawn into psychotherapy are highly similar. The end product is startlingly similar. Only the intervening years of expensive, highly complex training are different—different in ways that appear to have questionable relevance to the practice of psychotherapy, at least as seen by the psychotherapists themselves and as appears in the work activities of their subsequent professional lives.[23]

In the following section and remaining chapters, therefore, I will speak of psychotherapists indiscriminately, whether they are analysts, psychiatrists, social workers, or psychologists, and discussions of studies that have been done of one group—most often of psychiatrists, as it happens—might be assumed to be true of psychothera-

---

* One woman, a medical analytic candidate and the daughter of a Catholic psychoanalyst, recalled that in college she had a professor who told her that her father "couldn't possibly be any good as a psychoanalyst if he was a Catholic—it just didn't make sense."

My own father was a Catholic and a psychoanalyst, and I still have some letters that his befuddled midwestern hometown priest wrote to him in 1930. At the time my father was undergoing a training analysis with Helene Deutsch, and as was not uncommon then, to save time he followed her to Italy during her August vacation to continue his analysis there. The priest tried valiantly, but had a difficult time putting a favorable complexion on a project that entailed going to Italy with a woman to talk about sex.

pists in general except in those aspects, such as exact educational background or economic status, where common sense dictates otherwise.

The Patients*

The precise types of mental illness presented to psychotherapists for treatment have changed over the years, owing both to fads in mental illness and to a changing social environment. Among psychotics there was a period around the seventeenth and eighteenth centuries when believing one's limbs were made of glass and thinking that one had swallowed a snake were common afflictions, now mercifully seen no more, and the dawn of the radio age focused free-floating paranoid delusions on a fear of long-distance spying and manipulation by means of invisible rays. The less dramatic neurotic complaints have similarly varied. During Freud's most active years, the typical patient was a severe neurotic, with conspicuous obsessions, compulsions, and phobias or with hysterical conversions manifested in striking physical symptoms. Nowadays such flamboyant classical neurotics are mostly gone, owing to a changing society, less sexual repression, more open communication, and the general tenor of a culture homogenized by television, newspapers, and magazines. While the number of classical cases dwindled, the number of people seeking therapy has increased, and the types of problems that drive them to therapy have grown far more commonplace.

In 1980, according to a national study of medical care, 9,574,660 Americans, something less than half of 1 percent of the population, made one or more ambulatory mental health care visits. About half of these visits were to psychiatrists' or psychologists' offices. The remainder were to mental health or hospital outpatient clinics, or to the offices of social workers or physicians other than psychiatrists. In the same year the Epidemiologic Catchment Area Program of the National Institute of Mental Health conducted a massive diagnostic survey and estimated that about fifteen percent of the adult population suffered from a definable alcohol, drug, or mental disorder. Neither of these figures gives an accurate indication of the utilization of or need for

---

* It is convenient to use the word "patient" even though some psychiatrists and medical analysts may take one to task and strenuously object that they and only they have patients, whereas nonmedical therapists have "clients." It is too complicated always to use both terms. Moreover, the English language, as its words are defined by the *Oxford English Dictionary* and *Webster's Third New International Dictionary*, does not prohibit nonmedical therapists from calling their clients "patients."

psychotherapeutic services, as distinct from other forms of ambulatory mental health care, though they may indicate an order of magnitude of the problem.[24]

Another, 1975, study found that among psychiatric and analytic patients of private practitioners there was a very slight preponderance of women,* and that the average patient age was in the early mid-thirties. Of the patients, 29 percent were professional, technical, or kindred workers; 25 percent were housewives; 18 percent were students, and 28 percent were in other occupations. The rather vague initial diagnoses of all psychiatric and analytic patients were 23 percent depressive neurosis, 22 percent neurosis other than depressive, 18 percent personality disorders, 11 percent schizophrenia, and 6 percent affective psychosis. None of this is very informative or surprising, but the nature of therapeutic patients' problems is a subject that has been relatively neglected.[26]

The Therapeutic Attitude

The ideal psychotherapeutic attitude, articulated most clearly and thoroughly in the psychoanalytic literature, is that of the impartial mediator who helps patients grapple with their problems and find their true selves. Philosophically, this concept is related to one held by ancient healers, medieval theologians, and many eighteenth- and early-nineteenth-century alienists: that a person's soul cannot become sick, and that lunacy is a disorder afflicting the physical connection between a hypothetical pristine immortal soul and the rest of the material and spiritual world. Though modern therapists might balk at use of the word "soul," there remains an implicit assumption that there is an original potential for development into a normal, productive individual which, in the case of their patients, has been abnormally molded and perverted by passage through events of the material world, and that through therapeutic intervention these abnormal constraints can be removed. The therapist is to correct rather than construct.

Lawrence Kubie wrote that analysts ought not to trouble themselves with notions of ethics, except insofar as might pertain to their own behavior, because it is not their position to make value judgments on patients. The patient is simply a flawed process in need of repair, and the work the therapist performs is a psychic operation

---

* A somewhat deceptive figure, as an American Psychiatric Association study points out. Although 59 percent of psychiatrists' patients are women, 64 percent of primary care physicians' patients are women. Women are simply more likely to seek medical care.[25]

as objective and disinterested as the task of a surgeon or engineer. The basic substance of thought is a constant preconscious stream of data from inside and outside the body—sensations, bits of memory, and so on—but in the mentally sick individual, unconscious processes may disturb the representation of these data in the conscious mind and hamper its ability to manipulate and act upon that information. Analysis, therefore, aims "to broaden the domain of conscious awareness and control in human life and to shrink that darker empire in which unconscious processes play the dominant role, so that the essential freedom to change and to continue to change, which has been lost or impaired in various phases of each individual's development, can be regained and, with it, the freedom to learn, to mature, and to grow." Or as Freud more succinctly put it, "Where id was, there ego shall be," or again, though rather more dismally, "Much is won if we succeed in transforming hysterical misery into common unhappiness."[27]

The analyst frees the patient from enslavement to unconscious factors, pries apart the mental logjam and allows the stream of thought to resume its intended flow. It is implicitly assumed that the analyst will in some way be able to recognize when this state of freedom has been attained, and then his task will be done. What the patient chooses to do with himself once freed from unconscious constraints is not the concern of the psychoanalyst, but of the patient himself, or society, or, at worst, of the police. A common complaint heard from the children of psychoanalysts concerns this avowed willful amorality of their parents. "Everybody's potential, it seems to me," says one psychiatrist's son, "includes the potential to rape, murder, and burn down buildings, as well as to save lives and aid charitable organizations. If they truly believe that they need only *undo* and never *do*, that they can facilitate and never teach, then they are either wide-eyed pollyannas or hopeless idiots." The implication is that with work and training an analyst can correctly discriminate between those things that it is someone's nature to do and those things that they do due to unconscious, unchosen compulsion. This ideal analyst would not say that all bomb-throwing anarchists are bad, but would find that some were anarchists because of pathological compulsions, some were anarchists by nature but bomb-throwers through compulsion, and some were psychologically healthy individuals whose reasoned political beliefs led them to anarchistic revolt and the throwing of bombs.

In reality, whatever the theory may be, the therapist in the consulting room with a live patient before him is often denied the comfort of such nice, neat thoughts. An ophthalmic surgeon removing a cataract wishes to correct all refractive errors so that the full visual potential of the retina is achieved. A general surgeon operating on a stomach cancer wishes to remove the malignancy completely while minimizing the disruption of normal structures and functions, and however much the shape of individual tumors may vary, it is possible to distinguish between healthy and cancerous tissue. The psychotherapist, once he looks up from the textbook, sees no such discernible end point. People have different aspirations, different sources of satisfaction, and each has his own unique set of real-life circumstances that are only partially under his control and within which, however good, bad, just, or unjust they may be, he must manage to carry on. There is no common therapeutic terminus for the drug-abusing welfare mother whose ex-husband beats her and the middle-aged bank executive undergoing an identity crisis and contemplating a career change. There is no specific common goal, at any rate, merely a functional theme that in all cases certain human abilities must be mobilized in an attempt to cope with reality. In some cases it may not be possible to cope.

Often it is impossible for the analyst to limit his role to the discovery and reworking of past problems. Many psychological problems are not solely the result of isolated childhood trauma, and many that may once have been were subsequently so interlaced with other factors that simple removal of the original trauma's sequelae cannot compensate for all the related effects. For an analyst to limit himself to the pure domain of analysis would, in such cases, be like an educator who limits his role to discerning and correcting his students' mistakes while declining to teach anything new. But then once therapy admits some pedagogic function, it is impossible to exclude the therapist's values. One need only look at the American Psychiatric Association's changing views on whether homosexuality is a mental illness or merely a "condition" to see that diagnostic concepts, and the treatments they imply, are not independent of social values.

The mechanism of the abstract, pure form of psychoanalysis is well known. During therapy, an artificial situation is created in which the patient is invited to relinquish, as much as possible, all of the defensive mechanisms that have allowed him to conceal or control his inner disturbances and carry on with his life in the daily world. This situation is initiated through free association, by following the "fundamental rule of psychoanalysis" that "whatever comes into one's head must be reported without criticizing it."[28] Since the person is a psychological unit, what seems on the surface no more than a meaningless stream of memories, musings, daydreams, and thoughts turns out to have a definite internal structure and logic. Thoughts are linked by associations, and though the defensive mechanisms of the mind have contrived to obscure some of its more unpleasant workings, the mind never had to prepare itself against the subtle scrutiny and objective penetration of psychoanalysis. As isolated thoughts and strings of connectivity emerge over time, they coalesce into constellations and begin to form a full portrait of the patient's mind. The analyst perceives patterns not only in what is said, but in what is not said, or in how things are obscured, since the mechanisms of resisting free association are quite as revealing as the material that comes through.

In the idealized Freudian analytic situation, the analyst refrains from any interference during this free associative process, just as the physical scientist attempts objectively to observe a system that is not altered by his act of observation. Any steering on the part of the analyst would pervert the spontaneous emergence of the patient's thoughts, and any premature comments or interpretations would affect the factors that determine that emergence. Intervention is kept to the minimum necessary to maintain the production of material. In fact, the analyst is only supposed to listen in an impressionistic sort of way, with "evenly suspended attention," without specific concentration or expectations. Nor must the analyst identify with his patient, which would compromise his objectivity, though in order to accomplish the objective appreciation of the subjective entity that is the patient's mind, the analyst "introjects this object [the patient's mind] transiently, and projects the introject again onto the object," or, to use less jargonistic though even more distasteful language, "Any practical psychologist, analytic or nonanalytic, has to be able to perform this particular test just as quickly and reliably and as undisturbedly as, for example, the tea taster, who introjects materially a small sample only long enough to be able to taste it."[29]

The analyst's personality in the course of treatment is supposed to be as evenly suspended as his attention. What serves him as a personality outside the consulting room is in many ways nothing more than a prejudicial nuisance within the context of his practice. For the patient, the analyst should be a blank. This is important not solely so that the analyst does not interfere, but because a part of the analytic process is "transference," a phenomenon whereby elements of the patient's early affections and hostilities toward his parents are transferred to the analyst. Transference is the most difficult aspect of analysis, and was originally viewed as an obstacle, because it introduces a powerful set of emotional connections on the part of the patient, and makes tremendous demands on the emotional poise of the analyst. At the same time, however, transference came to be recognized as the most valuable element of the analytic process, since it enables the patient not only to remember past events that brought him to the present state, but to coax aspects of them into present reality and rework them with a maturity and wisdom previously unavailable.

Who is the person who should accomplish the analytic task? Freud, at some times, suggested that the analyst should be emotionally cold: "I cannot advise my colleagues too urgently to model themselves during psycho-analytic treatment on the surgeon, who puts aside all his feelings, even his human sympathy, and concentrates his mental forces on the single aim of performing the operation as skilfully as possible."[30] At other times he recommended a more humane and sympathetic approach, and in actual practice he is known to have talked quite openly about any number of topics, including himself, with many of his patients.

Some psychotherapists have been more Freudian than Freud,* averring that the analyst must maintain an inhuman silence throughout most of the analytic process. Others have moved toward the opposite extreme and advocated more equal, more human, and in some cases even passionate relations between patient and therapist. For the most part, however, it is held that the therapist is a professional, not a friend, and as such should perform the curative function with professional reserve and dignity, and afterward maintain no more intimate relationship with the client than a lawyer after the case has ended. Less, in fact, since lingering elements of the transference are supposed to make the patient unnaturally attached to the therapist, leading to a potentially unhealthy relationship that would be based upon things other than open friendship. As one therapist put it, the ideal would be if, years after therapy, the patient does not like or dislike his therapist, but is completely indifferent to him.

Becoming a psychotherapist is a difficult task, and if, as is often suggested, people go into therapy seeking answers and comfort to soothe their own inner turmoils, they encounter an unusually torturous phase in the course of professionalization.[31] Though all medical residents may have the sense that they are given too much respon-

---

* As Jung is said to have commented: "Thank God I am Jung and not a Jungian!"

sibility and too little knowledge to bear it properly, most have the consolation that the solid rules of anatomy, physiology, and biochemistry hold true and set some limit on the range of uncertainty. The psychiatric resident is denied this slim consolation and obliged to accept subjective impressions—which he has elsewhere been told to mistrust—as objective clinical data. He has, moreover, been required in this situation to abandon his "ordinary untrained good sense and adaptive capacities"[32] that might lead him to console the miserable patient or recoil from the angry one, in favor of acquired techniques that seem artificial and insincere, possibly even perverse and cruel. As one investigator said of the psychoanalytic candidate in the midst of his supervised analyses:

> Having some *information* and only a rudimentary grasp of the dynamics of the analytic situation of which his own behaviour is a part, the beginner looks for rules according to which his behaviour would be "appropriately analytic." Having lost his spontaneity, he now wonders about the appropriateness of each move he makes: should he smile; should he let the patient into the office first; respond to comments on the weather, etc.? Should he shake hands or wish the patient a Happy New Year? Should he answer some of the patient's questions? How austere should he be in his demeanour or expression? How uniform and stereotyped does his behaviour have to be to perform the analytic task adequately?[33]

However much the ideal therapist is supposed to remain neutral and hover above the therapeutic situation like a wraith that floats, seeing but not being, above the couch, the real therapist is a part of the process, and his personality, whatever he transforms it into, is the tool with which he works. The acquisition of a strong "therapeutic ego" involves a great deal of self scrutiny, of repression and diversion of natural impulses, and of frustration.

The most frustrating aspect of psychotherapy is the near total uncertainty of the job. Training seems inadequate or wholly irrelevant when the first patient walks into the consulting room. The documented appalling lack of diagnostic consistency between different therapists does not cast doubt on those therapists' ability to treat patients, but emphasizes the subjectivity of the therapist-patient relationship and the severe inability to identify and categorize significant factors, one of the first steps in any hard science. Meanwhile, practitioners from totally different schools, using different concepts and different techniques, may reach indistinguishable results.*

Patients may improve in spite of poor therapy or may obdurately remain sick despite the most brilliant and appropriate interventions. Since the original diagnosis, the process of treatment, and the end point called "cure" are all so ill-defined, the therapist can attribute success to his brilliance and failure to the patients' ironclad resistance or unwillingness to devote himself to the task of psychotherapy; or conversely, should he be so inclined, can elect to take blame for a failure wholly beyond his control.

Various studies have suggested that in at least some cases placebos (either drugs that did nothing or fictitious behavior modification techniques) are as effective as genuine therapy, implying that even more than with physiological disorders, *thinking* that one's emotional problems have been solved can be as effective as solving them. In one curious experiment, people who sought psychotherapy were assigned either to treatment by trained professional therapists with reputations for clinical expertise and an average of twenty-three years of counseling experience, or to treatment by college professors who had no therapeutic training at all, but who were reputed among students to be warm and trustworthy. The professors' patients showed as much improvement as did the therapists',[35] which appears to support the widespread allegation that most psychotherapy is at heart little more than baroque verbal embellishments superimposed upon (or sometimes replacing) common sense.†

Perhaps the most amusing indication of psychotherapy's amorphous aims and techniques is the fact that, in these litigious times, though psychotherapists are sometimes sued for malpractice—in cases, for example, when they take sexual advantage of patients—as of 1979 there were no reported negligence cases where a therapist was sued for what he had said. "As long as therapists restrict their practice

---

* Henri Ellenberger, in *The Discovery of the Unconscious*, remarks: "Those who undertake a Freudian analysis will soon develop an intensive transference neurosis, have Freudian dreams, and discover their Oedipus complex, child sexuality, and castration anxiety. Those who undertake a Jungian analysis will have Jungian dreams, confront their shadow, their anima, their archetypes, and pursue their individuation. A Freudian psychoanalyst who would undergo a Jungian analysis would feel as disoriented as Mephisto in the second part of *Faust,* when he comes to the Classical Walpurgis Night and discovers with amazement that 'there is another Hell with its own laws.' "[34]

† German psychiatrist Albert Moll related the story of a secret agent who came to him during the war asking to be coached so that he could assume the role of a doctor. Moll told the agent that this was impossible, since medicine was so complex, but that he could easily teach him to impersonate a psychoanalyst. After several days of training in the rudimentary concepts and jargon, the man went off and successfully passed the rest of the war as an analyst.[36]

to talk, interpretation, and advice, they will remain nearly immune from suit, no matter how poor their advice, how damaging their comments, or how incorrect their interpretations."*[37]

My intent with these pessimistic comments is not to cast doubt on the validity of psychotherapy. The investigators who questioned the significance of therapeutic technique intentionally selected subjects who would not be harmed by being deprived of psychotherapy, and in doing so, chose a population that did not really need it and whose troubles might really best be solved just by the chance to talk to someone, whether it be a therapist, a counselor, a friend, or a warm and trustworthy college professor. The point is, rather, that in psychotherapy, irrefutable proof of success is hard to find. People may not understand nuclear physics, but they must believe the physicist who says he has theories that are true, because he can point to tangible results. Psychotherapists have difficulty persuading doubters, because there is nothing for them to point to. If so inclined, they can doubt their own effectiveness, even when faced with apparent success. All in all, psychotherapy remains largely a matter of faith —faith in the technique, faith in the psychotherapist. And because it is a faith, it is difficult for someone not predisposed toward belief to be gradually persuaded through reason to believe, as a chemistry student who doubts the absurd notion of protons, neutrons, electrons, and orbitals might gradually be persuaded as he sees how this concept permits him to predict the reactivity of different elements. The psychotherapist-to-be must have a previous faith, or a strong desire or other motive, in order to seek out and persist in this baffling profession.

---

* On the other hand there was a recent court case, finally settled out of court, where a patient sued his psychiatrist for incorrectly diagnosing him and treating him with psychotherapy alone rather than with drugs.

3

A Child's-Eye
View of
Psychotherapy

> My father's a psychotherapist. You
> know what's really interesting
> about that? It starts with a "P."
>
> —A SIX-YEAR-OLD

For most people work is an unpleasant necessity that occupies a large part of their waking hours throughout the most active years of their adult lives. Work determines many things about them: when they leave home in the morning and return home at night, how much time and energy they have for other pursuits, their standard of living, and to some extent their living circumstances and circle of friends. "What do you do?" is a convenient question to ask a stranger. The answer may indicate some of his interests and suggest topics of conversation; it defines him economically, perhaps culturally, and sometimes in terms of more specific occupational stereotypes.

Nonetheless, most people view what they do for a living as clearly distinct from the rest of their lives. With few exceptions, when they think of themselves they think first of a body, a mind, a family, a home, a set of values and personality traits, not of an engineer, accountant, secretary, or short-order cook. Some years ago it was fashionable *not* to ask people what they did for a living, in recognition of the fact that this occupational pigeonholing unjustly ignored the individual person.

Children as well, with rare exceptions, do not think of their parents in terms of their jobs. They know what daddy or mommy does for a living, but pumping gas, running a corporation, driving a truck, painting pictures, even teaching school have next to nothing to do with child rearing, and play a negligible part in the child's sense of family identity. When adolescents rebel against their parents it is not their jobs they rebel against, but the values they hold or the social compromises they have made. Do dentists' children refuse to floss? Do taxi drivers' kids become reckless drivers? Do carpenters' children cultivate ineptitude in home repairs? Businessmen's children may revolt against materialism and a ruthless lust for power, but it is the underlying social philosophy they respond to, not the specific manufacture, distribution, and promotion of widgets. The parents' jobs certainly have great effects on the children, but rarely in such a direct and consistent way that one would group them according to parental profession and expect to find meaningful common denominators.

There are a few exceptions to this rule—conspicuous among them the children of clerics and psychotherapists.* Religion and psychotherapy are not merely occupations that have particular circumstances, economics, and demographics, nor are they professions easily left at the office when one goes home. Both are philosophical systems deeply concerned with the daily lives and social interactions of people; and in both cases their practitioners are expected, to a greater or lesser extent, to embody the principles they espouse. Their jobs become inseparable from their identities, and therefore become part of their families' identities as well.

Ministers are supposed to be good. They are not academics who merely teach about religion or anthropologists who have done field work on the moral behavior of congregants and can therefore address the subject with knowledge. Ministers are supposed to have been called by God, they have devoted themselves to God's purpose, and they lead lives of humility, piety, and benevolence. To society at large they are more than professionals who serve certain functions and conduct weekly ceremonies, they are the human incarnation of theological beliefs, ethics, and judgments. If a garage mechanic curses in front of a minister, he catches himself and says, "Oh, sorry, father." A priest who wears his collar while traveling by train or airplane invites peculiar confidences from people or else risks making his travel companions self-conscious and uncomfortable.

Ministers are even, sometimes to their exasperation, expected to embody the particular concept of goodness held by each individual

---

* "Army brats" are another group commonly segregated out by parental profession, but in their case so many powerful social factors—frequent relocation, paternal absence, the unusually regimented communal living experience of military bases, overseas assignments, and early paternal retirement—set them aside from their nonmilitary peers that any effects of professional values and personality are obscured.[1]

parishioner. One psychotherapist who used to be a Presbyterian minister in Princeton remarked, "This is a rapidly changing community with a lot of different types of people. When I was in the parish we had a bunch of corporate hotshots who commuted up to New York, and they expected me to sit up and shoot the breeze with them and solve the problems of the world till one or two in the morning, while my next door neighbor, the farmer, wanted to see the light on in my kitchen at 5:00 A.M. or else I was some kind of goof-off. It can get to you after a while when you have five or six hundred people watching you, and somebody wants you to drink tea, and somebody else wants you to have a belt with the boys."

Ministers' families are inevitably expected to support and extend the minister's role. Wives should be devoted and helpful. Children ought to behave, particularly since other parents in the congregation look to them as examples. "All the mothers kept a close watch on my daughter's clothes," one minister's wife told me. "If she went to school in a skirt that was above the knee, they figured it meant that God had okayed shorter skirts this year."

The burden of *goodness* can be unbearable for the minister's children, and may create insoluble problems. They must sing in the choir, participate in church functions, and generally conduct themselves like little adults. Disobedience is a more potent assault on the father than it would be in other families. Meanwhile, though the children are obliged to show public respect for their fathers and the church, in private they may know that the minister kicks the dog or drinks too much, that he despises certain congregants, or does not believe or practice what he preaches. In off-hours at the church, the children may enjoy running in the aisles, climbing on the altar, and generally raising hell; they may even, like one minister's son I spoke to, take particular delight in scratching obscenities in the pews with a pin and dropping Cheerios in the collection plate.

Among friends and classmates, ministers' children have a tremendous burden to overcome, which is a strong practical incentive for their notorious mischievous behavior. An Episcopalian minister, the son and grandson of ministers, told me rumor had it that "ministers' daughters are easy lays," something he had proved to his personal satisfaction during his youth. In general, his experience as a minister's son had been none too pleasant, since he never quite fit into the local life of the various parishes to which his father was assigned. In Pennsylvania steel towns he was the intellectual pansy who played the violin; on Philadelphia's wealthy Main Line he was on a cultural par with the local kids, but poverty-stricken in comparison. Worst was the loneliness of living alone, set off in the church—a weird place to live by any child's standards. The members of the family lived in a fishbowl where their behavior was constantly scrutinized or where they at least had to act as though it were. "Do you know how nauseating it is to be good *all the time?*" he asked bitterly. "It is awfully hard not to resent the life you are forced to lead." Little wonder that ministers' kids are supposed to be, and often are, brats.*

Whereas preachers' kids are supposed to be brats, psychotherapists' kids are supposed to be crazy. In many ways the social functions of ministers and therapists are the same, as are the opportunities for hypocrisy, the extraordinary expectations of the laity, and some of the peculiar pressures exerted upon the spouses and children. Religion and therapy are the two professions where the children's response, whether purposeful rebellion or unavoidable reaction, is supposed to be quite contrary to the profession's aim. Interesting comparisons, as well as interesting distinctions, can be drawn between the two populations.

One significant difference between ministers and psychotherapists is that, though the profound meaning of religion may elude the child's apprehension, its public manifestation and the clergyman's daily routine are clear to the point of theatricality. In fact, the lure of possessing a stage where one can hold an audience captive and show off all alone is often cited as one of the less appropriate attractions that draws people to the clergy.† Ministers' children have a better idea of what their fathers do for a living than the children of lawyers or accountants, and it is a more interesting sort of living, involving people and power, damnation and redemption, ceremony, history, and passion. They can see their fathers in the pulpit every Sunday morning and observe the responses of the congregation.

Psychotherapy, on the other hand, is inscrutable, willfully hidden, and tinged with the forbidden. There are no tools and there is no product. There is no process that can be watched. The patients are supposed never to be seen or identified. To the extent that the

* I am not sure whether the myth extends to rabbis' children as well, who would perhaps be more closely comparable to psychotherapists' children. I asked one orthodox rabbi at the Board of Rabbis of Greater Philadelphia whether rabbis' children are supposed to be brats, and he replied, "Only the children of reform rabbis."

† One psychologist I interviewed, a minister's son who began clerical training himself and now specializes in treating Episcopalian ministers, was so insistent about the theatrical power of the church that he wanted to arrange to have me read a lesson from the pulpit one Sunday, or at least to walk in the procession, in order to prove to my own satisfaction what an irresistible lure the role held. Interestingly, he also insisted that I switch places with him and sit in his comfortable leather therapist's chair while he perched on the couch, so that I could feel how much more powerful a position *that* was.

children are told about the work, which is often quite limited, the problems dealt with are purely adult problems and therefore virtually incomprehensible. Strangers respond to the parent's profession neither with indifference nor with the straightforward deference accorded a clergyman, but with an odd mixture of something indefinable but often distinctly apprehensive and sometimes overtly belligerent.

Interestingly, the PsyKs who are most comfortable in their knowledge of their parents' profession are the children—now usually much older—of institutional psychiatrists who lived on the grounds of state or private institutions and who had regular contact with severely disturbed patients. Sometimes their memories are extremely fond: the more innocuous patients acted as servants and gardeners for the resident medical staff and doted on their children. One man recalled that his first tennis instructor was a hospital inmate, though unfortunately a prefrontal lobotomy had ruined his game by excising his competitive spirit. An elderly woman whose father directed a state institution in Virginia mourned the loss of the "lovely, idyllic" surroundings she recalled, where her father looked lovingly after his "children," the patients—a curious picture in light of mental hospitals' current reputation, and retrospectively somewhat distasteful to the extent that such a devoted but captive and subservient staff reminds one of the lopsided joys of plantation life.

Some experiences were far less pleasant. One man, a sculptor, vividly described his unpleasant memories of eleven childhood years spent on the grounds of a private institution, where his psychoanalyst father worked to supplement his income from private practice. His mother had had nicknames for some of the most colorful inmates: "George from the Piggery," who was hunchbacked and smelled of tobacco juice and garbage, and "Tunk," a vast and powerful man who spent his days lifting and dropping a huge section of sewer pipe by the side of a lake near the bottom of the grounds. Most of all he remembered a huge four-story structure of porched cages. "Sick, sick men and women were in them, sitting in rocking chairs, quietly talking to themselves. But when we kids dared walk by, taking a shortcut for some urgent reason, they would all loom forward from the shadows up to the wire, and a din would pick up and rise to a scream. I suppose they could see how terrified we were. God, that was scary. It still gives me the creeps to think about it."

However unpleasant the memory may have been, nonetheless it was a robust and tangible unpleasantness with the fully comprehensible and even exciting feel of any other childhood adventure or persecution. In this open setting, the patients were conspicuously different from the staff and from normal people in the way they behaved and were treated. The psychiatrist parent could be seen interacting with them and could discuss them freely and by name. The whole process, even the terrors, remained within a manageable though strange perspective.

Questions are far less easily answered by the psychotherapist in private practice. What, precisely, does the parent do? Who are these patients who are never seen or named, and discussed in cryptic terms or not at all? What problems do they have? Those occasionally glimpsed through the window seem perfectly normal and there are only vague hints about embarrassing problems that lead them to skulk about and pay high prices to discuss their woes in secret.

"I had no clear impressions of what my parents did," says one man, "except that they went into rooms and talked to people. I do remember that when I was nine or ten someone explained to me that when you are grown up you have to work for a living, and when I looked around at what other people did, it struck me that my parents had it pretty easy, they had a very nice life."

A woman in her mid-thirties relates that the first time she gave serious thought to her psychiatrist father's profession was in first or second grade, when her teacher told the children to bring in something from their father's job to present at show and tell. Her classmates had fathers with real jobs, she says, and they brought in drainpipes, circuit breakers, machinery parts, blueprints, stethoscopes, and other paraphernalia. Her father gave her a pad of yellow legal paper, a pen, and a reflex hammer. She knew that he didn't even use the hammer and was just trying to make himself seem important. "I cried afterwards, because there was a long table covered with all these neat things, and I just had a piece of paper and a hammer. I was really upset. I decided that my father didn't do anything at all."

The therapist parents themselves have problems with the obscurity of their jobs. One psychoanalyst said that one of his more uncomfortable experiences was the reciprocal of the above. Parents were asked to come to their children's elementary school to discuss what they did for a living, and he found it impossible to think of anything interesting and coherent to say. Another less self-conscious analyst went to "Hobby Night" at his daughter's school, and after everyone else discussed stamp collecting, birdwatching, and golf, he undertook to explain the *meaning* of hobbies. "His talk made a very big impression," his daughter recalls. "Nobody had the *faintest* idea what he was talking about—not the grownups, not the children. They didn't understand a word he said all the time he was up there, but he went on and on, and probably thought he was the hit of the evening. I was very embarrassed by the whole thing."

The fact that their children do not understand their work and are not impressed by it bothers some psychotherapists. One successful and respected psychiatrist I interviewed seemed sad that his children were not interested in what he did. When they were very young, they occasionally came to the office with him on Saturday mornings when he had paperwork to do. They played with his check-writing machine and his calculator, sat in his chair, lay on the couch, looked out of the thirty-sixth floor window, but they tired of the boring little room very quickly and did not want to come back. He found himself envying the fathers whose jobs made a more vital and favorable impression on their children. Despite his very real importance and success in his field, there was no way to convey it.

Sometimes parents can point out the families of their children's classmates as people undergoing the divorces, mournings, and other catastrophes that may lead people to psychotherapy, but for the child such problems remain elusive and certainly much less tangible than the bumps, breaks, and colds that take people to "real doctors." There are no X-ray machines, no needles, no examining tables, no tools of the trade. Presenting the fundamental concepts of psycho-analysis in a form comprehensible to a six-year-old is beyond the ability of most people, even if they felt it would be useful. Vague talk about dream interpretations and the unconscious mind tends to be misleading, meaningless, or incredible, and perhaps ultimately em-barrassing to the parent. One thirteen-year-old, commenting upon a dream analysis her lay analyst mother had proudly related to her, said that she had been very impressed. "It's wonderful that you can just make something up and your patients will believe it. I think it's neat that you can just sit in your nice chair, make up some mumbo jumbo, and have a lot of people say 'Wow, I never realized that before!' and make $60 an hour—*a dollar a minute!*—just for that."

Some therapists tell their kids that they are "feeling doctors," or that they just spend their time talking to people about problems, which makes their professional function seem curiously close to their parental one. "I think I thought that my [psychiatrist] father was able to be a father to people who didn't have strong fathers. And I thought that my [child analyst] mother probably played with the kids whose mothers didn't play with them. They were rich kids whose mothers were too busy doing something else, so my mother played the part of a sophisticated kind of nanny. I was very envious of those kids, because my mother had play therapy toys in her office that *I* never had—Scandinavian dollhouses and all sorts of great stuff. Basically I thought people came to get yelled at by my father and to play with my mother, just like me. Except that when *my* mother was too busy to play with me, I just went to my room."

The most striking feature of the childhoods of many PsyKs is the home office. More therapists have offices at home than almost any other type of professional: space requirements are minimal, there is no need for elaborate equipment or for more than a single, usually part-time employee and, even on an unusually heavy workday, patient traffic is limited to nine or ten people. Thus a room is set aside in the house or apartment, or an extension constructed with a separate path and entrance: "It's a very odd thing when you bring over your friends. You say, 'This is my father's office,' and the doors are all soundproofed and padded."

The home office is quiet, soft, rich, and soothing, both to present an ideal therapeutic environment and to make the therapist's long hours there as comfortable as possible. There are many books—an inordinate number of them by some guy named "Frood," thought one analyst's daughter as she helped her father pack for a move—perhaps an assortment of art objects and an iconic portrait of Freud. Therapeutic consultation rooms often have a curious air of anonymous intimacy: to maintain the disinterestedness of the psychotherapist's role they should not speak too strongly of any particular taste or preference nor show children's drawings or family photographs, yet when a therapist spends so many hours in one place, sitting, thinking, listening, and looking, he can scarcely refrain from gradually molding it into a complement of his real or contrived personality that helps make him seem the way he would like to be seen.

Special rules govern the home office. Children must be very quiet. They should not listen at doors. Most of them do, anyway, though what they overhear tends to be disappointingly plain old boring grown-up talk, and it is difficult to believe that so much fuss is made over so little. In my own house, where both parents' offices were on the ground floor, we were simply forbidden to enter or leave between ten minutes before the hour and the hour—the changing of the patients. Precautions were also taken to shelter them from one another, and I recall complex routines where four arriving and departing patients had to be shunted into various waiting rooms and offices while the others were hurried invisibly down the hall.

In other houses, such separations were not always possible, but one did the best one could. A New York analyst's son, now an analyst himself, practicing out of the apartment where he grew up, showed me the small vestibule that served as a waiting room. A dozen feet to the left of the front entrance is a door leading to the apartment and office. Half a dozen feet to the right is a back door that leads to the kitchen. It was impossible to prevent him from encountering patients at all as a child, short of barring him from ever coming home, and as the best compromise he was told to take the shorter route through the back door, thus minimizing this unwanted contact, though at the expense of giving him a longer path to his room once he got inside. He agrees that it was absurd, more symbolic than rational, but considered necessary nonetheless. It was never definitively settled whether he should or should not say hello to the patients as he passed.

The reasons for not disturbing therapeutic sessions may never be clearly articulated, but the children have a strong sense of taboo that is quite distinctive. A psychotherapist whose father was a gastroenterologist and whose mother was a psychoanalyst recalls the dramatic difference between her perception of their two working situations. Both had offices at home, though her father's was filled with specialized equipment that, while different from what she saw in her pediatrician's office, was perfectly clear in its general purpose. Her father had friends who were patients and patients who became friends, and there was nothing covert about his job or the least bit secret about the patients' arrival. She was expected to respect their privacy, of course, but it was in the ordinary way that children are generally supposed to behave, and keep out of the way, and not disturb their parents while they are working.

Quite different was her attitude toward her mother's office, located in the back of the house behind the kitchen, with a separate path, an entrance concealed from view by the landscaping, and soundproofed double doors that by their very existence implied that people should yearn to listen:

> I remember her coming out fiercely once or twice saying "You are being too noisy!" It was very much a sacred place, like a chapel, and the idea that I had intruded there *terrified* me. I don't remember her ever saying anything so blunt as "Something very special is going on in here and you are ruining it," I just remember having the absolute, certain knowledge that it was terribly private and you had to stay out. There was no question. It would never have occurred to me to disobey.

Once I brought a friend home, and we went into the kitchen to eat, and for some reason this guy was horsing around and he charged through the door to my mother's office. I had the sense that he had crossed the *Boundary* and something apocalyptic would happen. There was a waiting room and then a hall and then the office, so fortunately he hadn't actually penetrated to the inner chamber, but just *seeing* him cross through that door made my heart stop. Some incredible taboo had been violated.

My mother's work was certainly more intriguing to me than my father's, in large part because of the mystery. What *did* she do in that office? What went on? We sometimes played shrink when we were kids, as probably most shrinks' kids do. That consisted of going into her office on occasions when she wasn't there, and either my friend or I lying down on the couch and doing whatever we thought the patients did. The problem was that we didn't know what they did. I'm sure I asked my mother, and no doubt she told me something, so I had the broad strokes of it, but no meaningful detail. The only thing I knew with certainty was that my mother knitted profusely. She had a little cushion that she would hide her knitting behind when the patients entered and left, and she used plastic needles, which clicked less. Since most of her hours were analytic, the patients were facing away from her and apparently didn't know what she was doing. Reams and reams of baby things and often sweaters for ourselves came pouring out of her office. I suppose that since knitting was the only part of it I knew for certain, it was that that I fixed on in some strange way. I had a fantasy that one day I would be wearing one of those sweaters and suddenly I would start *feeling* something, one of the patient's dreams or associations that had become ravelled up in the material.

The son of two psychiatrists recalls:

My father's profession was pretty enigmatic. Here's a guy in this profession where *he shuts the door*. If it's time off and you go in and sit down to talk to him, you see two chairs, and you realize that this is where your father does his job. In these two chairs. Chair, desk, little space, another chair. But as for what the job entails, all I knew was that he talked to somebody. I probably asked if there was anything else, because of course it is a little curious—even suspect. We had this white brick colonial thing in the suburbs, not a very memorable house in itself, and my father had built an adjoining rectangle for his office. It didn't lie flush with the main façade of the house, so there was a real sense of an addendum—that around which one walks quietly, that around which one makes no noise. Inevitably it got to be a little mysterious. It naturally resembled a church in some sense, or the theater or the ballet or the movies. So I suppose I thought there was something mysterious going on, because of the magic associated with the theater, ballet, or movies, or a church.

The deep mystery of the situation was compounded by the fact that, for analysts' children in particular, other, even more incredible reasons were given for avoiding contact with the patients. It was not simply a question of privacy; it was actually essential to the cure. "My mother gave me some primitive explanation of transference—that these patients passed through a stage where they saw her as their mother, and it would upset them if they ran into me, her real child. So I was never allowed to play on the lawn when patients were coming, and if I was out shopping with my mother and she saw one of her patients we had to quick go the other way. I never knew *exactly* what would happen to them if they saw me, but I knew that it would be an unbelievable disaster."

A psychoanalyst's son found this aspect particularly intriguing. "I was curious about them. My father and mother both told me that the patients would be really interested in me, that they would want to see *me*, and that this was, in fact, associated with their problem." He laughed. "That was why they were coming to see my father in the first place. So I felt very shy and self-conscious, but also very interested, because I wanted to see these people who were so eager to scrutinize me and my family and environment, and whose mental stability in some way apparently hinged upon their impressions of me."

The analysts themselves sometimes took exceptional precautions against meeting their patients outside the analytic setting. One psychoanalyst refused to attend concerts, though he was passionately devoted to music, because somewhere in the audience might lurk one of his patients. When the family went to the seashore in the summer he scarcely ventured outside the house, telling his sons that he dared not let some stray patient glimpse him in a bathing suit and sun hat playing in the waves. On those rare occasions when he attended a dinner party, his wife had to telephone the hostess beforehand for a guest list so that he could make sure that none of his patients, nor even someone who was close to a patient, was going to be there as well. Fortunately, few analysts were quite so extreme, and over the years this obsessive passion for anonymity has subsided to more commonsense levels.

However protected patients were from children and children from patients, the children did inevitably learn some things. Parents tell stories at the dinner table about the patient who is so fat that he can't fit into the chair, or about the girl who almost never eats, or who eats too much, and how these problems relate to some thoughts that seem unrelated. Phobias, compulsions, and hideous disasters make wonderful stories, though they are little more than just that. "Tell me a story, Mommy, a *juicy* story," one girl regularly pleaded, and she relished such tales as homosexual couples living together, with children in the house who did not know. A few patients come to be part of the family lore. The son of two psychiatrists remembers: "My mother had one patient named Mrs. Hiss. I have no idea who she was, but she would call my mother, not infrequently, for *years*, and just give her hell. My mother would leave the dinner table for three-quarters of an hour, and we would all sit there getting irritated, and we would hear her saying, 'Yes Mrs. Hiss, yes, Mrs. Hiss, yes.' She told us that Mrs. Hiss needed to give somebody hell, it was a release for her, and that she ended up as the whipping boy. But then three days a week my mother worked late, and my *father* would answer the phone, and he would say, 'No, Mrs. Hiss, that is *not* so. No, I'm sorry, you're wrong. Good-bye.' Boom. Then the next week it was back to my mother again."

Other PsyKs have more direct contact with patients. Says one young man, the son of two psychoanalysts:

Over the years I heard various scraps of conversation over the dinner table, and formed a very impressionistic sense of these people who needed psychoanalysis. But then there was one where I knew exactly what was wrong. We had a big bulldog when I was growing up, a wonderfully friendly dog, but the classically ugly, ugly, drooling, fanged bulldog. Apparently my father was seeing someone who was severely phobic of dogs, and one day our dog got lonesome down in the kitchen and decided she wanted some company. So she walked up the stairs, muscled open the door, strolled into the living room, and sat down, wagging her tail, waiting to be petted by this person who was terrified of dogs. My mother and I were on the third floor with the doors closed, but we heard these screams reminiscent of an Alfred Hitchcock movie. Everybody ran, and here we found this person standing on a chair, absolutely livid, the picture of terror, screaming hysterically, and there was the dog. Well, even I could put two and two together and come up with a diagnosis: that person is afraid of dogs.

After hearing dramatic stories about patients and perhaps reading exciting case histories in the readily accessible psychiatry books, it can be disconcerting to learn how insidious mental illness can be. "I was puzzled for a long time by the people I saw looking out the window," says a painter in his mid-thirties, "the guy in a suit and a normal overcoat, someone dressed the way my father did, or my teachers or I did. Or women, very normal, so neat, and with straight makeup on. It was hard to believe that there was something extreme going on inside them, and there was some confusion in my mind as to the point at which mental illness becomes legible on the face of a person in its grip. You would think there should be telltale signs. I was constitutionally a little reserved and nervous myself, so I didn't read things like just a little physical tension in a walk as indicative of something which would make somebody have to go to a doctor. So I was mystified. I wondered: were they coming for themselves, or for somebody that they knew?"

A young woman whose father first worked at a mental institution, where she grew accustomed to the obviously disturbed patients, was rather puzzled after he went over into exclusively private practice. "I was fifteen or sixteen when we went out to the theater one night, and this schoolteacher walked up and said, 'Oh, hello, Dr. Peel.' And later I asked, 'How do you know her?' because she had never taught me, and my mother said, 'She's one of your father's patients.' It was only then that it really struck me that these very normal people could be seeing a psychiatrist: before that I thought the only people who saw psychiatrists were really visibly crazy people. After that I was more and more aware of the fact that an awful lot of my own friends were anorexic and so on—middle-class girls right in my school—and a lot of them were seeing my father's colleagues. It meant that it was no longer *them* and *us:* it was just sort of everybody and anybody who could be psychiatrists' patients."

Sometimes the encounters can be profoundly disturbing:

I don't know exactly how old I was when, one day, on my way home from school, I sat in on a session that my father was having. My father worked at a psychiatric institute near my school, and the school bus dropped me off there and I would wait for him to take me home. It was a pretty interesting place. People in neighboring offices included anthropologists and people in other fields, and I have fond memories of them, because they used to play nice games with me after school. But for some reason, on one occasion—this will be enigmatic to me till the day that I die, and I sometimes tell it to people who are interested in just how crazy it was growing up that way—one day, while waiting to go home, my father said that either "I could" or "Did I want to," or that "It didn't matter if I" sat in while he talked to a painter who, because of some shock he'd experienced in the military, was behaving in what I think would be termed a near catatonic manner. He was accompanied by a sister who brought him to the sessions, and he would, in response to all my father's questions, say nothing except "Sit on the bed." Those were his exact words, "Sit on the bed," and he would repeat that in various modulations. I remember his sister as large—of course I was very little—but I remember her as pretty and sort of tallish, and he as a sizeable man who was reduced to very few physical movements and this one phrase. And my father said: "Sit on the bed how?" or "Sit on the bed like a prostitute?"—which of course was my father the psychiatrist, always thinking of the nicest possible explanation. And to each of these inquiries, the painter would reply, "Sit on the bed." And my father said to me, "That's what artists are like."

I remember that what impressed me at the time was not anything about how my father was handling the situation, but how impenetrable the guy was. I was aware that I was in the presence of—not some neurosis that was just going to get well. I remember being aware that I was looking at something that might not change. I was beginning to learn that there are shocks in life so profound that they can interrupt the normal course of consciousness.

The fantasies that PsyKs have about what goes on in the consulting room can be exceptionally bizarre, fueled by the cryptic arrangement of the office and the profession's steamy reputation. David Reiser, a psychiatrist and the son of an analyst, relates in an unpublished paper his deep curiosity about what his father did—a curiosity that he believes to be a compelling reason why he followed his father into the profession.

Between the ages of 9 and 18, my father maintained an office in the home. This was the inner sanctum, a proscribed area at the far end of the apartment with its own separate entrance. Not inconsequentially for me, the lay-out of the apartment was basically this: there was my sister's bedroom, my bedroom, then my parents' bedroom. Beyond my parents' bedroom lay the sanctus sanctorum—my father's office with its separate waiting room, mysterious books on the shelves, pictures of Freud, and—above all—the couch. I knew that people laid down on that thing and that it had something important to do with what happened between them and my father. There is very little doubt in my mind that much of my curiosity regarding the parental bedroom got displaced, so to speak, down the hall. This is a theme that I hear over and over among children of analysts—memories of intense curiosity about what went on behind that closed door. The connection of this curiosity to fantasies of the primal scene was graphically brought home in my case by an episode of snooping when I was sixteen. One Saturday, when my father was out at work, I was snooping in his study (not unusual at that time). In his desk I found a series of spiral notebooks which had been written in his unmistakable handwriting. For some reason, I decided on this occasion that these process notes were actually his diary. Therefore it was with some horror as well as titillation that I read a verbatim first person account about the details of sexual intercourse. "Boy—it was never like that; it's never been this good before!" The narrative had gone on to describe, in very graphic and colorful language, details of a very lively love-making session indeed.

Drenched with sweat, I found myself flooded with a mix of emotions. They (my parents) really did do it. Should I be happy for them that it was so great? But what the hell was he doing writing it down in a diary anyway? Some ill-intentioned and unscrupulous person might even be snooping in his office and find it![2]

A thirty-two-year-old New Mexico astrologer recalls:

I went through a period where I wanted to play psychiatrist with my father. I would go in and sit in the chair and make up problems. I had one running story about my husband and our unhappy marriage. My husband worked in a tuna canning factory, and he'd lost his finger and I didn't love him anymore. Hello, Dr. Freud? It was pretty corny stuff. I was fascinated with it all. I always looked at all the books; I *loved* abnormality, abnormality of any kind, deformity . . . I think that to some extent I cultivated a certain abnormal streak in myself. I think I thought that if I'd be weird, I'd get attention. It was logical. If your parents pay attention to weird people, then they'd pay more attention to you if you were weird. But it went the other way, too, because I was also very afraid that I really was insane, and that if they ever found out they would lock me up. Later on, when I was seeing a therapist, the therapist asked what I thought would happen if I did exactly what I wanted all the time. It came out that I was afraid that I'd get locked up. That was really my greatest fear.

It is scarcely surprising that envy and resentment of patients should be fairly common among psychotherapists' children. Edward Futterman, a child psychiatrist who participated in the 1979 and 1980 American Psychiatric Association discussions on psychiatrists as parents remarks that one of the main concerns expressed by the children involved the feeling of exclusion.[3] Intellectually the children understood very well that the work was important and that privacy and confidentiality were essential. Nonetheless they felt left out—not merely neglected, as the children of all busy professionals may feel, but left out of something that is unquestionably an intimate and powerful human interaction.

Some children act out in protest against the exclusive intimacy between parent and patient, most often in ways calculated to embarrass one or both of them. Margaret Mahler, in a paper called *"Les enfants terribles,"* recounts several cases of children who went out of their way to insult patients or, in one instance, to humiliate an analyst mother by running through the house shouting, "Mooommmy, come out of the bathroom, hurry up, the patient has arrived!"[4] I have heard numerous stories of children who burst into the consulting room, purposely called on the telephone during office hours, went out of their way to make loud noises; one even wore a sign while cutting the grass—"Shrink your head: $5 an hour."

"There is something weird about the feeling of sharing your parents with so many people you don't know," says a woman in her early thirties, the daughter of two clinical psychologists, who has become one herself and married another. "When it's Christmas time there is all this mail, and you are not supposed to read the signatures on the cards. Or some new object will appear in the house under mysterious circumstances, a gift from a secret admirer. Sometimes there were telephone calls—usually they had meant to call the service, and they just left a message and got off, but sometimes they were persistent and even threatening. So I had this weird idea that my parents were important to this imagined legion of people, and you never know who they are, and you know that some of them might be dangerous."

The potential danger of psychotherapy was a recurring theme in my interviews. Many PsyKs had simply worried about it because of what the movies and newspapers had taught them about the homicidally insane, but a disconcerting number reported unpleasant personal experiences. One girl's family was persecuted for months by a woman who called to make threatening or obscene remarks, and every time her father went out for the evening she had nightmares of him being murdered. One man's therapist mother had a patient who habitually flew into rages and began hurling stone sculptures around her office; she asked her son to remain in the house so that if the patient grew really dangerous and needed to be subdued, he would be there to help. "I began to think that *my mother* was crazy, being paid $30 an hour so that some fucking lunatic could throw rocks at her."

A few people, notably the children of child therapists, unavoidably come into contact with their parents' patients:

My mother treated the most popular girl in the class ahead of me in high school, who took me under her wing and made me her best friend. I couldn't figure out why until she told me that my mother was treating her after her fourth abortion or something like that. So Sally and I became friends. My mother, to this day, never comes right out and says that she was her patient, but she will say "Oh, I had lunch with Sally the other day," and Sally would come over to my house and she would say, "Hi, Dr. Babbage." I knew. And my mom knew I knew. And Sally knew I knew. And Sally knew my mom knew I knew, and the whole bit, but nobody ever said anything.

It was also nice that my mother was so popular and accommodating with everyone; other kids always wanted to play at my house. And when my friend Zelda, whose parents were Zionists to the point of ridiculousness, was going out with Jim the football player, who wasn't Jewish, and Zelda's parents found out and she ran away from home, she ran to my mom's office and stayed there, and my mom was the one who mediated between Zelda and her mom to get Zelda to be allowed to live at home and go to the prom with Jim. When any of my friends had problems, or their parents had problems . . . I can't count how many times my girlfriends' mothers called my mother.

Mostly it wasn't a disadvantage at all. Sally never would have noticed I was alive if she hadn't been my mother's patient. And it was nice to know that the popular kids were so screwed up that they needed to go to a shrink. I know that she treats the mother of another good friend of mine from high school, and it's sort of nice to know that Sharon's mom is so screwed up. It was comforting in a way. I felt sort of like I could lord it over them, but I wouldn't, because I realized that there was nothing wrong with going to a psychiatrist.

One man in his late thirties found himself in a slightly different and somewhat awkward position:

I knew a lot of my mother's patients. In fact, at one point when I was in college, four of my friends were seeing her. They all knew each other, so in part they went through each other's recommendations, but one of them told me she went because of me: she thought that I was sufficiently intriguing or whatever that if my mother had produced me she wanted to see what my mother could do for her. She knew from me that my mother was a wonderful mother as well as a therapist, whereas her own parents were an utter mess, by anyone's standards. At one point I was sleeping with one of these friends who was my mother's patient, and her boyfriend was a patient, too. I don't know whether she told my mother about her relationship with me—if you're in therapy and a large part of your problem is your relationship with your boyfriend, which it was in her case, it would be hard not to mention the fact that you were having a wild affair with somebody else. On the other hand, it would be hard *to* mention it when the person you were having the wild affair with was your therapist's son. All I know is that my mother never mentioned anything about it to me, though if she knew about my involvement she must have thought it pretty harmful to the girl's other relationships and also rather swinish on my part, which I have to admit it was. She never breathed a word about having them in therapy, and when they were at the house visiting me I wasn't aware of any sign of unusual recognition between them. It was a while before I learned they were all in therapy with her, and it was they who told me. I have to admit that I worried about it for a while after I found out, because I wondered, jeez, what if this girl had been telling my mother about what kinds of things I did in bed? That was unthinkable, sort of oedipus vicariously come true.

One of the most common stories about psychotherapists' children is that if you ask them what they want to be when they grow up they will respond, "a patient." Having wondered about the mysteries of the consultation room, envied the intimacy patients have with the parent, idealized the warmth and help the parent can give in this obscure alternate role, they, too, want to enjoy the benefits of therapy. A college-age man in New York whose father is an analyst and whose mother teaches underprivileged children commented, "My brother and I used to joke that in order to get attention from our parents we would have to do poorly in school, wet the bed, throw things around the room, hit our parents, have no friends, be terribly shy, et cetera. As a joke we used to curl our back and drool or 'make like the elephant man,' saying that that was the only way to get attention. Though it was in jest, there was certainly an element of seriousness to the whole thing."

A psychiatrist voiced this concern to me about just this subject:

I've always wondered about the wish to get close to a parent who is involved with emotionally troubled people. Since that parent seems to appreciate emotional problems, one of the ways of getting close to him is to have them yourself. When my son was very little he used to ask me what I did today. He would say, "Before I go to sleep, tell me one of your patients' problems." And I would make up a little story about someone who was very thin and didn't want to eat, or something like that. To the extent that my son has a few little problems of his own, I've always wondered whether there was some jealousy and competitiveness, some need to reach me through the medium of something that I was interested in. A roommate of mine in college was the son of an internist, and the only time that his father really spent any time with him was when the kid was really sick. That was the only time he was even very interested in him. If he had a cold his father would ask what color the phlegm was, and dote on all the details. He developed asthma as a young kid, and his father was always involved.

Nonetheless this is not, at least in its most literal form, something I have found in the course of my research. It is true that the children envy the time and imagined intimacy with their parents; they like to play patient when little. Yet though many do have a near religious belief in the powers of psychotherapy, very few would admit to having actually wanted to be a patient. Counteracting this possible desire in some cases is the fact that the parents may be condescending toward patients: patients are troublesome, patients are troubled. However benevolent the parent may be, a superiority is implied by the very fact of the relationship, and the child, by virtue of his blood ties with the therapist, is included in this envelope of superiority. To become a patient, in that case, is to become one of those who are ignorant and need help, rather than one who knows and helps.

One man described his emotional attitude toward the patients in these revealing terms:

> I knew that these were people who had a certain amount of money, because I knew it took money to go to a psychiatrist. I had heard enough about some of them to know that they held important positions—there were lawyers and businessmen and big wheels in society—yet they had these horrible dirty little things in their lives that they couldn't talk to anybody else about, and they had to come to some specialized person and *pay* them to listen to their problems while they were shut away in a little room where nobody could overhear. There was some fundamental weakness in these people that they were concealing and that they hadn't a clue how to handle on their own. When I heard about some of their problems, it was amazing to know they could be so blind. I'm sure that I felt superior to them, because *I* didn't have such shameful little problems. Of course one doesn't, as a child. But at the same time I would never have let on that I felt so superior to them, because my parents set this example of compassionate understanding. So I probably felt very compassionate and understanding, too, in a paternalistic, condescending, snide sort of way.

Overall, the circumstances of being a psychotherapist's child do not seem to produce unilaterally good or bad results. Depending upon how the issues are handled, familiarity with the concepts and the nature of human problems can be an enlightening experience or a source of secret worry. Many analysts with whom I have spoken say it would be fascinating to speculate on the developmental implications of the obscure parental function, but such considerations are a bit too ethereal for the present study, and in general I am inclined to believe that though the mystery leaves room for fantasy, those fantasies, too, can be harmful, beneficial, or completely benign depending upon the child's predisposition and the parents' response. Envy of patients, and certainly the fear of dangerous patients, are clearly undesirable, but other people's children have their own special fears.

Viewed on the surface, the practical day-to-day world into which the hypothetical magical psychotherapist of chapter 1 would be dropped is curious in many respects, but not, on its own, sufficiently strange to account for any systematic difference in the therapists' children. For that, it is necessary to look more closely at the motives that bring psychotherapists to therapy, the meaning they find there, and the assimilation of this faith and these concepts by their children.

The most unusual, and certainly the most pleasing, PsyK response to the obscurity of the parental profession is that of a man who, when I asked what effect his psychoanalyst father's profession had had, replied cheerfully:

> It made me rich. People used to ask me, "Oh, your dad's a shrink: is he a Freudian?" I didn't know. So I asked him. I said, "Are you a Freudian?" And he said. "That's a silly question." "Why?" He said, "Because it is no more possible to discuss the history of psychoanalysis without starting with Freud than it is to discuss the history of the discovery of America without starting with Columbus. But to suppose that nothing has happened since Columbus, and to suppose that nothing has happened since Freud, is to be extremely rigid and doctrinaire." And he went on to explain just how an analyst went about his job. "When a patient comes to me, I listen to what he says, I listen to how he says it, I try to hear what he does *not* say. I look at what he is wearing, I observe his physical language, his body language. I am, in short, searching for clues from him as to why he is not happy. And against this I try to apply a background of some clinical experience." And I said at the time, "Gee, that sounds like detective work." He said, "It is *exactly* like detective work."

Some two decades later this young man, Nicholas Meyer, wrote *The Seven-Per-Cent Solution*, in which Sherlock Holmes meets Sigmund Freud. It was a best-selling book and successful movie. Moreover, he received enthusiastic praise from psychoanalysts. "They seemed to particularly enjoy the part where Freud was shoveling coal into the maw of this locomotive. Make of that what you will."[5]

4

The Wounded Healer and the Helping Professions

What asylum doctor has not had
his own attack of madness by dint
of continual association with
madmen? . . . But before that,
what obscure inclination, what
dreadful fascination had made him
choose that subject?

—MARCEL PROUST

I think that my parents were crazy,
and I think that, somehow, being
psychiatrists kept them in line.
They used it as a protection.
They're both *quite* crazy, but their
job gave them a really good cover.

—A PSYCHIATRISTS' CHILD

Alfred Adler, according to his son, once said, "I think I could make out of a sadist a good butcher—perhaps even a good surgeon."[1] All he would need was to imbue the sadist with social interest, modify certain patterns of behavior, and he would end up with a constructive member of society who nonetheless retained the sadist's underlying personality pattern and motivations. One might wonder what sort of pathological type Adler would have selected as raw material for a psychotherapist.

One does not need to search for pathology behind every career choice any more than one must seek underlying scatological or sexual explanations for every innocuous bit of behavior. It seems vicious to say that altruistic people, who work hard to help others, should be suspected ipso facto of harboring ulterior selfish motives. Nonetheless it is true that the "helping professions," such as nursing, charitable work, the clergy, and psychotherapy, attract people for curious and often psychologically suspect reasons. There is something a bit odd about people who proclaim, "I want to help other people," with its underlying assumption that they are in a position to help and that others want to be helped by them. They may be lured, knowingly or unknowingly, by the position of authority, by the dependence of others, by the image of benevolence, by the promise of adulation, or by a hope of vicariously helping themselves through the process of helping others. Though some helping professionals have humbly and realistically perceived that they have something to offer and are willing to take on the responsibility of doing so, there are others who use the role to manipulate their world in a convenient, simplistic manner, ultimately not taking responsibility in a meaningful way at all, but using authority precisely to avoid it. For such people, psychotherapy is not merely a way to earn a living: it is in itself the essence of their lives.

In its most trivial form, once again, the statement is made that psychotherapists are crazy and that this is probably the stimulus that led them to their jobs. "What still strikes me," says one PsyK woman, "is I'll go to a party in New York, and inevitably the craziest person there is a psychiatrist. I mean the person who is literally doing childish, antisocial things, making a fool of himself and embarrassing everyone else. I just shrug. That's the way it is." A president of the American Academy of Psychotherapists once said, in an address to the members of his organization: "When I first visited a national psychiatric convention in 1943, I was dismayed to find the greatest collection of odd balls, Christ beards, and psychotics that I had ever seen outside a hospital. Yet this is to be expected: Psychotherapists are those of us who are driven by our own emotional hunger."[2]

Psychotherapists often take a perverse delight in criticizing their peers, and the amount of abuse I have heard them heap upon each other in the course of my research was truly astounding. Psychiatrists say that analysts are crazy. Analysts say that psychiatrists, being unanalyzed, are crazy. Both of them say that social workers and psychologists, with lower training standards and fewer controls to weed out the bad ones, are crazy, and particularly harmful because armed with that little bit of knowledge that is such a dangerous thing. Social workers and psychologists accuse psychiatrists and analysts of being pompous asses—pompous *crazy* asses, so puffed up with theoretical abstractions that they have lost track of down-to-earth clinical considerations.

"I very rarely have found a healthy, well-integrated, happy person *seeking* this profession," says one training psychoanalyst, and another man, a clinical psychologist, remarked, "I questioned your calling it a myth that therapists are crazy, because the *fact* is that most of them *are*. If you needed any proof, let me tell you that every patient who comes into this office who has had a previous experience with some other therapist has some kind of horror story to tell, some *major* failing on the therapist's part, including, quite often, sexual abuse, verbal abuse, things that cross the boundary of mere bad technique and come pretty damn close to the criminal."

Various statistical surveys of the psychopathology of therapists have been published, but this literature yields inconclusive results. In one study, 90.7 percent of psychiatrists surveyed reported that members of their profession had "emotional difficulties that are special to them and their work as contrasted with non-psychiatrists," though they said that some of these problems were related to the personalities of people who went into the field and others stemmed from the nature of the work, and it was not at all clear how many would be willing to elevate "emotional difficulties" to the level of diagnosable clinical problems.[3] On the other hand, an interesting Swiss study found that when one compared the military conscription records of people who subsequently became psychiatrists to the records of those who became surgeons and internists, significantly more of the eventual psychiatrists had been declared unfit for military service because of psychiatric disorders.[4]

In another survey, this one of psychologists, social workers, counselors, and other nonmedical psychotherapists, 82 percent of respondents claimed to have relationship difficulties, 57 percent had experienced depression, 11 percent admitted substance abuse, and 2 percent had attempted suicide.[5] Again, it is not clear how serious the relationship difficulties and depression were. No comparable figures are given for a nontherapist population,* and even if there were, one might quite reasonably expect therapists to apply different, possibly more liberal, standards than the lay population in judging the presence or absence of emotional problems.

In alcohol and drug abuse, a more concrete measure of emotional problems, physicians in general show a higher incidence than non-

---

* This lack of control groups is an almost universal flaw in all research conducted on the personalities of psychotherapists. In this, I fear, my own research is no exception.

physicians. A study of 98 physician members of Alcoholics Anonymous found that 17 percent were psychiatrists, who constituted only 7.8 percent of physicians at the time. This was interpreted to mean that there is a disproportionate number of alcoholic psychiatrists, though it might equally mean that out of the total population of alcoholic physicians, psychiatrists are more likely to seek help. Other studies have found therapists to have alcohol abuse rates between 6 and 11 percent, but there is little consistency or proper control, and it is difficult to draw any intelligent conclusion from them. When therapists are asked about themselves, 4 percent report drug or alcohol abuse serious enough to affect their work. When asked about their colleagues, they report that 18 percent of them are similarly impaired.[6]

Studies of suicide among psychiatrists also furnish contradictory results. As long ago as 1964, in a leading article in the *British Medical Journal* on suicide among physicians, the remark was made that "[a]mong the specialties, psychiatry appears to yield a disproportionate number of suicides. The explanation may lie in the choosing of the specialty rather than in meeting its demands, for some who take up psychiatry probably do so for morbid reasons."[7]

Physicians in general do not seem to commit suicide at a significantly different rate than their nonmedical peers, though given their knowledge and access to drugs, they understandably do choose different methods to accomplish the deed: doctors poison themselves more than twice as often as the lay public, and shoot themselves less frequently.* Psychiatrists, on the other hand, show a markedly greater tendency to commit suicide than the population at large or their medical peers. Following the publication of several conflicting and methodologically flawed studies of suicide among psychiatrists, the Task Force on Suicide Prevention of the American Psychiatric Association instigated its own study of psychiatrist suicides. Investigators examined nearly 19,000 physician deaths between 1967 and 1972 and calculated the ratio of suicides to members for each medical specialty. They found that psychiatrists killed themselves about twice as frequently as other physicians. No other specialty showed a frequency greater than expected. Moreover, when individual years in this span were examined, the rate was found to be constant, "indicating a relatively stable over-supply of depressed psychiatrists from which the suicides are produced."[9]

---

* Interestingly, several studies have shown that doctors' wives are much more prone to suicide than the wives of other professionals and that they tend to be unusually depressed and dependent on drugs or alcohol. No study has looked at psychiatrists' wives in isolation.[8]

Some people have tried to explain away psychiatrist suicides on rational grounds.* Perhaps they are more likely to kill themselves when they are terminally ill than are most other people, since they take a more realistic and enlightened view of human life and suffering. This was true of some of the prominent early analysts: Paul Federn shot himself when he was dying of cancer, and Wilhelm Stekel, faced with declining health, poisoned himself. Nonetheless, as a general explanation, this is no more than a fanciful supposition.

Others suggest that the strains of the profession, whether practical or emotional, may drive practitioners to despair. Marmor points out that the burden of constantly associating with depressed people, the stress of the transference-countertransference situation, the problems of role uncertainty, the burden of continuing education, and economic difficulties might be expected to take their toll on anyone.[11] Fritz Wittels, originally an antagonist of psychoanalysis, though later an ardent supporter, wrote of analysts who "involve their own unconscious in the dreams of others as in a distorting mirror; so that a gremlin catches them and drives them to death. Weininger was one of those who became involved in a bit of self-analysis, saw a distorted image of his unconscious that pressed a revolver into his hand. I have known three brilliant analysts, Shrötter, Tausk, Silberer, who voluntarily ended their lives. And in Vienna alone. Others will follow." After Wittels changed his opinion of psychoanalysis he retracted this view, saying that Weininger was not really a qualified psychoanalyst, that the others had not been properly analyzed, and that this, in the end, was to blame. "An analyst who has not himself been analyzed is in danger, be it suicide or otherwise."[12]

On balance, with the significant exception of an apparent high suicide rate, there is only slight evidence that psychotherapists are *impaired* as compared to their professional and nonprofessional colleagues, and it would be folly to accuse them en masse of gross psychopathology. Therapists are not crazy. Nonetheless, in terms of personality types, emotional weaknesses, and psychological motivations, a substantial majority of them may show a drift away from the general population in ways more subtle than full-blown pathology yet more important than mere stylistic differences. More significantly,

---

* One writer dismisses the relevance of suicides among psychiatrists with an analogy: "whether or not allergists have the highest hay fever rate of any professional group has absolutely nothing to do with the validity of immunological teachings; and whether or not psychiatrists have the highest suicide rate of any professional group has absolutely nothing to do with the validity of psychiatric teachings." True, it may not necessarily reflect poorly upon psychiatry, but it reflects very curiously upon the psychiatrists.[10]

the relationship of therapists to their profession is very interesting, as is the gratification they expect and actually derive from the exercise of their jobs.

What draws people to become psychotherapists? About this, not surprisingly, data are sparse, poorly controlled, open to wide interpretation, and generally anecdotal, as is psychotherapy itself. Henry, Sims, and Spray's study, *The Fifth Profession*, presents hard statistical data that are diverting but scarcely enlightening. Presented with a multiple-choice questionnaire asking why they had become interested in the field of psychotherapy, 15.8 percent of all polled therapists said they wanted "to help people," 14.4 percent wanted "to understand people," and 9.6 percent wanted "to gain professional status." Psychoanalysts and psychiatrists, considered as separate groups, were more interested in "gaining an identity," whatever that means, than in any of the other choices, whereas this was a negligible concern to the clinical psychologists and social workers. Of all therapists, 24.4 percent gave an "other" reason for their interest.[13]

Once one gets past the more or less beauty contestant type of responses that invoke benevolence and civic-mindedness, the reasons one finds tend to involve the search for compensations and cures for the therapist's own personal unhappiness. Freud theorized that a strong desire to help others stemmed from longings resulting from childhood losses. Indeed, several authors state, on the basis of their personal knowledge of therapists, whether through friendship, in training, in therapy, or during interviews, that many therapists grew up in rejecting or inadequate families, which led them to what Karl Menninger has called a "professional interest in lonely, eccentric and unloved people."[14]

One detailed study of the lives of twelve psychotherapists concludes that the majority were given heavy responsibilities for maintaining family happiness during their youths. The mothers of those authors studied were seen as pallid or uninspired women, notably indifferent to their children except insofar as they could be manipulated for the mother's gratification. The fathers were weak and estranged, though admired by the child. "Since every study shows that [therapists] mostly come from disrupted or disjointed families, often with the father physically and psychically absent, the therapists-to-be were delegated the task of assuring the fate and fulfillment of the family. They became, and are, the family nurturer."[15]*

---

* It is, admittedly, difficult to find all of these studies "every" one of which concurs in such a simple conclusion. One statistical survey of a very small population found that every single therapist had had at least one family member with a "physical or behavioral difficulty involving

Often the secret goal in psychotherapy is to continue in the role of family supporter. Just the reciprocal of analytic transference, where the analyst comes to represent aspects of the patient's parents, here the patients represent aspects of the therapist's earlier life. Unfortunately, however, patients are not trained to manipulate this curious relationship, nor is that what they have come and paid money to do. Meanwhile, the therapist treats a succession of patients not quite for their own problems, but for other problems, belonging to another time and place, that haunt his consultation room. One study describes a series of therapists in which this was quite clearly the case. A female psychiatrist undergoing analysis became depressed when she realized that she would not be able to cure her mother, an idea that lay in the back of her mind and had been almost her sole motive in entering psychiatry. A male psychiatrist, who in childhood had been saddled with the burden of maintaining family harmony, was found on close scrutiny to harbor the fantasy of one day finding his father and mother happy together as a result of his efforts. Meanwhile, it was particularly trying for him as a therapist to treat patients with irreconcilable marital difficulties, and his own marriage suffered from his tendency to treat his wife like a patient. In a third case, a medical student embarking upon his psychiatric residency broke under the strain of caring for his emotionally disturbed mother and dependent psychiatrist father: he had planned to work in child psychiatry, and was especially interested in helping doctors' families.[17] From my own research experience, I could mention the psychoanalyst who scolded me when I suggested that therapists might choose the field because of their own problems, saying that he had chosen it in hopes of curing his psychosomatic mother.

In speaking to the children of psychotherapists, I have been forcibly struck by the number that bring up their parents' emotionally dismal childhood. They paint portraits of their therapist parents as exceptionally lonely and unhappy, socially ostracized at school and abused at home, either psychologically or, sometimes, physically. They were people who had been ill at ease with themselves and with others, who sought through association with the world of adults and

presumed psychogenic factors," although the list of what was admitted as such a difficulty was extraordinarily broad—including heart attack, high blood pressure, diabetes, and asthma—and the majority of the therapists examined had at least one parent with some sort of psychological difficulty, though the severity of the difficulties is difficult to assess since not one of the parents had been in psychotherapy. A much larger statistical study, on the other hand, found that the incidence of traumatic separations from parents during childhood and of family mental illness were slightly higher than in the general population, but not enough to set these families clearly apart.[16]

a retreat into the world of the intellect, and ultimately through the field of psychotherapy to understand and manage their misery and to protect themselves and, later, their families. In many cases the parents themselves had invoked their unhappy early lives as the primary motivation for their ultimate career choice, while in others the story seemed sufficiently clear that the children drew the conclusion on their own. These children usually love their parents, and almost invariably admire them, yet quite often there is also the sense of something a little pathetic about it all, something sad and vulnerable and in need of protection.

A host of other less-than-selfless motives may enter into the benevolent wish to become a psychotherapist—sublimated sexual curiosity, forms of aggression, the problem-solving pleasure of making confused issues clear, and a voyeuristic interest in the lives of others. These factors, which have been discussed by other authors,[18] very likely do play some part, but they seem like secondary rather than determining causes and will be considered here only insofar as they enter into what I believe to be the most important characteristic: that of the wounded healer.

In Greek mythology, Chiron, the centaur who taught medicine to Asklepios, suffered an incurable wound at the hands of Hercules. St. Augustine was conspicuous but not alone among the Christian saints for having used his early weaknesses and his struggles against them to help him find compassion and strength. Mythology and religion are fraught with figures who must learn to heal themselves before healing others and to recognize and forgive their own sins before earning the humility and genuine sympathy to forgive anyone else.

Many of Freud's most significant early discoveries came from the scrutiny of his own unconscious mind and a heroic confrontation of the painful things he found. In case histories of his patients he draws upon his personal experience often enough to prove how extensively his own flaws had been put at the service of the empathic process. Psychoanalysts in training are required to undergo analysis for two complementary reasons. First, they must try to rid themselves of their own psychological problems, so that they will be less likely to project their own preoccupations onto their patients and then mistake what they perceive in them for objective fact. Second, it is instructive for them to endure the painful analytic process themselves: if an analyst is to venture into the patient's world, it is useful for him to have been there before, to know how analysis can hurt and how it can help, and to recognize that he and his patients are made of the same mortal stuff. Having emotional problems of one's own may not actually be a prerequisite or an advantage for a psychotherapist, but it is clear that having had problems is not in itself a handicap, as long as these problems have been recognized, confronted, and successfully resolved.

The danger occurs when the wounded healer has not resolved, or cannot control, his own injury. There is, I believe, a bifurcated path in the course of the helping professional's career. The more difficult, but ultimately more satisfying, road leads to a painful confrontation with his own problems and weaknesses, and ultimately to self-knowledge. Ideally, he can overcome the difficulties; at worst, he may be forced to resign himself to insuperable handicaps. In either case, though, the end result is a clearer perception of his ambitions and needs and their relationship to the task at hand. He can approach others with honesty, compassion, and humility, knowing that he is motivated by genuine concern, not by some ulterior motive.

The other path is an easier and more disastrous one. In the case of the psychotherapist, he comes, consciously or unconsciously, to recognize the profession as a means of *avoiding* the need to deal with his problems. He gains authority and power to compensate for his weakness and vulnerability. He acquires a set of slippery dialectic techniques that enable him to justify his own actions in almost all circumstances, perhaps even to shift the blame onto somebody else. In his work with his patients, the entire therapeutic relationship is perverted and turned to the service of his own hidden purpose. The therapist is ultimately not there to treat the patient but, via a circuitous and well-concealed route, to treat or protect or comfort himself. The patient is not an object of empathy and altruism, but an unsuspecting victim who is taken into the therapist's realm of personal needs and subjective impressions, and assigned a role there that he does not recognize, and which is far from the one that he ideally wants.

In adopting the profession of psychotherapy, the therapist-to-be may even make his problems much worse, because he discovers a justification for divorcing himself from the emotions that have caused him so much pain. He is to become a cold, accurate instrument instead of a sloppily warm and vulnerable human being. He may console himself with the heady deceit that he is martyring himself for the good of others: rather than live a happy and self-interested life, he says, he will deny his own satisfaction in order to transform himself into someone who can do greater good. The flaw in this formula is that he is not being selfless at all, but seeking, through the very medium of ostentatious self-denial, a perverse gratification of his personal needs. For these therapists the wound has become *encapsulated* and been walled off both from causing pain and from susceptibility to healing. Since their energy is directed toward defending the status quo, they are diverted from the arduous and humbling process of self-examination and personal reconstruction that might otherwise have made them whole, and are forced, continuously and forever, to work just to stay where they are. With this encapsulated problem now forming a foundation stone of their personal and professional lives, the farther along they go, the more difficult and costly it becomes to attempt to correct the mistake. It is an almost Faustian tragedy, in which they have sold their hopes of future redemption for temporary power, comfort, and knowledge.

The parallels to the world of religion are conspicuous and instructive. The church has often been regarded as a haven for the exalted emotionally disturbed. Like the research on the mental state of psychotherapists, the studies that have been done on the clergy are contradictory and emotionally charged, but overall they suggest a high incidence of family problems and narcissistic disorders,[19] and a host of other problems involving interpersonal relations and questions of self-esteem. In the course of my research I spoke to several psychotherapists who had begun their careers as clergymen, and who now specialize in treating the emotional problems of the clergy.* Some of these problems are incidental to the occupation, or result from its peculiar pressures and strains, but others are a common enough recurrent theme to rate as a mild but prevalent clergy pathology.

One type of clergyman, like one type of psychotherapist, is the repentant sinner who has recognized his weakness and can therefore align himself with other mortal men in the process of seeking salvation. Another kind, the encapsulated sinner in his most extreme form, is the rigid and damning preacher who exhorts and chastises his flock from above, who has no sympathy for their weaknesses and may hurt rather than help his congregants by condemning their transgressions instead of leading them to righteousness with new understanding. These preachers are not ones who have gotten true religion or brought their own lives under proper control: they are people so beset by uncertainty and unresolved problems that they have marshalled external life into shape through sheer brute force and imposture, leaving the inside untouched. They cannot understand their

---

* It is noteworthy, though hardly surprising, that many people who leave the church for one reason or another find in psychotherapy the nearest secular occupational equivalent.

congregants because they cannot understand themselves, and they cannot constructively help with problems because the solution they have adopted themselves is to cap them tightly and hold them unseen.

Perhaps the most interesting and significant problem, described by a number of therapists, is that of the person, often a firstborn or only child, who was rushed through childhood too quickly, without the warmth, protection, and love children deserve, and obliged to become a premature Little Adult.* Such people are imbued with the belief that hard work and responsibility are the only things that give them value in others' eyes. They have a chronically low sense of self-worth, a stunted ability to receive genuine love or friendship from others, and only their selfishly selfless labors make them feel satisfied with themselves. As a result they are driven into a veritable frenzy of wholesale helping, motivated not by altruism but by a desperate need to fill an inner vacancy—an effort that ultimately helps little at all, since, like trying to fill a bucket with a hole in the bottom, it can never succeed until they have attended to the necessary repairs.[21]

As one man, a Jungian analyst and Episcopalian minister who has treated many clergymen, describes it:

They give too much, without knowing how to take, and it has an effect upon them, as well as on their families. They build up even more of an inhibition against being able to appropriately take things for themselves, which is taboo. They can justify this attitude with all sorts of theological jargon that says "It is better to give than to receive" and so on. They are into loving their God and loving their neighbor, but they forget that little, crucial, additional thing: "as thyself."

These people are pathological givers, and so they become servers, pastoral counselors, and so on, and they can even be good at it, to a degree, but they become impoverished after a while. They have given so much that they finally run out of spiritual and nervous energy, and what remains is the underlying resentment. You find a great deal of resentment and sourness among the clergy. Just go and interview your garden variety Catholic priest in the parish. Get to know him a little bit and you will find a lot of anger and bitterness, even though he will

---

* A 1945 study of the lives of three prominent American psychotherapists, Austin Riggs, Thomas Salmon, and S. Weir Mitchell, observed that "[a]ll were burdened by an extreme degree of responsibility beginning early and all through life." Interestingly, all three also suffered from tuberculosis in late adolescence and had long periods of inactivity and depletion.[20]

maintain a façade of benevolence and contentment. And their problem is themselves: they have given more than they had to give, and they've gotten very little back. They get a salary of $11,000 a year, the manse thrown in, and 5¢ a mile car allowance. And they're called upon day and night.[22]

All these are people who, in choosing a profession, have embarked upon an ultimately doomed quest, and one that perverts the purpose of their position. One bishop summed the issues up quite neatly in his comment that, when screening candidates for the ministry, "One of the things I look for is: is this a whole person seeking to express his wholeness through the ministry? Or is this a person trying to *find* his wholeness in the ministry?"[23]

William Dewart, a clinical psychologist who works primarily with the ministry, points out another interesting problem that afflicts many of the clergy he sees. One of the lures the church, and the priesthood in particular, holds is that of a position of authority that would help them compensate for their feelings of inadequacy and emptiness and escape from the painful imposition of others.

For some, they go into the clergy believing that "In the end, I answer only to God." That is a very nice arrangement, they suppose, because God is a spiritual entity, after all, and His love is unconditional. They won't have to deal with a foreman or boss, no changes of administration. It's just you and God, who, after all, called you in the first place. At least that's what they believe when they begin. But before they know it, they find themselves running up against authority and issues of power everywhere, from the vestry of their own small parish all the way up to the bishop of the diocese. For example, in the Episcopal church, the canons provide for the bishop to make the final decision regarding the very question of one's calling to an ordained priesthood. So the poor individual unconsciously seeking the priesthood in hopes of circumventing issues of authority and power will certainly find himself walking straight into one of the more authoritative, political organizations in the world.[24]

Among psychotherapists this is rarely a problem—with the exception of those entering a psychoanalytic institute, who may feel that the teachers and training analysts hold despotic power over their fates.[25] Indeed, the problem is rather the reciprocal, for the psychotherapist in private practice has no authority over him, in fact no outside awareness of what he does except for what he chooses to tell and the perceptions of his own patients, who are by their nature subordinate to his personality and mistrustful of their own judgment. The therapist truly has the independence that the clergyman does not, and rather than being subject to authority, he is the only authority in his microcosmic domain. This unusual circumstance tends to exacerbate the existing problem and to add novel difficulties.

In an important 1913 paper entitled "The God Complex," Ernest Jones, a pioneer psychoanalyst now best remembered as Freud's biographer and chief English-language ambassador, described a set of character traits resulting from a pathological unconscious belief that one is god. This does not mean that people with this complex actually wander the streets proclaiming themselves as the deity, but that a better concealed, more insidious faith in their own importance and entitlement, and an inability to conceive of others as comparably important, tinges every aspect of their relations with the world:[26]

> . . . the type in question is characterized by a desire for aloofness, inaccessibility, and mysteriousness, often also by a modesty and self-effacement. They are happiest in their own home, in privacy and seclusion, and like to withdraw to a distance. They surround themselves and their opinions with a cloud of mystery, exert only an indirect influence on external affairs, never join in any common action, and are generally unsocial. They take great interest in psychology, particularly in the so-called objective methods of mind-study that are eclectic and which dispense with the necessity for intuition. Phantasies of power are common, especially the idea of possessing great wealth. They believe themselves to be omniscient, and tend to reject all new knowledge. . . . The subjects of language and religion greatly interest them . . . Constant, but less characteristic, attributes are the desire for appreciation, the wish to protect the weak, the belief in their own immortality, the fondness for creative schemes, e.g., for social reform, and above all, a pronounced castration complex.*

Oddly enough, this comes very close to a description of many psychotherapists, or even a job description for psychotherapy. Some of the qualities are ones psychotherapists go out of their way to cultivate as part of their professional persona, and the training process

---

* The castration complex might appear as fear and jealousy of younger rivals and manifest itself as a desire to help and protect them as a patron and benefactor, as long as they are suitably abject and grateful and adhere to the party line.

may encourage them.[27] Indeed, Jones says that people with god complexes are more likely than others to go into psychology and related professions. He hastened to add that they are not drawn to psychoanalysis, his own specialty, which requires intuition and an ability to empathize with others that is outside the reach of their self-centered grasp. One must say, however that there are only too many analysts and analytically oriented therapists who plod through their job on the basis of dogma, with little empathy at all. Jones himself was notable for his lack of psychological intuition,[28] and was a curious mixture of radicalism and conservatism. He broke away from the medical and national tendencies that threatened to hold power over him, yet once he had converted to Freudian psychoanalysis he became its most inflexible defender, just as he remained a devoted Welshman and monarchist.* His belief in the powers of psychoanalysis bordered, by his own admission, on grandiosity:

> Perhaps, indeed, in centuries to be, the medical psychologist may, like the priest of ancient times, come to serve as a source of practical wisdom and a stabilising influence in this chaotic world, whom the community would consult before embarking on any important social or political enterprise. Mere megalomania, it may be said. Perhaps, but it is my living faith none the less, and only our descendants will be able to say if it was a misplaced one.[29]

Freud himself had a strong element of grandiosity, and readily admitted that he was not a man of science, an observer, an experimenter or a thinker, but rather a conquistador.[30] His bitter relations with Jung, Adler, Rank, and others who strayed from his patronage and guidance are in keeping with Jones's image of the man who can tolerate no god but himself. But grandiosity is clearly essential in someone who is to discover a new theory and defend it against strong opposition.

In any psychotherapist, for that matter, an unusual degree of self-assurance is necessary. After all, his patients are people whose attempts to conduct their own lives have failed, and who are seeking help from another. However much the therapist may wish to play the part merely of mediator rather than guide, the situation forces him into a position of superiority where, by whatever direct or subtle

---

* Jones was very distressed by the abdication of Edward VIII and the damage it did to the prestige of the monarchy. He wrote a letter to the London *Times* suggesting that in future, potential kings should be psychologically tested in order to avoid later embarrassment to the nation. The letter was not published.[31]

means, he must assert his notion of what is good for the patient above what the patient may believe to be proper in the management of his own life. Moreover, a substantial amount of self-confidence and poise, combined with a great deal of humility, is required for the therapist to withstand the emotional onslaught of the patient's unreasonable attitude toward him. Patients force therapists into superior positions through their idealization—the therapist's marriage must be wonderful, his children perfect, his interests cultured and profound, his understanding of issues clear and correct. Many patients want to be like their therapist, they adopt facets of his tastes and mannerisms, and many patients do go on to become therapists or counselors themselves, since it has emerged in their minds as the most perfect of all occupations. Patients do not simply want advice from their therapists: as children they expected magic from their parents. And thanks to the transference, they often entertain similarly unrealistic hopes that the therapist will soothe their fears and miraculously resolve their problems.

The field of psychotherapy attracts people with God complexes in the first place, and is nearly custom designed to exacerbate such a condition when it exists. Psychiatrists are often expected by others and by themselves to address questions that lie quite outside the range of their expertise, simply because they study human beings, and, by erroneous implication, are therefore supposed to understand all things human. Psychiatrists comment on the law, politics, art, literature, and ethical questions that nothing in their training has qualified them to comprehend any better than any other intelligent and educated person.* Above all, within the therapeutic situation itself, those therapists who do not have the personal strength and equilibrium to resist the temptations of power and to see the patients' adoration as the epiphenomenon of their actions that it is, are offered free range to run amok with their notions of self-importance:

Each profession carries its respective difficulties, and the danger of analysis is that of becoming infected by transference projections, in particular by archetypal contents. When the patient assumes that his analyst is the fulfilment of his dreams, that he is

---

* Three different psychiatrists I spoke to angrily mentioned the incident during the 1964 presidential campaign when a magazine asked a number of psychiatrists to pass judgment on Barry Goldwater's mental health, and they willingly, without ever having met Goldwater, tendered very definite "professional" conclusions. In criminal court cases, the role of psychiatry has been bitterly debated for decades, because the psychiatric witness's "expert" testimony so rapidly strays from the domain of his expertise and into the area of conclusory legal or ethical judgments.[32]

not an ordinary doctor but a spiritual hero and a sort of saviour, of course the analyst will say, "What nonsense! This is just morbid. It is a hysterical exaggeration." Yet—it tickles him; it is just too nice. And moreover, he has the same archetypes in himself. So he begins to feel, "If there are saviours, well, perhaps it is just possible that I am one," and he will fall for it, at first hesitantly, and then it will become more and more plain to him that he really is a sort of extraordinary individual. Slowly he becomes fascinated and exclusive. He is terribly touchy, susceptible, and perhaps makes himself a nuisance in medical societies. He cannot talk with his colleagues any more because he is—I don't know what. He becomes very disagreeable or withdraws from human contacts, isolates himself, and then it becomes more and more clear to him that he is a very important chap really and of great spiritual significance, probably an equal of the Mahatmas in the Himalayas, and it is quite likely that he also belongs to the great brotherhood. And then he is lost to the profession.

We have very unfortunate examples of this kind. I know quite a number of colleagues who have gone that way.[33]

This description by Carl Jung is more exaggerated than what one generally finds, which is fortunate in one obvious sense, though unfortunate in another, since these people are not necessarily lost to the profession, but continue to practice. They can justify their attitude to themselves and to others. It is always potentially treacherous when someone wields power in the name of some perceived ultimate good: the zealot can find a moral excuse for oppressing others that is unavailable to the mere bully or charlatan.

Reduced to a more clinical entity, the God complex can be related to the concept of narcissism, a personality disorder the chief features of which are well established.[34] Those with narcissistic personality disorders have a grandiose self-image, often entertain unrealistic notions about their abilities, power, wealth, intelligence, or appearance, and feel entitled to things without earning them, simply by virtue of their inherent greatness. Nonetheless, this exalted view of themselves, lacking the comfortable and certain support of reality, is very fragile. Narcissists constantly need admiration and praise from others and can be incongruously devastated by relatively unimportant failures, which threaten the fragile tissue of their belief. This paradoxical indifference to the wishes and feelings of others, combined with a simultaneous dependency upon their praise, is a particularly striking feature of narcissists. Many of them have the deep-seated sense that they are frauds, as, indeed, in many ways they are.

Narcissists are much more concerned with the appearance of things than with the reality; thus their ambitions tend to have a driven quality but to be empty of genuine sustained interest or pleasure. Stunted superego development leaves them "ethically empty," though their fundamental immorality is often masked by an intense though superficial show of morality and social, political, or aesthetic concern.[35] Since these cosmetic ethics do not touch them personally, however, narcissists may readily change their stance or entertain conflicting ethical beliefs.

Their relations with others tend to be emotionally hollow and exploitative, since narcissists are ultimately interested only in themselves (and in a profound way, do not even perceive other people as separate from themselves) and are thus unable to maintain equal give-and-take relationships. They are insensitive and lacking in empathy, and their view of others is more a projection from within themselves, and therefore vacillates between idealization and debasement. Frequently they believe other people to be basically unscrupulous, unreliable, false, and opportunistic. Despite this, they may make extravagant shows of generosity and concern for others, but ultimately it will be found to be just that, a show, that serves to polish the fine image they strive to hold of themselves.

Various schools of psychoanalytic thought postulate different etiologies of narcissistic disorders but they all agree on the fundamental outlines. Like both the clergy and the psychotherapists described above, narcissists were deprived, in infancy and childhood, of appropriate affection and meaningful emotional interactions with their parents that would have allowed normal development of a distinct sense of the difference between self and other and a feeling of personal value. According to Kohut and Miller, in particular,[36] pathology in the parents—often narcissistic as well, since it tends to be a self-perpetuating disorder—kept them from treating the child as an independent person and responding to it on its own merits, and led them instead to use the child for their own gratification. As a result, the child's sense of self was stunted, while simultaneously his sense of value was structured around his ability to comprehend and satisfy the parents' wishes. The parents looked to the child for a sense of worth, and the child, wanting to be appreciated and loved, developed an unconscious ability to intuit or divine the needs of the parents and respond to them. As Alice Miller comments:

This ability is then extended and perfected. Later, these children not only become mothers (confidantes, comforters, advisers, supporters) of their own mothers, but also take over the responsibility for their siblings and eventually develop a special sensitivity to unconscious signals manifesting the needs of others. No wonder that they often choose the psychoanalytic profession later on. Who else, without this previous history, would muster sufficient interest to spend the whole day trying to discover what is happening in the other person's unconscious?[37]

Thus the peculiar miseries of the narcissist's childhood will have encouraged him to develop a sensitivity and quasi-empathic intuitive knack for anticipating and dextrously catering to others' needs that are extraordinarily useful in the practice of psychotherapy, as well as a need to exercise these talents and to achieve the approval of others that drive him into the profession. But the very same factors ultimately hinder his ability to help his patients or, as will be seen in subsequent chapters, to raise children who are free of his own emotional problems, since his empathy and altruism are basically false. Meanwhile, the profession he has slipped into presses him further than ever from the chance of cure.

One of the best ways to avoid or counteract feelings of grandiosity is through the cultivation of genuine human loves and friendships. By dealing with people as equals, in symmetrical relationships where the corners tend to get knocked off of one's fantastic monuments to oneself, and where one may grow comfortable with one's own shortcomings through others' acceptance of them, one learns to be a real, solid human being who can take true pride in his genuine strengths and learn to recognize and deal with his genuine weaknesses. A healthy, loving marriage, in particular, might wean one from his lonely grandiosity, and also mitigate the effects of his particular problems on his children.

Unfortunately, this is not the sort of marriage many psychotherapists seem to have or to seek out. Though when measured in superficial statistical terms psychiatrists, at least, have a divorce rate insignificantly higher than other medical specialists, and considerably *lower* than the general professional population, under closer scrutiny their marriages appear to be unusually distant and formal, based on shared intellectual and recreational activities rather than on affectionate personal interaction.[38] Moreover, there is considerable anecdotal evidence that therapists, both men and women, tend to marry troubled and dependent partners who will not counteract their narcissistic disturbances, but contribute more of the admiration they crave.

"They marry their patients," it is said—which is sometimes even literally true—and end up in relationships that are anything but equal. Psychiatrist Richard Robertiello, speaking from professional and personal experience, says:

[Therapists] tend to be drawn to partners who have rather serious emotional problems and who are looking for a wise understanding person who will help, support and perhaps "cure" them. . . . They are drawn by their own feeling of grandiosity and omnipotence. They think they will be able, by their love and caring and wisdom, to make this person happy, especially one who has frustrated several previous therapists in their efforts to accomplish this. Of course, the therapists feel very noble and generous and altruistic in this endeavor.

But their satisfactions are hardly only altruistic. They start off having tremendous adulation and admiration from their "sick" mates. They begin in an unchallenged position of superiority and control. They are always "right" or "healthy" and their mate is always "wrong" or "sick." In addition to all of the narcissistic gratification this provides, it also gives a perfect assurance of acceptability and a near-guarantee against being abandoned.[39]

Ultimately, this sort of relationship is not very profitable for either person. If the therapist grows, he (or she) may outgrow his wife (or her husband) and come to resent the dependence that had originally brought them together. "I used to complain that I saw out-patients all week long, and then had an in-patient on my hands every weekend," says Robertiello.[40] If the spouse grows, on the other hand, it can pose a threat to the therapist. They may end up in a stale relationship, where even the gratification of the one's adoration and the other's dependence eventually wears thin. Meanwhile, the whole household revolves around the initial narcissistic demand of the therapist, and the subordinate spouse may come to function more as a part of this pattern than as an autonomous entity. "My father was very shy and insecure," says one woman, a lawyer and the daughter of an analyst, "and he insisted that the family provide him with a lot of reassurance all the time. He stayed very close to home in every way—his office was in the house—and there was this ritual that my mother had to tell him how wonderful he was even though he wasn't, and how great the things he did were even when they weren't. That seems to be why he needed her."

Close friendships, the other curative alternative, are also rarely found. Psychotherapists tend to have very few friends.[41] It is depressing to speak with PsyKs and hear their descriptions of their parents' bleak social lives. Therapists explain this away as a result of the tremendous demands of their professional lives—long hours, the teaching, society meetings—but such rationalizations seem forced when one looks at the figures and finds that psychiatrists have more free time than almost any other medical specialists, and that compared to many lawyers and businessmen—people not noted for a paucity of friends—psychotherapists have relatively undemanding schedules. Moreover, having little time does not automatically mean that one cannot find time to make friends.

The real reason often appears to be much more unpleasant, if unconscious. Many therapists do not need friends, because they have begun to live vicariously through their patients, just as the clergyman vicariously seeks love and self-worth through devotion to his congregation. For people who are uncomfortable with others and with themselves, the therapeutic situation offers an unparalleled opportunity for asymmetrical intimacy. The rules of therapy demand that the patient tell the therapist everything, while the therapist is under no obligation to reveal anything at all and thus open himself to the painful risks incurred in normal human relationships. Life in the office can be exciting—more exciting, socially redeeming, and financially rewarding than watching soap operas. One therapist related the story of an analyst who retired and looked forward to the joy of reading novels, but by the end of a few months he was dreadfully bored, because fiction did not possess the immediacy and veracity of clinical cases. And at the same time that they are allowed admission into their patients' lives, these therapists are repaid for this privilege in the patients' grateful adoration.* "My father had an inability to relate with his family or other people," says an analyst and son of an analyst, "and his way of being close was through his patients. It was

---

* As if to prove the vicarious gratification and lopsided intimacy that is offered to the narcissistically impaired, healthier analysts may suffer from the opposite problem. Willard Gaylin, for example, comments that "I *don't* think psychoanalysis is an intimate profession. It's as lonely as being a streetcar motorman or toll booth collector. You do not communicate with your patients, though you must listen. As a matter of fact I remember when I heard that my mother had died, I had a very sick patient coming, and I knew that I could not share this information, which would have been too much of a burden at that stage, nor could I cancel the patient. So I just had to sit there. This may be why a lot of psychoanalysts become depressed later in life; I think they are people who are *looking* for communication and contact, but it's a very isolated existence. You are *not* free. Even a lawyer is free to turn to his secretary and say 'I'm just miserable. My wife's been giving me a hard time and my children are on drugs.' A psychoanalyst is cloistered all day long without even a secretary, with only patients, and he *dare* not share his miseries with them."[42]

a way for him to have an interaction, but there was always a wall, or a desk, or a couch, to protect him."

Swiss psychotherapist Adolf Guggenbühl-Craig describes the tragic consequences to the therapist of this form of vicarious living:

> His own private life takes a back seat to the problems and difficulties of his patients. But a point may be reached where the patients might actually live for the analyst, so to speak, where they are expected to fill the gap left by the analyst's own loss of contact with warm, dynamic life. The analyst no longer has his own friends; his patients' friendships and enmities are as his own. The analyst's sex life may be stunted; his patients' sexual problems provide a substitute. . . . His own psychic development comes to a standstill. Even in his non-professional life he can talk of nothing but his patients and their problems. He is no longer able to love and hate, to invest himself in life, to win and lose. His own affective life becomes a surrogate. Acting thus as a quack who draws his sustenance from the lives of his patients, the analyst may seem momentarily to flourish psychically. But in reality he loses his own vitality and creative originality. The advantage of such vicarious living, of course, is that the analyst is also spared any genuine suffering. In a sense this function too is exercised for him by others.[43]

The therapeutic situation can become a refuge for both the therapist and the patients. Both enjoy a form of intimacy and vitality that is difficult to replicate in the world outside. "It's a very tricky situation," remarked one PsyK who is a psychologist. "It seems as though you've had all this intense personal contact, and then you go out and who are your friends on the outside? Well it turns out you don't have a lot of friends, and this is very surprising, because it *seems* as though you have forty very close friends. But you can't socialize with them, you can't have them over to dinner, you can't go stay at their house in the mountains."

The particular danger to the patient against which therapists must be vigilant, but often are not, is that the therapy begins to settle in as part of the patient's life rather than remaining an active process whereby he can reintegrate himself into living.[44] The patient may begin to look forward to sessions and live his life for the unacknowledged purpose of interesting and pleasing the therapist. Problems may be apparently resolved and changes made because the patient feels that is what the therapist wants, and have no profound or permanent effect because performed more for the dramatic value or the therapist's approval than from a sense of inner need. Patients do not want to leave the idealized therapist, and in the pathological relationship described above, neither is it in the therapist's interest to help the patient leave. In the worst case the entire therapy is poisoned by the fact that ultimately, unconsciously, the therapist cannot bear to cure the patient because then he would lose him, and he therefore perpetuates the curious relationship that he may have had with his parents, and that he may inflict not only on his patients but on his own children.

I have heard such stories again and again. One of the first and most dramatic accounts came from a respected psychoanalyst who had always admired and sought to emulate his own analyst father, had gone to the same medical school and analytic institute, and set up his practice in the same city. He dated the beginning of his most significant personal growth from the time he foolishly agreed when his father, during a period of illness, asked him to take over certain psychotherapeutic cases.

"I agreed. I wasn't that busy. I was in analytic training and was getting some supervision analyzing, and I thought this would be more grist for the mill. Besides, I figured I could do it as well as anybody else, and I never thought about the possible consequences of this kind of involvement with him. But in the course of doing this two or three times, I began to realize that he had a number of patients who were very dependent on him. He charged them low fees, for one thing. His fees were quite reasonable anyway—too reasonable, in a way—and there was this cadre of patients from the old days whom he charged exceptionally low fees. That should have been a clue. But then, more important, with a number of his patients it seemed clear that he had no good idea of the difference between maintenance, support, and cure. With some of them there seemed to be a kind of *collusion;* they needed him, and he needed them."

What ultimately both alarmed and helped this man most of all was that he came to recognize the same factors operating in the relationship between his father and himself. He idolized his father and his father depended on this idolization in a manner very analogous to his relationship with his patients, and though his father was willing to help him grow to a certain degree, and though he benefitted in many ways from his closeness to his father, there was a point at which his increasing independence worked against his father's interests, both the father's selfish interests and his inappropriate wishes for his son. "I saw the contrast in the relationships between my psychoanalyst and me and my father and me. My analyst was providing me with an opportunity to grow up, while my father was not providing me with the same kind of opportunity. It was as though he didn't want me to go through the same sort of pain he did when he had to grow up." Gradually the son established his own independence: he divorced his wife, having married in part to please his father, moved out of the state, and eventually abandoned full-time psychoanalysis in favor of a psychiatric practice altogether removed in its orientation from that of his father.

Several teaching analysts and psychotherapists readily agree that what poses as enthusiasm and professional dedication is often at heart a morbid addiction. A training analyst in New York discussed the unwillingness of analysts to leave their practice.

They may say that they can't give up the income, or offer some other explanation, but what they really miss is feeling needed. Personally I think that it is unethical and immoral for analysts to practice beyond a certain time in life. You can say a word for experience, but how much experience is experience? You can't really say that a seventy-year-old's experience is better than that of someone who is fifty-five. There comes a time when you are simply repeating the same experiences. Yet analysts will not retire. They *won't*. I do consultations or see an occasional ex-patient, and mostly do teaching or supervising. But an analyst who is in his eighties said to me the other day, "I have time," meaning that he wanted some referrals. I told a friend, and she said I should have replied, "Not much." What is someone like that doing for his patients? He can't see as well, he can't remember as well, he can't hear as well, but he's still in there, and nobody's going to tell him what to do, and since there are no rules or laws or need for operating room privileges, nobody can stop him, and he'll just keep doing it. And, transferential feelings being what they are, the patient doesn't have enough sense to move on, or move up. Sometimes patients actually stay because they feel sorry for the therapist. I've known cases like that.

The forty-year-old son of one analyst remarks:

I don't know what personal gratification my father derived from helping people—seeing someone come into his office and then go out, forty years later, better adjusted to the world. He may get some satisfaction out of that, I don't know. What it did do was to give him a world; it gave my father a life. He grew up unhappy, with an awful father—a father so terrible that not a single kind word was said about him even at his funeral. My father's childhood was just dreadful: he was on his own, and he didn't have many people to relate to in life. His patients gave him a world, they were people to relate to, whether emotionally or unemotionally, as the case may be. And even if he was unemotionally involved in their problems—it didn't personally affect him that So-and-So had this terrible sexual problem with her boyfriend—he could still react emotionally to the fact that this person was telling him that, and that he was saying something back. His world was defined by his hours of practice. I don't know whether people who dig ditches find that ditch-digging gives them a world. It gives them a job, makes them some money, but at the end of the day they get out of that ditch. I don't know if my father, when he came home from his world, ever stepped *into* another world. He may have left that other world behind and stepped into some middle region, but I'm not really sure that he ever stepped into the world where his family lived. I contend that this was all because of the person he was. Being an analyst didn't make him any different, except that perhaps, over the years, it may have dulled his senses, inured him, dulled his ability to deal with his family. He could look forward to tomorrow, when he would go back to the world where he really belonged.

For most patients the problems of these psychotherapists are irrelevant. Most of the people who seek therapeutic help need the benefit of knowledge, experience, and objectivity, and the opportunity to devote a specific amount of time to the careful scrutiny of whatever is wrong with their lives, and the narcissistic therapist's encapsulated wound and secret self-centered agenda may have no discernible effect on this simple program. But in cases that demand more from the therapist, or tread close to his own problems, or issue challenges that his therapeutic persona cannot easily handle, serious difficulties may arise. In such a therapist's family, difficulties almost invariably arise, since one's family is inextricably tied to one's sense of identity and is relentlessly present to throw back an image of what one's life is.

One man I interviewed, a commercial artist in his fifties and the son of an early American psychoanalyst, told horror stories of his early emotional abuse at the hands of his father. "It was Christina Crawford, but without Beverly Hills," he said. At his father's funeral his stepmother, who had silently witnessed years of unbearable family life, acknowledged for the first time that there had been something strange. She asked him:

> "Why is it that a guy who would work fourteen hours a day, take a sleeping pill at nine o'clock, then at eleven o'clock get a phone call from a patient who was drunk and was going to commit suicide, and who would get up and drag himself back out of the Seconal and go out into the night for some son of a bitch who at his analyzed best would be a prick—why would a guy do that and yet destroy his own children?" Those aren't her exact words, but the sentiment is there.

I answered her by telling her a story. Years ago, when I was living in Greenwich Village, I got a call about one o'clock in the morning from this friend of mine whose chick was going bananas. Her shrink, whom she had fallen in love with, had gone on vacation. He was going to this place, Nantucket or Martha's Vineyard or wherever shrinks went, and the DC-3 he was on went down and killed twenty-six psychiatrists all at once. That's kind of a funny thought. One of them was hers, and she was terribly upset, drinking, inconsolable, and her boyfriend asked me to come over and do something, because she and I liked each other. So I went over and we bullshitted awhile, and at one point she said, "You know, you're very good at this." And I said, "Well I love you." She said, "No, no, it's not that. You're very good at this because basically, way down deep, you don't give a shit." I thought to myself, you know, she's right. So when my stepmother asked how my father could be such a saint to his patients and such a fiend to his children, I told her, "Basically, way down deep, he didn't give a shit about his patients. Us kids maybe he cared about. He was emotionally involved with us; he was involved all wrong, but he was involved, and that's why he was so terrible."

For many psychotherapists who adversely affect their children's lives, the fault is not neglect or malice. They care a great deal and they try very hard, perhaps too hard, but in not quite the right way.

5

Child Rearing:
How and Why?

The ideal condition
Would be, I admit, that men
  should be
    right by instinct;
But since we are all likely to go
  astray,
The reasonable thing is to learn
  from those who can teach.
—SOPHOCLES, *ANTIGONE*

The more people have studied
different methods of bringing up
children the more they have come
to the conclusion that what good
mothers and fathers instinctively
feel like doing for their babies is
the best after all.
—BENJAMIN SPOCK

It is meaningless to ask whether, over the past few thousand years, we have learned to be better mothers and fathers to our children. The nature of society, of the family, of parenthood, and the concept of what skills and ethics parents should instill in their children and which responsibilities for them they ought to assume have changed so radically, and differ so still from place to place, that it is almost impossible even to define one's terms. The best one can say is that the child must in some way be taken from a state of near total physical and mental dependence to one of relatively complete personal independence and appropriate integration into the structure of society.

The concepts of childhood and family that most of us take so much for granted are, historically, a recent development. According to Philippe Ariès, a pioneer in this area of study, until the end of the

Middle Ages there was scarcely a distinction between childhood and the remainder of life. Children were regarded as diminutive and somewhat backward adults, more quantitatively than qualitatively different, who were given more duties and responsibilities in the same way that they were given larger clothes: as their size and experience grew. The family determined such practical matters as lineage, social class, and property rights but did not represent the emotionally knit entity that now encloses and nurtures the child for sixteen to eighteen years.[1]

Many children succeeded or failed and grew up or died much more at random than they do nowadays, with neither family nor state making concerted efforts to guarantee their proper nourishment, clothing, good care, or education. Children were often sent away from their natural parents and put straight to work. Childhood, it may be claimed, did not exist because there was no time for it. People moved directly from infancy to useful labor, after which adulthood was signalled by marrying and having children of one's own. In times when there was little social or job mobility, which is to say during most of civilization, the routes open to a child were narrowly predetermined, and parents had few ways of helping to guide their children. Clearly there was little point in helping a child blossom into the void to "find itself," to realize some unsuspected potential, or to attain fulfillment. These ethereal concepts did not exist. The incentives were quite in the opposite direction: the better the child could be disciplined or instructed to fit within the constrained space that was its future, the better suited to life it would be. Even mandatory education, at its inception, was not justified through some benevolent wish to improve the quality of the child's mind, but in the general social interest, as a way to help each individual bear his share of civic responsibility and reduce the likelihood of his becoming a burden on the state.

Childhood, in the sense that we know it, was born of increasing wealth and leisure. In the absence of material pressures that hastened the change from infancy to mature responsibility, childhood could grow longer and more intricate. The notion emerged that children were fragile innocents who needed intellectual and spiritual guidance, and they were held in a sort of "quarantine," as Ariès puts it, until discipline, education, and moral instruction had fully prepared them to join the adult world. They had opportunities to contemplate abstract ideals amidst only attenuated contacts with reality, freedom to entertain uncertainty, to postpone the need to make concrete decisions or commitments. Erik Erikson wrote, "It is human to have a long childhood; it is civilized to have an ever longer childhood. Long childhood makes a technical and mental virtuoso out of man, but it also leaves a lifelong residue of emotional immaturity in him."[2]

Parents have always influenced their children as they grew, whether through training, discipline, or more subtle manipulation, but well over a century ago the notion began to emerge that one could institute a systematic program of character formation. An 1807 manual entitled *The Importance of Domestic Discipline* contains the following bit of sinister and quite sophisticated psychological manipulation, a precursor of more modern childrearing gambits:

> A pious friend of mine has four sons. Like other children, they often do wrong. The father used to employ the rod, but a better acquaintance with human nature, taught him to lay it aside, and to adopt other measures infinitely more effectual. The little offender is called into his father's closet, and the door is shut so that no one may overhear what is said; for we naturally resist reproof that is given before others, and feel a propensity to justify ourselves. The pious father begins to inquire the reason of his conduct, in order that he may show that circumstances were not sufficient to justify the crime. He then informs him how sinful the action is in the sight of God; when he has silenced the young offender, he falls down upon his knees, and makes his son do the same; and there he confesses the sin before the all-seeing God, and implores mercy for his son, and weeps over him, till his heart begins to relent, and he bursts into tears also, and feels his crime most acutely. —This method is most effectual. It secures the two grand aims at which parents ought always to aim, I mean, filial fear, and filial love. Many parents are dreaded, but not loved. But it is difficult to say whether my friend is more feared or venerated—for their love rises to a sort of veneration. Such a mode of treatment suits all dispositions. This will awe the most inflexible mind, and affect the tenderest.[3]

The question that remained amidst the increasing flood of advice about how to raise one's children, how to solve various types of problems, how to sway them from this way of thinking or acting to that, was: What ultimate purpose was this training to serve? What was the aim of child rearing? With the rapidly relaxing predetermination of a child's role and station in life, there was less emphasis on grooming him to fit into a specific slot, and parents were freer to form subjective notions of what they wanted their child to be. Do we model our children strictly after our personal ideals, which may quite possibly have been inherited wholesale from our parents, their parents, and a sluggishly evolving ancestral tradition? Or do we attempt to design them according to some intellectually conceived plan that leads them closer to ultimate perfection?

Dr. Boris Sidis was a Russian-born psychiatrist who enjoyed considerable prestige in the late nineteenth and early twentieth centuries; some placed him on a par with Pierre Janet and Morton Prince.[4] His use of a form of cathartic hypnosis he called "hypnoidization" to cure psychoneurotic disorders by bringing out their unconscious causes, was not dissimilar to the methods Freud used before he abandoned hypnosis for free association. Sidis's most memorable accomplishment, however, was his son, William James Sidis, a precocious and ultimately pathetic child prodigy, who burst onto the public scene in 1910 when, aged eleven, he gave a lecture to the Harvard University mathematics department on four-dimensional bodies. He graduated from Harvard four years later, and withdrew from the law school three years after that, just short of earning his degree.

Dr. Sidis categorically rejected the suggestion that his son was naturally gifted: he took full credit for the phenomenon himself and averred that the same could be done with any child of normal intelligence, if only one began early and continued with unswerving devotion. Dr. Sidis's child-rearing theories were based on the idea of his mentor, William James, that humans possess untapped reserves of psychic energy, and that if they press on, rather than flagging at the first sign of mental exhaustion, they will get a "second wind" and find additional levels of mental energy. From the earliest age, therefore, Sidis concentrated on teaching his son reading, mathematics, languages, logical analysis, and avoiding childish games and utterances. In a book on child rearing he published, entitled *Philistine and Genius*, Dr. Sidis railed against frivolous and wasteful things, such as fairy tales and athletics. There was a puritanical zeal to his recommendations, but no high moral or even human aspiration, nothing except a driven quest to accomplish for accomplishment's sake, which led to a spartan, intellectually gorged yet emotionally exsanguinated existence.[5]

Dr. Sidis may have succeeded in raising a brilliant child, but he failed in raising a child. William James Sidis was desperately unhappy for most of his life and had no concept of pleasure or play. He derived no real satisfaction from his intellectual accomplishments, which were motivated neither by childhood curiosity nor the pursuit of fun, nor indeed by anything within him at all, but by the fact that these were the only things that elicited interest and approval from his parents.

After his auspicious beginning, he purposefully sank into obscurity, working at one menial job after another and fleeing the dogged attention of journalists. In 1925 he published a derivative philosophical study claiming that life was a manifestation of negative entropy, and the following year a peculiar and highly original pseudonymous work on his personal hobby of "peridromophily," or the collecting of streetcar transfers.* In 1937 James Thurber wrote an article in *The New Yorker* holding the ex-prodigy up to public ridicule, for which Sidis sued the magazine in federal district and appeals courts and the U.S. Supreme Court for malicious libel and invasion of privacy.[6]

Man's increasing knowledge of human behavior and behavior manipulating techniques brought further attention to the possibilities of making one's children as one wants. John B. Watson, the founder of behaviorism and later a highly influential writer on child rearing wrote the famous claim, "Give me a dozen healthy infants, well-formed, and my own specified world to bring them up in, and I'll guarantee to take any one at random and train him to become any type of specialist I might select—doctor, lawyer, artist, merchant chief and, yes, even beggarman and thief, regardless of his talents, penchants, tendencies, abilities, vocations, and race of his ancestors."[7] This gives one the creeps. But what is really frightening about it? Nothing explicit in this grandiose boast is alarming: absolute certainty of achieving desired results is by no means inherently bad. What is frightening is the promise of absolute power without any indication of the purpose to which it will be applied. When Watson says he can train any child to become any specialist he might select, one wonders what specialists he *would* select, and why, and where he would draw the line in this limitless foray into social engineering, and what on earth gives him the idea that, however fine a behavioral scientist he might be, he is the least bit qualified to determine people's destinies.

---

* *Notes on the Collection of Transfers,* a unique and understandably rare book, tells everything one might ever care to know about transfers: their history, descriptions of the various lines, types of transfers, and transfer procedures for a large number of cities. There are entire sections on the coloration and dating methods of transfers, instructions for patching and repairing damaged transfers one has retrieved from the ground, advice on trolley and bus riding, a section of maps and timetables, and a chapter of anecdotes and verse (mostly his own) about transfers and public transportation. The book was not a publishing success. From a personal point of view, it may be significant that public transportation had been one of the few childhood pleasures he was allowed. He enjoyed riding on streetcars with his parents. Before he was five he had memorized the hours and stations on several timetables, and "would occasionally recite timetables for guests as other children recite Mother Goose rhymes or sing little songs"— something that, being complex and numerical, must have slipped past Dr. Sidis's censorship of juvenile foolishness.

In Watson's own case, one is particularly appalled when one finds that he conducted downright barbarous experiments on children,* and was often cruel and inhuman in his detachment toward his own and the rather bizarre situations to which he subjected them in his unending quest for scientific knowledge. His wife, who had assisted him in much of his psychological research, was forced by her maternal instincts to subvert some of his efforts at home.[8]

Attempting to define a happy child, Watson, the most authoritative expert on child rearing in the late 1920s, gives a pathetic description that indicates he was far more concerned with parental convenience and gratification than with any present or ultimate good for the child itself:

> The happy child? A child who never cries unless actually stuck with a pin,† illustratively speaking; who loses himself in work and play; who quickly learns to overcome the small difficulties in his environment without running to mother, father, nurse, or some other adult; who builds up a wealth of habits that tides him over dark and rainy days; who puts on such habits of politeness and neatness and cleanness that adults are willing to be around him, at least part of the day; a child who is willing to be around adults without fighting incessantly for notice; who eats what is set before him and "asks no questions for conscience's sake"; who puts away two-year-old habits when the third year has to be faced; who passes into adolescence so well-equipped that adolescence is just a stretch of fertile years, and who finally enters manhood so bulwarked with stable work and emotional habits that no adversity can quite overwhelm him.[10]

Most people, if offered the chance to determine absolutely their child's total development, would reject it. As in any field of human endeavor, the more refined the means become, the more clearly defined the end must be, and though benevolent tyranny might be an ideal form of both political and parental rule, we recognize our lack of omniscience, total foresight, absolute goodness, and self-control and always, quite rightly, shy away from this treacherous avenue. This leaves us in the paradoxical position of wanting to have *less* control over what our children become or, phrased in a more positive man-

---

* While studying the learning process in children, Watson allowed babies, from the age of five months, to reach out for candles. At five-and-a-half months one subject continued to reach for the flame "regardless of the fact that her fingers were often scorched," but by six months "definite progress in avoidance was noted."[9]

† A definite possibility around Watson, it would seem.

ner, of cherishing their right to grow up according to their own design, yet to do so only within certain guidelines. But what is the appropriate balance to strike? Psychoanalyst O. Spurgeon English likes to relate the story of the woman who won a Mother of the Year award. After the ceremony the reporters swarmed around, clamoring, "How did you do it, Mrs. Smith? What is your secret? What method do you use?" and Mrs. Smith replied, "Well, I just saw that they got what was coming to them."

When someone tries to raise his child according to a system, as Boris Sidis, John Watson and, less extravagantly, those parents who try to raise superbabies today, it often follows that they are trying to prove something, and this something is usually in their own interests rather than in those of the child. When one seeks to satisfy selfish ambitions through the instrument of the child, it will generally lead to unfortunate results, since one ignores the child's interests and protests and genuine predilections and abilities, rushes on oblivious of the child's sense of gratification and accomplishment, and strives toward an—to the child—arbitrary goal that may well be inappropriate for the child at that particular stage or even harmful for a child at any stage. Moreover, the effort is doomed even from the pathological point of view, since no degree of success by the child will altogether satisfy the parent's need, which lies buried somewhere in the parent's past.

The right thing is often done for the wrong reason, so that the consequences of such perverse motivations may not be immediately apparent. A man driven by a pathological need to win can be an excellent high school football coach. Someone can put his lust for power and sadistic tendencies at the service of the Resistance and become a wartime hero. Yet circumstances can and often do arise that separate people according to their motives—when a coach puts winning before the rules of good sportsmanship or the physical health of his players, or when the heroic resistant is captured and finds it convenient to put his talents to work as a collaborator or when, in peacetime, crime offers the closest parallel to his wartime occupation, which is suddenly revealed to have been patriotic only by coincidence.

In parenthood the intermingling of good and bad motives is much more insidious. It is quite natural to project one's likes and needs upon one's children. This projective attraction forms a basis of the parent-child relationship and makes one fonder of this random young personality that has been deposited in one's family than one would be of any other stranger. Your children belong to you, and you invest a great deal in them. They go out into the world bearing your name and representation. It is only natural that you should expect them to give something back, to admire you, to perform for you, and to earn you credit. Only the most obnoxious and mercenary parents would consciously think of their children in these terms, but the forces, couched in more pleasant and circuitous ways, are there. You love your children, and who would not rather that his child be attractive, intelligent, popular, strong, and successful?

This is the basic theoretical and practical problem in raising children: when is one acting in the child's interest, and when in one's own? When a parent "watches his language" in front of a child, is it because he, poor sinner, the incurable victim of his shortcomings, has managed to see the error of his ways sufficiently to resolve that his child will not also succumb? Or is it an attempt to persuade himself, through the molded mirror of his child who mimics him, that he does not really do those unpleasant things that he does? Is the father who roots for his son at bat, and is so crestfallen when his son strikes out, just benevolently concerned for his son's happiness and self-image, or for the public impression his young plenipotentiary is making of him?

Parents do not want to recognize their own needs in child rearing. One psychiatrist ran a three-week seminar for parents on how to handle conflicts with their chldren. The class was packed the first week. Attendance was way down the second week. By the third week, 70 percent of the people were gone. The reason appeared to be that he was trying to explain that the *parents'* needs and problems accounted for fully half of the conflicts and had to be handled as well. This, alas, was not what the audience had come to hear: they wanted to learn how to manage and control and get their way better, not to be told that perhaps they should examine their ways and learn that it was not, after all, the case that the parents were always right and the children, hardheaded little beasts, were always obstinately wrong.[11]

Where does one learn to be a good parent like the hypothetical Mrs. Smith? It is all well and good for Dr. Spock to advise that what good mothers and fathers instinctively do is generally the best, but how does one know whether one is a good mother or father? And what if one isn't and wishes to become one? The very people who read this sensible statement are quite possibly, at that very moment, reading Spock's *Common Sense Book of Baby and Child Care* precisely because they do not trust their instincts, or do not have any, and want someone else to advise them about "common sense." And, indeed, Spock's advice was so sensible and persuasive that a whole generation of parents totally ignored its own instincts and followed

Spock to the letter. So much so that there is a whole class of people labeled "Spock children," whether it is right or wrong to lay blame for their problems at Spock's feet.

Most parents muddle along as best they can. Usually they do the right thing, sometimes they make mistakes, and often the mistakes don't really much matter. To err is human, and so are parents. When they do not know something, they seek advice, most often from relatives or friends, sometimes from experts or books. As long as they incorporate their new knowledge into their normal lives, things probably work out for the best. Problems may arise, however, when the parents completely substitute new knowledge and theory for old instinct and experience, and try to raise their children according to a rigid, alien program. An artificial structure is imposed upon home life that does not allow for the normal give and take. There is a split between the way the parent is as a human being and the way he or she is as a parent, as though the parents had gone out and bought scripts, and every time they were called upon to play the parental role they snatched up sheets of paper and began declaiming someone else's text.

It is even worse when the system parents follow is flawed. In an article on the "Spock Children," psychiatrist Richard Robertiello wrote that parents influenced by Dr. Spock tried to bring their children up without the trauma and complexes they themselves had suffered. They did this by emphasizing a loving, demonstrative, indulgent attitude rather than following a more traditional, rigidly autocratic role, so that the children would be happier and healthier, and less socially, sexually, and intellectually inhibited. This attitude was rather a misunderstanding of Spock and his interpretation of psychoanalysis, since he recognized quite clearly the dangers of overpermissiveness, but it has nonetheless been linked to his name. As Robertiello says:

In many ways these child-rearing methods worked. These young men are very open, friendly, get on easily with people, have wholesome relationships with their male peers and with the opposite sex. They are warm, loving and lovable. They are not anxious about sex or about being liked and accepted by people. They expect to be well-liked and have none of the social or sexual anxieties that so many people had in their parents' generation. So far, so good. So "Spock" worked. Yes, it did work and very well. Except that there is a fly in the ointment. These young men do not seem to be able to choose a profession, to earn a decent living, to channel their considerable intellectual ability and talents into some meaningful career. They come to us therapists lost and floundering. They are still emotionally and financially supported by their parents. They feel defeated by their inability to cope with the challenge of carving a niche for themselves in the world.[12]

The problem, Robertiello says, is that these children were *too* well raised, treated too liberally, loved too indiscriminately, and never exposed to any challenges or hardships that would have helped them develop into mature, capable adults. This is by no means a phenomenon restricted to children raised in the heyday of Benjamin Spock. It is, however, a phenomenon that one finds with unfortunate frequency among the children of psychotherapists.

It is an unfortunate fact that the therapeutic image of parents is largely negative. What the therapist sees in his office are the remains of the hypothetical unsullied potential being that the child once was, after it has been bashed about by misunderstandings, poorly explained or handled situations, avoidable traumas that were not avoided, and sometimes by outright abuse. This is, after all, much of why people see psychotherapists. They do not come in because of their parents' success in raising them well. It is no wonder that some therapists then, through a rather perverse interpretation of the facts, try to limit their own parental role to a blandly positive one, or else to a more active one where they give carefully weighed responses after considering all possible ramifications. Others, particularly those many whose own childhoods were unhappy, dare to hope that their knowledge and training will enable them to spare their own children from the same misfortunes.

One child psychiatrist reported with befuddlement the behavior of an analytically oriented colleague and his wife, who had dedicated the first year of their son's life to making sure that, during this theoretically critical preverbal period, the child experience no disappointments, frustrations, or stress. "The lengths to which they went, going out of their way and denying themselves in order to spare this little kid some moderate doses of life, was excessive." He said that in this case, in spite of appearances, he felt no real concern for the future of the child. I find it hard to be so sanguine about people who, for so long, ignored the realities of life—both their own and their son's—in favor of theoretical abstractions. Freud himself, when considering the possible prophylactic virtues of child analysis, concluded that rather than using preventive techniques with the children, it was probably more efficacious and less difficult to analyze the parents and teachers instead.[13] This, after all, is where the problems originate.

The ultimate aim in raising a child is to produce a contented and productive adult, whatever our definition of those terms might be. If we are satisfied with our own personal ideals, then "contented" and "productive" will be just what we ourselves are or had hoped to become. Or we may take a more philosophical approach—one closer to that of the therapist in the consultation room, who serves as a mediator freeing his patient from the perverting constraints of his past—and try to raise "omni-potential" children, so to speak, in whom we have not inculcated our prejudiced values, to whom we will give freedom to discern and choose the principles that should guide their lives. We will expose them to opportunities without defining their path, help them without pushing, correct them without repressing.

It is not easy to figure out where to draw the appropriate lines. When is the child's rebellion a healthy striving for autonomy and when is it incipient criminality? When does the child need to grapple with his problems on his own and when should a grown-up step in and help? When is a child holding back because he is genuinely not ready for something, and when is he irrationally stuck and in need of a firm, kindly nudge? There is never a clear, prescriptive answer, since each situation encountered is unique. Parents must exercise some judgment and make use of their natural ability to empathize. To have empathy, they must be able to draw on their own recollected childhood and make use of their personal experience and their memories of happiness and sorrow and of what helped them or hurt.

Parents are not psychotherapists to their children, because they do not have the requisite emotional detachment. Nor should they. Yet in some ultimate way, the function of being a parent very closely resembles that of a therapist in that the parent must help the child outgrow him. Parents want their children always to love them, but for affection to be meaningful and mature it must pass through difficult phases, possibly estrangement, and be freely given without need or guilt. For the child to become an adult he must cease to be a child. In this sense parenthood is far more difficult than being a psychotherapist. The loss of patients for the therapist who depends upon them is hard, but the loss of a child by a parent can be terrible, since one's sense of identity is so much more closely allied to one's family than to even the most interminable analytic patient.

A key aspect of the problems of many psychotherapists as parents is that they bring into their family lives the same problems they bring to their practices—the same problems that led them to their profession in the first place. Whether one regards them as "narcissistically impaired," "pathological helping professionals," people with "God complexes," or, to use D. W. Winnicott's disarmingly innocent phrase, "not good-enough" parents,[14] they are people whose low sense of true self-esteem, discomfort with themselves and with others, compensatory grandiosity, and flight into the curious profession of psychotherapy leads them to seek gratification and admiration through others, primarily patients and children.

The intention of the parent is certainly not hostile, nor even conscious, which makes it more difficult for the child to defend himself against the parent's subtle directives. Conscious manipulation is fairly easily handled, sooner or later, but this more insidious form of desperate unconscious manipulation is more imperceptible. Many such parents seem to get along particularly openly and well with their children. They are close, spend time together, talk a great deal: one commonly hears what a good, mature relationship a PsyK has with his or her therapist parent. Yet as Kohut points out, "the appearance is deceptive, for these parents are unable to respond to their children's changing narcissistic requirements, are unable to obtain narcissistic fulfillment by participating in their children's growth, because they are using their children for their own narcissistic needs."[15] They get along so well with their children because they cannot afford to get along without them.

One woman lawyer said of her analyst father, "I don't think he really recognized that I was a person and that I had feelings of my own or a separate identity. He really didn't think that I was anything but his daughter. He got unreasonably upset whenever I was not doing what he wanted."

"A helping relationship ultimately ought to lead to the other person being more independent," says a forty-year-old painter and psychiatrist's daughter, "which means that you're losing them. I think a healthy person will see that happening, but many people can't allow it to happen. They can't see that they have helped, and that that should be the gratification, but instead it may seem that, after all the help and encouragement you've given, after all the things you've done, they just don't need you anymore. That's very tragic to some people: they feel wounded and betrayed, when in fact what happened was that they succeeded, they did good. I have seen this all happening within my family at many points. It's a pattern that is only recently being broken, and it is interesting to see the changes, the feelings of rejection. I need to reassure my father that I still love him even though I don't need him."

An unusually painful case is that of a woman, an artist in her fifties, who spent most of her life under her analyst father's control:

I was my father's favorite. I was adored. I could have become a psychiatrist and been like the little Anna Freud trotting around after him. Thank God there was some thread of common sense telling me to find another field.* As it was, though, we were tremendously close, he confided in me about my mother: she was the villain, while I was the Pygmalion figure whom he could shape as he wished. I never rebelled; I suppose I was getting too much out of it. What I object to in retrospect was his using me as a confidante, almost as an in-house mistress, though without any physical thing, but definitely overstepping the parent-child relationship and his role as a father, treating me as an equal when I never should have been. This continued through my marriage until his death. We talked on the phone every day. I never questioned it because there were no strings attached, I could do as I liked, though of course there was every conceivable string. He gave me money, he would stuff hundred-dollar bills in my hand, paid for child care. I think for him my husband was just this pleasant little person, but no threat. I was married to *him* for life, and that was that. My brother, meanwhile, was totally squashed, has had endless problems with identity. My mother has blossomed since his death. "Destroyed" is perhaps too strong a word, but he certainly had strong harmful effects on everyone, and in the end even on me. He died just before I turned forty, and I had a nervous breakdown, because I think one of the things he did was really to infantilize me. He made me feel like he was the world. His death was a turning point in my adult life that turned out to be good. It turned out that life went on without him. In fact, it went on a lot better.

The child has a need to be perceived and respected for the person that he really is, because only in this way can he develop as an individual. The good parent, or Winnicott's "good-enough" parent, responds to the child's spontaneous acts, and gradually weans it from its infantile sense of omnipotence into a healthy recognition of the

---

* At one point during our conversation she stopped, gazed around the room where we sat, and commented that, after all, it looked very much the way her father's office had: a desk, a few chairs, a couch, many books, some primitive sculptures. She found this recognition a little disconcerting.

differences between itself and the rest, between reality and imagination—without, nonetheless, sacrificing its sense of spontaneity. The "not good-enough mother" (or father), on the other hand, "repeatedly fails to meet the infant gesture; instead she substitutes her own gesture which is to be given sense by the compliance of the infant. This compliance on the part of the infant is the earliest stage of the False Self, and belongs to the mother's inability to sense her infant's needs."[16]

In other words, instead of the child seeing himself mirrored in the response of his parent, an appropriate process that would help his nascent True Self flourish and grow, the child of the not good-enough parent sees only the visage of a needful parent who is searching for his or her *own* image in the child. In an unwitting attempt to please, the child gradually comes to neglect, here and there, his own spontaneous action, and constructs a self-conscious self dedicated to the service of the parent's demands and expectations. This False Self is a sort of artificial personality that may function more or less successfully, and sometimes extremely well, but it cuts the child and subsequent adult off from his spontaneous self. It is an emotional puppet or automaton that does a pretty fair imposture of a normal human being, but lacks its own inner motivation. Such children end up, as Kohut described, feeling vaguely unreal, lacking emotions, without meaning and vitality in their lives. They have spent so much time and effort devoting themselves to the parent, and to those things the parent represents, that they are drained of life and have very little sense of independent self.

"They have all developed the art of not experiencing feelings," remarks Alice Miller, "for a child can only experience his feelings when there is somebody there who accepts him fully, understands and supports him. If that is missing, if the child must risk losing the [parent's] love, . . . then he cannot experience these feelings secretly 'just for himself' but fails to experience them at all. But nevertheless . . . something remains."[17]

These not good-enough parents would like to do the right thing for their children, but at those points where they need intuitive judgment and empathy, where they should draw on the memory of their own childhood experience, they run into a blank—the blank of their own stunted and unhappy emotional past. They are therefore left with external standards and a detached, intellectual, scarcely spontaneous sense of what is right and wrong. As one PsyK phrased it, "it's a little like being raised in a finishing school." The children of such parents tend to be intelligent and perceptive, and they seem to have a great deal of empathy, though it may really be more of an intellectual facsimile. They are charming, polite, and a credit to their parents. They appear to be independent and responsible, for that is what their parents want, but at the heart of it all lies a fundamental vacancy, because their parents have infected them with the same impoverished childhood and diminished sense of self-worth that they themselves experienced. It is doubtless better concealed, sometimes behind a compensatory show of closeness and interest, but the affection may be inappropriate or lacking.

Says the son of two psychiatrists:

> My parents tried to love me. I do think that they tried to love me, and they still do try, but for one reason or another, they do not love. I don't know how many people really do experience love, but it is like a musical performance, and you can tell when there is real spirit behind it. If a musician or composer has inspiration as well as the technical means to transform it into sound, he convinces you that he is feeling something, whereas the technique without the feeling will produce something you might, perhaps, admire, but which does not touch you personally. In the same way, I believe that a human being who loves you can make you aware, and my parents did not. I may have been an extremely difficult child. No doubt I was extremely difficult. But where did it all begin?

This much would apply to any narcissistically impaired parent; in fact psychiatrist David Reiser, who has noted that analysts' kids are often so amazingly good, bright, and charismatic, ventured to say very tentatively that quite similar goodness, perfectionism, and superficial excellence, coupled with chronic anxiety and feelings of inadequacy and rottenness, is to be found in the children of alcoholics and bulimics, possibly for comparable reasons. They, too, had to grow up too quickly and assume emotional responsibility for a fragile, ego-impaired parent.[18]

In what way, one might justifiably ask, could the profession of psychotherapy enhance this narcissistic effect? It can do so in two ways. First, it provides the impaired parent with a profession that resonates with and partially legitimizes his or her personality flaws. It gives improved means of protection, concealment, and rationalization, and provides an alternate route for dealing with emotional issues through purely intellectual methods, like wearing gloves to avoid the contaminating touch of real things. Psychotherapy can be construed to condone a lack of spontaneity, a calm examination and weighing of issues, a very tentative form of living in which one waits and observes without clearly acting. Therapeutic training also offers the therapist parent effective techniques, and sometimes more important, the *appearance* of having techniques, to manipulate his patients, his children, and his world into giving back the psychic nourishment he needs.

Second, the profession of psychotherapy exerts an effect upon the children, through osmosis if not through direct instruction, by giving them a prematurely intellectual way of regarding themselves as they pass through the early stages of life. Coupled with their own incipient parentally inspired impairment, this cognitive approach to living may exacerbate the children's sense of uncertainty, unreality, and emotional stuntedness. The need to please the narcissistic parent already undermines their sense of spontaneity. The analytic notion that something *else*, some unacknowledged and perhaps unknown and unknowable motive always underlies their acts, can further aggravate this flaw. The man quoted earlier said that his parents had never been able really to love him, but rather than inciting him to resentment, this realization promptly led him to speculate about how much he had contributed by being a difficult child. It is a double curse: first he was wronged, and then he took the blame for it.

Even in the absence of particular impairment of the therapist, the learning and practice of psychotherapy do supply the parent with certain powerful information. The more one knows about people and is accustomed to dealing with them, and the more defenses and techniques one understands, the greater the effect one can have upon another. To deny this is to deny that there is any value to psychotherapy, or that umpteen years of psychiatric or analytic training do anything at all. The most benevolent parent in the world may make mistakes, and though the therapist's training does, in the best cases, help him avoid errors, in other cases it may make errors worse. Moreover, for the children, as for the patients, the therapist's opinions and statements carry more weight, because the therapist is someone who is supposed to know. This makes it all the more difficult for PsyKs to feel truly certain of themselves when they rebel against their parents, or to persuade themselves that their parents are wrong. In choosing the profession, a therapist has placed himself in a position of authority that extends both directly and indirectly beyond the consulting room door, and he must consequently accept the added responsibility this position imposes and try to be a better parent than most, to understand himself better and ensure that his aims are clear.

*   *   *

The following case illustrates in a general way some of the problems just discussed, when a parent tries to compensate for the lacks in his own past through the things that he does for his children, and when the child's devotion to his parent's ideals and anticipated approval undermined his ultimate sense of self. Many years into this PsyK's life he still has great difficulty determining what, exactly, he wants and feels.

An acquaintance of mine met David at a party, and in the course of a brief conversation learned that his father was a psychiatrist. She thought that a thirty-one-year-old man whose father's profession was so present in his mind that it would emerge so readily, without provocation, would be interesting for me to meet. David was a professional juggler and performer, and I tracked him down with some difficulty. When I found him, he was out of work owing to a physical injury, temporarily supporting himself as a salesman. It was not a cheerful phase of his life, he said, and he assigned the cause of many of his emotional difficulties to his relationship with his father, something he had thought about considerably in recent times and was pleased to be able to discuss. As soon as we sat down, he told me he would relate his life story twice: first as he had perceived it at the time, second from his present viewpoint.

It was extraordinary to hear the intensity with which David spoke of his father. "I grew up worshipping him. He was the center of my universe. He was the one who made the world make sense, and made me feel there was some sort of justice. He clearly loved me, and since I thought he was the most wonderful person on earth, that made me feel worthwhile."

David's mother, on the other hand, was unstable and moody—in many ways, he said, one of his father's most chronic patients. She did not enjoy what he saw as typical maternal activities, resented the demands her son made on her time, and maintained such a compulsively neat, repressive atmosphere in the house that David's friends called it "the museum" and rarely wanted to visit.

David's father, despite his busy professional schedule, spent a great deal of time with his son, and there was almost no activity David would not gladly abandon if given the opportunity to be with his father. When David grew interested in athletics, it was his father, who was neither particularly athletic nor interested in athletics himself, who accompanied him to games and who helped out at the refreshment stand alongside the mothers. When David reached the point where he did virtually nothing but play sports, watch sports, or read books about athletes, and his mother and others in the family expressed concern that he was growing too one-dimensional, David's father said, "No, if you enjoy it, you do it. You do what you think is best."

Everything that his father said made a tremendous impression on him. When he explained, for example, why he thought smoking was bad, David began to dislike all his television heroes who smoked. Later, he had a recurring nightmare that he walked into a room and found his father smoking; he was tremendously relieved when he woke up and found that his father was still his hero. "Doubtless that is fraught with all kinds of Freudian significance, whatever it may be."

David's father always told him that it did not matter what sort of work he did in life; the important thing was to find a job that challenged him, that made a contribution to society, and in which he felt he could do good work and derive a sense of personal satisfaction. It was not important to become a psychiatrist, a doctor, a lawyer, or to make a lot of money. Money had been set aside for college, and even for graduate school if that was what he wanted, so he should never worry about money, or obligations, or about what other people thought, but only about what he wanted to do and what he could do well. The constellation of power in his life was such that this was the final word.

When David had problems, his father dealt with them. Once he was falsely accused of stealing some microphones from their temple and was going to be denied the right to have a bar mitzvah as a result. "But in this case, as in every other case where something terrible happened and it seemed like I would hit bottom, there was this cushion, and it was him. Even if everything else went to hell, I still had a wonderful father who still really loved me, so it would all work out." His father persuaded the rabbi that if David, until then one of the worst Hebrew school students, could get exceptional grades, it would somehow prove that he was a person of integrity, unlikely to commit crimes, and that he deserved a bar mitzvah. "And then, to make *sure* that this happened, *he* was my tutor. It was twenty or thirty years since he had even thought about Hebrew, yet he was so intelligent that he still remembered enough that, once he got out the book, he was able to tutor it. Not only that, but though it was something I genuinely hated to do, he made it fun. We would go out in the backyard together, and forty-five minutes later I walked away not having learned a lot, but feeling that I'd had a great time. Lo and behold, I quickly went from being virtually the dumbest to the very top of the class. Everyone wanted to know whether I had taken some kind of miracle intelligence pills, but I knew it was my wonderful father.

"My father was my Rock of Gibraltar. I always had this feeling that at the bottom of who I was, at the core of my identity, the base, the bedrock, was him. How could I be too bad if he was so wonderful? And if I was, according to him and to so many others, a chip off the old block, surely even if I had these downfalls, I would end up having a very wonderful life. And that, to some degree, happened, for a while."

David so much internalized aspects of his father that, contrary to his own expectation, he did not miss him even when he went away for two months to summer camp. He felt his father within him, he thought about him, and he talked about him. "Whenever I met anyone, one of the first things I would talk about was my *wonderful* relationship with my father, and I loved telling anecdotes about the things he could do."

In school, David was not the most popular person in class, which he wanted to be, and which he fantasized his father must have been; nor was he the smartest, which his father had in fact been. Nonetheless he did well enough to gain early admission to the University of Pennsylvania, and when he set off for college his father drove him there, spent a few days in Philadelphia helping him get himself comfortably installed, and upon leaving once again left David with an internalized sense of his presence that made the shock of starting college much less than it is for many students.

David discussed all of his major decisions quite openly with his father. Throughout high school he drank moderately, with his father's knowledge and permission. Toward the end of high school he felt he wanted to try marijuana and, typically, told his father that he felt ready to do so. They discussed it, and after his father had heard his reasoning he said that he felt confident David knew what he was doing, and that he would trust his judgment. "That gave me a clear conscience, and made me feel that I had the Good Housekeeping Seal of Approval. If this very learned psychiatrist, who dealt with many other people's psyches, thought that mine was sturdy enough to deal with a few stimulants, I felt more secure that in fact I could. I became very fond of smoking pot. I probably smoked once a day for the next seven or eight years."

David enjoyed his college years because his father endorsed whatever he chose to do. While other students worried about finding a career, he felt free to pursue whatever interested him. His individualized major was in cultural pluralism, with specific emphasis on black aesthetics and how it related to American folklore and culture—not, as he willingly admits, a field that easily leads to constructive employment. "Again, my father's attitude was, 'Why do you want to do this?' and once I had explained, of accepting this strange choice, and therefore tacitly approving of it." He spent a year abroad, and after graduation returned to Europe, with his father's blessing and in spite of his mother's trepidation, for an extended hitchhiking tour. It was during this trip that he first became involved in juggling and street performing, and when he returned to the United States he announced to his mother and other worried relatives that he was going to be a street performer. They were relieved to hear that he would also attend graduate school to study folklore, and thus turn this curious interest into a serious academic pursuit.

While in Europe he also fell in love, and he returned with the understanding that the woman would follow immediately and live with him in the United States. "Under tragic whatever, it didn't work out, star-crossed lovers that we were, and I felt terrifically hurt. This will seem strange to you, but that was the *first* real disappointment I had to deal with that my father could not diminish. No matter how consoling he was, no matter how much of a pep talk he gave me about how he knew I would meet other women, or that this would all work out, it *crushed* me. It crushed me, and I was utterly unprepared to cope with it—which relates to what I will say later about how I view my life in retrospect."

At that point, David said, he sank into a debilitating depression. He dropped out of graduate school and began performing full time, but even that did not satisfy him. "The crowds were applauding, but inside me there were boos and jeers: 'You're no good. This is a sham. How can you pretend to entertain children at a hospital when you're such a wreck you should be hospitalized yourself?' " He reached the point where he could not perform any more. Though he did not need hospitalization, he did enter psychotherapy.

Therapy was very helpful, in large part simply because the therapist pointed out that, whatever David's father said and whatever David professed to believe about money being unimportant, it seemed clear that if he were ever to develop a sense of self-worth, then before worrying about making meaning in life, he should demonstrate his ability to do what everyone else did and go out and earn a living. David got a job as a busboy and a waiter, and soon, as a way to make some extra cash, began performing again on the side. He regained his confidence, and was soon making twice as much performing as he was at his job, so he quit and returned to performing full time. On the occasion of a tour he also quit therapy, after only three or four months, something that he retrospectively believes to have been a serious mistake.

For several years he was very successful, juggling, playing music, and telling stories. He was on the road a good deal of the time and felt talented, full of energy, and excited about life. His family was pleased that he was back to his normal, cheerful self, and even his mother, who had done some amateur acting in her youth, felt a new kinship with him now that some of her seemed to be surfacing in him. At several performances that his parents attended, he invited his father on stage as a storyteller, and his father captivated the audience.

But then after about three years of doing this, my father's attitude noticeably changed to essentially one of: "This is all well and good, but when are you going to get serious?" At the time I was too defensive to fully grasp how much of a betrayal that was of what he had always led me to believe. Here I was doing something that challenged and thrilled me, something that I felt made a contribution—being able to make people laugh, to create a performance that in some way portrayed and interpreted the human condition—and something I was genuinely good at. What's more, I was making money. I was able to pay all my bills, and even to set some money aside. But he told me I could never support a family.

His disapproval was awfully hard to take. I think, in retrospect, that one of the reasons I got injured was that I worked myself so fucking hard in order to prove him wrong. I wanted to be vindicated, to prove that my judgment was sound, and to show him that, smart as he was, this was a field he knew nothing about and he was dead wrong. And if he was going to say that a rolling stone gathers no moss, that never having a family would be one of the penalties I would have to pay if I spent my life as an itinerant troubadour, I was going to prove him wrong on that, too. So I got married.

David loves his wife, but admits that he married her for all the wrong reasons, not because of what he wanted or felt ready for, but because of what he wanted to prove to others. She was beautiful, like his mother, and just as his mother had been dependent upon his father, he tried to have power over his wife, to support and console her, and to make her dependent on him. She was Jewish, which pleased his family. She was a juggler and tightrope walker, so that in marrying her he got not only a wife, but a husband-wife team, which is far more marketable to schools, civic organizations, cruise ships, and the like than a single performer, no matter how talented.

Not long afterward, everything began to fall apart. At a Renaissance festival in Kansas City, an allergic reaction to a particular type of ragweed gave him such a bad case of asthma that he was constantly coughing, had difficulty sleeping, and could barely catch his breath after his juggling act. At the same time he drove himself ever harder in his attempt to prove himself. He prided himself on being a juggler's juggler, doing routines that were harder and more complex, though inconspicuously different except to a trained performer's eye. He grew obsessed with creating a one-man juggling rendition of *Hamlet*, illustrating the play with different kinds of juggling, and introducing comical plays on words. He constantly wrote, rewrote, revised, and started over, often going straight from his act to his room to write, working through the night until six o'clock the next morning, then with scarcely any sleep going back out to juggle, breathe rag-weed pollen, and cough. One day he was stricken with severe back pains and could scarcely move.

David was forced to abandon several thousand dollars of contracted work, leave his wife in Kansas City to pack up and drive back on her own, and fly to New York for emergency treatment. At that point his father stepped in, in his most nurturing capacity, and did his utmost to find the best people, have all necessary tests, and do everything possible to diagnose the mysterious, excruciating pain. After CAT scans and electromyograms, the problem was finally, though not conclusively, identified as a severely pinched nerve, and he ended up with his neck in a brace, a regimen of analgesic and anti-inflammatory drugs, and regular visits to a chiropractor and an acupuncturist.

At this point, with his health and profession seemingly gone, and with a dawning realization of the problems in his marriage, David again sank into a profound depression and began thinking back over his life, first alone, then with the help of a therapist. At the heart of it all he ran up against his father, whom he blamed for many of his problems. It was curious to hear David describe his relationship with his father, in many ways so idyllic, in tones of bitterness and resentment. But from the vantage point of the present he saw the unquestioning love and support that had been lavished upon him for his first twenty-five years as having undermined his ability to form his own sense of values, values centered upon himself rather than upon gratifying his father. As a child, his father had been at the base of his sense of identity. As an adult, he felt hampered in trying to establish his own base. When his father turned and challenged what life he had made for himself, he was crushed:

> When I thought about it, I finally realized that my father needs to be in a very dominant position, and he managed to construct a set of relationships in which he *was* the dominant person. He certainly was with my mother, always consoling her and making her feel she was all right as a mother. Unquestionably he was with his children, which is fine to a point, but then he was unwilling to play any other kind of role, which means that as long as you're father and child it's okay, but if the child tries to grow up, the father is reluctant to allow it and to relinquish his position of control. I'm sure the same thing is true in his work. He thrives on the fact that one person after another walks in and pays him for the privilege of depending upon him. I suppose that's one reason why he really loves to get up each morning and go off to his job.
>
> I ended up analyzing the analyst and I figured that perhaps as a child he had not had very much power, that he couldn't make decisions, and that there was no one he felt important to. I finally talked to him about it and it turned out that this was true. Essentially he had been the runt of the family. His eldest sister was the prima donna everyone doted on, and his older brother was the strong, funny, zany one whom everyone liked, while he was the one his brother always picked on and whom everyone blamed for everything. He was the last one to be chosen in games, and he grew up in a rough Italian neighborhood where the other kids called him "Jew boy" or "kike" and used to beat him up. So he sought refuge in the library, and came to what I think was in some way an unavoidable realization, which I can sum up as: "I'm not going to beat them with my body, but maybe there's power in knowledge, and maybe the one thing that's left in me is my brain. Maybe here in the quiet of the library I'll soak up enough knowledge that some day I'll get even, or at least things will go better for me."

David's father also acknowledged in a recent conversation that he had thought that the training he went through and the knowledge he gained as a psychiatrist would enable him to help his own children grow up without the misery he had felt. As a more or less conscious plan he had set out to rectify the problems of his own life in theirs. From David's point of view, however, the result was a total disaster.

He finds it particularly disturbing since his father has spent the past forty years as a successful and highly respected psychiatrist who really ought to know better.

I've discussed my feelings about all this with my father, and he's been willing to sit down and talk. He is very candid and open, but at the same time very winning. It's a knack he has: he won't boast about what he did, or even necessarily try to persuade you that he was right, but he will explain his actions as a master apologist might explain them, so that at the end you certainly wouldn't want to find him guilty of anything and could feel nothing but a certain amount of sympathy and respect for the way he'd dealt with a difficult situation. His favorite phrase is "I did the best I know how." Now that's *good,* except that falls short of admitting to someone "Hey, I'm really disappointed that I failed. I know how much this has meant to you, and I really feel bad. I want to search my soul and see if maybe next time I can do better." *That* is very different from just saying, "Well, look, I messed up, but I'm human, I did my best, can't ask more than that." A lot of our impasses have ended with him saying, "Well, the best we can do is agree to disagree." That's a pretty swift bit of Orwellian semantics.

My father pays lip service to having regrets, but I don't *feel* it. He's not a real feeling man. He lives so much in his head that he can speak about things in a calm, reasonable way that is totally disconnected from real flesh-and-blood feelings. Perhaps that is a side effect of being a shrink—maybe sitting in that office and listening to people and listening to other people's torments while keeping his own feelings out of it has given him a personality disorder. But as his son, being in the position I'm in, I need to *feel* that he is sorry, and see, through his actions, that he is not just mouthing platitudes. When I was in the pits—marriage falling apart, didn't know what I could do to earn any money—he was very supportive and tried hard to help me figure things out, but it really was clear that the minute he hung up the phone or the minute he drove home, I was gone. It was as though the next patient had walked into the room.

I don't know how to reconcile this with the warm feeling I had growing up. It is like a juggling or a magic trick, a conjuring act. It *seems* that he can allow himself to feel happy feelings. It seems that he can get in touch with things that are warm and winning and fun. But anything that comes from the dark side, he seals off. A lot of times when I was growing up I said to him, "You know, I feel as if whenever we talk I tell my troubles to you, but you never say anything back to me. Is anything troubling you?" And he would say, "No, nothing's troubling me." As I got older I said, "This can't be. Is there really nothing that ever troubles you?" And he said, "Look, if something is troubling me, believe me, you'll be the first to know. I'll tell you about it." Well, there were some pretty horrendous things that happened in his life, yet he never did talk. It was more "I've got to be strong, I've got to look after everybody else and make sure that they're able to deal with this. I don't need anybody, because I'm a psychiatrist. I can counsel myself. I've been through analysis. I've worked out all the things that could trouble me."

I still wrestle with how much influence he has over me. I still—even though I know it probably wasn't healthy from the start—have moments of incredible yearning for the kind of love that we shared when I was growing up. I sometimes see him and wish that we could go back to those times when he was so proud of me and happy with who I was, and I felt so lucky that he was my dad, and the greatest thing of all was just to go down to the hardware store with him. Now there's a void, an incredible void. I think we each know, in our rational minds, that we can't go back, but it's appalling how much of me still misses that childhood attachment and still craves it. The other side of it is, of course, that sometimes I feel really furious that some of the stuff that has been so painful for me to deal with might not have been so painful if I'd had a more realistic childhood and if I'd been given a little more chance to learn to cope with things that are not so pretty. If there had not been so much denial. The first time I got sad and depressed, no one acknowledged that it was something I would really have to work at and deal with. Instead, as soon as the worst of the depression lifted, it was "Great! Let's get back to having fun and happy times again. Let's not think about this dark side. Let's not deal with any of this despair." And for an experienced psychiatrist to see how deeply depressed I was and not say a word when I announced, after three or four months of therapy, that I didn't need help anymore and felt fine, that strikes me as a gross error in judgment.

Our relationship now is certainly strained, to say the least. It's not *es*tranged. The firmament of love is so deep that I'm sure no matter what happens we'll always love each other, right until we die. But in terms of being able to have a healthy relationship, I've got to constantly guard against the ways in which his meddling—and it's not really meddling, it's his well-intentioned efforts to try to smooth over situations and pave the way for me to be able to have a happier existence—they trap me in being a child. Half of what I'm dealing with is, how can you be married and be a husband if, at the same time, you're still a boy? And when it comes down to my dad, he wants to treat me like a boy. We're stuck. We're like Willy Loman and Biff, and it's hard for both of us to get away from that.

His attitude is that he really wants, of course, for us to get out of whatever had been unhealthy, he really wants to acknowledge his share of the responsibility, and he's really willing to be called to task and to—for a while—stay out of things. But in some insidious way, his craving for power, or for someone to be dependent on him, is something that it's hard for him to control. I think a lot of times he may say those words, but his actions still end up being those of someone who really wants to be such an all-powerful figure to his son. I don't think that he knows how to love or receive love in another mode.

It's just as hard for me not to take from him in the same old way. He's wise and knowledgeable and willing to help, and when I have all these things I'm trying to grapple with, it's tough not to go back to what had for so many years been my Rock of Gibraltar. Sometimes I'll be at a family gathering and I'll see people drawn to him because he's such a funny guy and a good conversationalist, and I'll kind of get on the periphery, and I'll remember how much I wanted to be close to him. It's like being next to the sun, getting next to the source of so much good stuff. I look up to him still, though hopefully there is not quite as much worship. Time and a lot of pain has taken some of the shine off of the statue on the pedestal, but there still seems to be this reverence, this kind of respect for his knowledge, respect for his efficiency. The guy is so efficient. He's just incredible. He gets so much stuff done.

I think that is probably a problem for a lot of sons of psychiatrists: it's a tough act to follow. I end up inadvertently comparing my own efficiency with his efficiency. During the time when I was so driven to write the *Hamlet* routine, I must in some unconscious way have been competing with another ghost of a father. I hoped that this could be something I could feel would measure up with his work. Somehow this could give me a feeling of having achieved something like what he's achieved, or to have reached a level of craft similar to the kind of honors that are conferred on someone who gets through college and medical school and then analysis and residency and all that stuff. I remember hearing about a son of a psychiatrist who wound up being a mechanic. At the time I thought what a disappointment that must have been to the father. But now when I consider it, I think that, hell, that may have been the only thing that guy could do to get his own turf. You can't compete with these giants in their own field.

6

"Does Your Father Analyze You?"

DOTTY (*off*): Help!
(BONES reacts. ARCHIE *restrains him.*)
ARCHIE: It's all right—just
  exhibitionism: what we
  psychiatrists call "a cry for
  help."
BONES: But it *was* a cry for help.
ARCHIE: Perhaps I'm not making
  myself clear. *All* exhibitionism is
  a cry for help, but a cry for help
  as such is only exhibitionism.

—TOM STOPPARD, *JUMPERS*

"The womenfolk do not back me in my investigations," Sigmund Freud lamented to Wilhelm Fliess in 1897. He had been barred from making empirical studies in the nursery to determine the developmental stage at which babies first show disgust for excrement. "The answer would be interesting theoretically," Freud believed. Mrs. Freud did not agree. She had always been surprised by some aspects of her husband's work, had remained almost purposefully ignorant of it, and was apparently determined that it should not be inflicted upon her unsuspecting family. "Psychoanalysis stops at the door to the children's room," she said.[1]

Psychoanalysis may never have entered the children's room, but when the children came out, analysis was everywhere throughout the apartment, just as it permeated their father's thinking. If they were never made the objects of analytic experimentation, analysis eventually, ineluctably, albeit erratically, affected their lives in other ways. Freud could scarcely avoid using professional understanding of certain behavior any more than he could or would suddenly disregard the law of gravity or forget that fire was hot or ignore the whole host of self-evident facts that form the foundation for understanding and functioning in the real world around.

The first question anyone asks of a psychoanalyst's child, and quite often of any other therapists' child, is "Did your father (or mother) analyze you?" It is not always clear, even to the asker, what is meant by this question. Did the father bring to bear his analytic understanding on the daily happenings of the household? Did he analyze his child's dreams and slips of the tongue and use this unfairly gleaned knowledge to control the child, or file his observations away for future reference or to use in a book? Did he lay his kid down on a couch in his office and make him free associate and spill out his heart for fifty minutes by the clock?

The last case is rarely ever, but not never, found; the second is quite frequent, the first nearly universal. Not unexpectedly, introduction of analysis into the home was much more common in the earlier days of psychoanalysis, when it was even more of a passion than a job. Every aspect of human nature was an unexplored field of potential discoveries, and it was only natural that analysts should take every opportunity to expand their preoccupation. Many of Freud's greatest discoveries were made first through introspection and self-analysis, and only later confirmed or embellished through the reported experiences of others. *The Interpretation of Dreams* is filled with analyses of Freud's own dreams. It also contains two of his children's dreams, both, admittedly, simple cases of wish-fulfillment that do not reveal intimate details of the children's secret lives. Freud apparently regretted that he had not been prepared to make better use of his children for analytic study on other issues; when writing of the hostility that children feel upon the arrival of an infant brother or sister, he commented that "In the case of my own children, who followed each other in rapid succession, I neglected the opportunity of carrying out observations of this kind; but I am now making up for this neglect by observing a small nephew, whose autocratic rule was upset, after lasting for fifteen months, by the appearance of a female rival."[2]

In *The Psychopathology of Everyday Life* Freud wrote, "When a member of my family complains to me of having bitten his tongue, pinched a finger, or the like, he does not get the sympathy he hopes for, but instead the question: 'Why did you do that?' " His children themselves inevitably absorbed this method of interpreting themselves:

One of my boys, whose lively temperament used to make it difficult to nurse him when he was ill, had a fit of anger one day because he was ordered to spend the morning in bed, and threatened to kill himself, a possibility that was familiar to him from the newspapers. In the evening he showed me a swelling on one side of his chest which he had got by bumping against a door-handle. To my ironical question as to why he had done it and what he meant by it, the eleven-year-old child answered as though it had suddenly dawned on him: "That was my attempt at suicide that I threatened this morning." I do not think, by the way, that my views on self-injury were accessible to my children at the time.[3]

For the most part, though, Freud left his children alone. It would have been surprising in a nineteenth-century Viennese professional household if he had not, since between seeing patients from eight o'clock in the morning until nine or ten o'clock in the evening, writing, reading, carrying on his correspondence, lecturing, and attending meetings, there was little time left outside the midday and evening meals and a brief afternoon walk to see members of his family. Even on Sunday, when he saw no patients, Freud often wrote or entertained analytic colleagues from abroad. He enjoyed vacations in the mountains with his children, but also took extended vacations abroad by himself. Nonetheless, when Freud did spend time with his children he was a loving father who enjoyed their company.

Theodor Reik had a similar attenuated relationship with his eldest child owing to the pressures and preoccupations of work. His son Arthur says that, "Up to the age of four he used to go out with me and walk with me and ask me questions, and he was amused by my cute sayings. But after that, during my formative years, from the age of four to about sixteen, he really was not interested in me at all. He was busy in his office from morning to night with his analytic patients— and these were not forty-five minute hours as they are today, but hour long hours, he came out and went right back, without a coffee break or anything—and then in the evening he wrote. He didn't have time for me, and I suspect he didn't believe a noisy little boy with his childish concerns really had anything to say that would interest him anyway. Then when I was sixteen I started to smoke, and that brought us together, because he was a chain smoker, and he supplied me with cigarettes. Smoking gave us something to talk about."*

* Theodor Reik also became very emotionally involved with his son around the time of the latter's high-school graduation, for a very curious reason. Owing to guilt feelings over his own

Rather different was Jung's relationship with his children. Jung spent even less time than Freud or Reik with his family; as one biographer commented, "[h]is family, much of the time, was more of an abstract idea than a living reality for him." He worked long hours, and cherished his solitude the rest of the time. He was often caustic and mocking, or flew into rages, and his children felt alternately abandoned and terrified. One of his daughters was afraid to say her bedtime prayers because she feared his ridicule, and another worried that he might not remember her name if he were not reminded of it. Jung justified his neglect of his children on quasi-theoretical grounds, saying that he did not want to smother his children with his powerful personality and hoped to spare them from father complexes.[5]

To the extent that Sigmund Freud had a philosophy toward raising his own children, he was liberal, at least for that time. He believed in letting children develop freely with a minimum of restraint or reprimand, and was particularly concerned that they not be troubled by anxieties about money, which had marked his own childhood. On the other hand he objected to over-tenderness from parents, believing that it might foster homosexual tendencies, or that inadvertent Oedipal seduction might create other neurotic problems.[6]

Freud is the greatest and most startling exception to the statement that analysts do not formally analyze their own children: he actually did analyze his youngest child Anna, who later pioneered in the field of child psychoanalysis and was the only of Freud's children to follow her father into the field he created. The fact of the analysis, which stretched over a period of several years, is now certain, though no details are known: Freud never wrote about it, and Anna Freud was notorious for her reluctance to speak of her own or her father's personal lives. As late as 1977, when she was asked directly, Anna Freud replied:

---

father's death, Theodor Reik was plagued with fears about when he would die. As he went through life he set various limits on himself: he would die when he was the same age as this person or that. At one stage, for obscure reasons, he believed he would die when he was the age of Mussolini's brother. When he lived past forty-eight, he switched to Gustav Mahler, who had died just short of fifty-one. The worst hurdle for Reik was the fact that his own father died just before he passed his final high school examinations. "So this was his great worry: that he would have to die when I finished high school. Unfortunately, due to circumstances beyond anybody's control—we moved back and forth between Vienna and Berlin, and there were different school programs and I fell behind—I failed on my first attempt and had to take the exams again a half a year later. This was a *terrible* time for my father. When I finally finished and he was still alive, out of deep gratitude to me, he gave me a motorcar—in Europe at that time it was simply unheard of to give an eighteen year old boy a car. It was a Ford, a green Ford. I remember it well."[4]

Speculations regarding my own analyst have always abounded and I could give you a whole list of people who have been suggested for that role in the course of time. I have always claimed the privilege of neither denying nor confirming what has been written, and I should like to keep to that line, even if it would be useful for your paper if I said either yes or no.[7]

How extensive the analysis was is a subject of conjecture. There is evidence that Anna was in analysis with her father in 1918, when she was twenty-three, and that in the spring of 1921 she was still, or again, going into his study for analytic sessions.[8] How deeply the analysis probed and what unusual effects it may have wrought will doubtless never be known. It served as a training analysis that permitted Anna Freud to become an important and original lay analyst, though many would aver, in light of her personal idiosyncrasies and her fanatical devotion to her father, that it clearly had not properly dealt, nor could it, with the crucial issues of her relationship with her father. That Freud should have analyzed his own daughter deeply shocked psychoanalysts when the fact became known years after his death. By then there was an implied interdiction against analyzing people with whom one was closely involved, and the prospect of analyzing one's own child would have been unthinkable. Freud, though he had some very real reservations about the practice, never took such a categorical stand. When, in 1935, toward the end of Freud's life, a colleague asked for advice on the issue, Freud replied:

Concerning the analysis of your hopeful son, that is certainly a ticklish business. With a younger, promising brother it might be done more easily. With [my] own daughter I succeeded well. There are special difficulties and doubts with a son.

Not that I really would warn you against a danger; obviously everything depends upon the two people and their relationship to each other. You know the difficulties. It would not surprise me if you were successful in spite of them. It is difficult for an outsider to decide. I would not advise you to do it and have no right to forbid it.[9]

The field of child analysis itself began with the analysis of a child by his parent: its recognized origin was the case of "Little Hans," reported by Freud, but actually carried out by Little Hans's own father under Freud's supervision.[10] Little Hans, who was in fact Herbert Graf, later the stage director of New York's Metropolitan Opera Company and general manager of the Municipal Opera House of

Geneva, was the son of Max Graf, a musicologist and critic who met Freud in 1900 and subsequently became a regular member of the Wednesday evening meetings at Freud's house. When Herbert Graf was five, he developed a fear of horses* and was afraid to go out in the street lest a horse bite him. "[T]his fear seems somehow to be connected with his having been frightened by a large penis," his father wrote to Freud in 1908, when he sought advice on how to deal with his son's disturbing and baffling phobia. Fortunately for analytic interpretation, Professor Graf had kept extensive notes on his son's sexual development and preoccupation with penises, and this material was very useful to Freud, not only in helping the father treat his son but in developing a more general theory of infantile sexuality.

Freud diagnosed Little Hans, "a positive paragon of all the vices," as a neurotic child with anxiety hysteria, and recommended a course of informal therapy to be implemented by Professor Graf himself. The father questioned his son about the issues that troubled him, made interpretations, and gave the boy a dose of honest sex education in order to correct some of the misapprehensions about men, women, childbearing, and excretion that had contributed to his phobia. The analysis succeeded in ridding Herbert of his symptoms, and Freud published his case history the following year. This first child analysis was attacked by many people, who believed that Little Hans would turn out badly "because he had been 'robbed of his innocence' at such a tender age and had been made the victim of a psychoanalysis."[12] This apparently was not the case, as shown by Herbert Graf's successful and seemingly trauma-free adult life. Years after his analysis, at nineteen, Graf went to visit Freud. He remembered nothing of the analysis, nor had his father spoken to him of it, but he had found a copy of Freud's article in his father's office and, recognizing some of the names and places that Freud had not changed in reporting the case, had a glimmering recognition that it concerned himself. Freud was delighted to find his theory and actions vindicated by the healthy youth before him.[13]

Many other early analysts derived analytic material from observations of their own children, as was only to be expected, and some of them did not hesitate to go farther. Karl Abraham, inspired by Freud's paper on Little Hans, used analytic techniques during walks with his daughter to help her cope with certain minor problems, such

---

* It is a rather sick coincidence that for Herbert Graf's third birthday Sigmund Freud had given him a rocking horse.[11]

as a proclivity to daydream and inattentiveness in class.* He also wrote, in disguised form, about some of his observations of her.[14]

One of Helene Deutsch's first papers, published in 1919, was based on observations of her two-year-old son Martin's reaction to the departure of a favorite nursemaid. Under the pseudonymous disguise of "Rudi" she described her son's temporary regression in certain toilet and eating habits, his sudden and uncharacteristic clinging to her and incessant demands for affection—relatively minor disturbances that assumed particular importance only under the scrutiny of psychoanalysis, where they were illustrative of the relationship in the child between eroticism, eating, and excretion. In less than two weeks Deutsch's son recovered from his disappointment about the nurse, with no active analytic intervention needed or imposed. Nonetheless the mother ominously speculated: "The completion of this task represented a major step in his adjustment to his external environment. We do not know how this first great accomplishment will influence the future of his psychic functions, the vicissitudes of his life, and his further strivings.† As analysts, however, we cannot help but engage in some conjectures."[16]

Ernst Simmel analyzed castration anxiety aroused in his young son by a strange early incident. At two-and-a-half, the boy suffered from inflammatory phimosis, a stricture of the foreskin, and was taken to a surgeon for corrective treatment. At the end of the procedure, while complimenting the child on his bravery, the surgeon took a pair of scissors from his drawer and joked—an ironic bit of attempted humor in front of a psychoanalyst—"Next time you come I will cut the whole thing off for you with these," a jest that served to terrify the poor boy utterly. A year later, when the father asked about the occurrence, the boy remembered all of the smallest details, but nothing about the

---

* Interestingly, Abraham was not altogether consistent in his roles of father and analyst. In June 1913 he expounded a very liberal psychoanalytic view of masturbation in an address to the Berlin Medical Society, while in November of that year he more prudishly counseled his daughter against the practice.[15]

† It is rather amusing that Martin Deutsch dates his liberation from the persecution of incessant analysis to another, later, somewhat similar incident. Helene Deutsch was never able to keep household help of any kind for very long. "She would hire a housekeeper, she would think she was wonderful, there would be a few weeks of a sort of honeymoon, and then after a while that housekeeper would become the enemy, it would slowly get worse and worse, then the housekeeper was fired. I found it painful because, for me, the housekeeper was the woman of the house: when I came home from school and I wanted a cookie, that's where I went. My mother was depriving me of a person to whom I had developed an attachment, and it happened repeatedly as I grew up. Then one day at the table, when I was ten or eleven or thereabouts, my mother again said that so and so had to be fired, and I blew up. I said 'Just because you have never resolved your sibling rivalry is no reason why we can't keep a housekeeper.' There was a moment of silence, and I was free. I had learned the game."[17]

frightening incident with the scissors. Pressed more strongly by his father, he remembered the scissors but not the poor joke about them. "Didn't he say in fun he would cut something off you?" "Oh yes, he said he would cut *my hair* off!" Simmel was fascinated by this striking example of child amnesia and symbol formation.[18]

Melanie Klein actively analyzed all three of her children. Her son was the undisguised subject of her first publication and the pseudonymous subject of several subsequent papers. She believed that an analytic approach to child rearing, by which she seems to have meant a lack of strict rules, letting the child develop at its own pace, and candid discussion of all matters, particularly sex, would work miracles for children, and lay "the foundation for a perfect uninhibited development of one's mind in every direction." She was so impressed with her ideas that she abandoned her earliest sporadic efforts at interpretation in favor of systematic daily hour-long analytic sessions with her five-year-old son, something he later looked back upon with displeasure, and which, at the time, far from fulfilling her hopes of making him even healthier, turned him into a troubled and withdrawn little boy.[19]

Another son was subjected to 370 analytic hours, conducted sporadically during school holidays and spread throughout a period of more than three years in his mid-teens. It is bizarre to note that in these sessions with his mother he was apparently obliged to discuss the subjects of masturbation and his early exposure to intercourse between his parents. What the results of these curious analyses may have been, aside from leaving a uniformly distasteful impression on the children, is unclear, as is whether or not Melanie Klein herself had later misgivings about her acts, though her biographer concludes that "all her future work was based not only upon her insights into her children's anxiety but on her realization of the mistakes she had made while analyzing them."[20]

No others among the early analysts are publicly known to have systematically analyzed their own children.* The very idea is now shrouded in an almost inviolable taboo, and analysts today are even more reluctant than they were to use their children so freely and intimately as raw material for discussion in papers. I have encoun-

---

* J. L. Moreno, the founder of psychodrama, conducted much of his personal life in terms of psychodramatic principles, though these are in many ways almost the reciprocal of psychoanalytic techniques. Instead of looking inward and back toward the cause of an action, psychodrama attempts to foster spontaneity and resolve disagreements and misunderstandings through role reversal, in which one acts out the other person's part and tries fully to understand the other's point of view. A curious little book entitled *The First Psychodramatic Family* describes the use of this method within the Moreno family, for example, to resolve dinner table argu-

tered a single psychotherapist who actually treated his own child, and that was a teen-age son in a group therapy setting, where interaction with peers counted for more of the therapy than intimate contact with the moderating father and therapist. Interestingly, this therapist said that when he presented a paper on his experience in the early 1970s, the response from colleagues was far from opprobrious; rather, other therapists were extremely curious and, he believes, even slightly envious.[22]

The analysis in the home that one does find tends to be of a subtler, more insidious, frequently unintentional, and quite often innocuous variety. The therapist parent brings some aspects of his technique to bear on problems and circumstances found in the family. He interprets and understands the hidden import of bits of behavior, statements, or dreams that would suggest nothing to the untrained parent. He teaches, either openly or implicitly, certain methods of understanding oneself and others in terms of underlying causes. In an effort to avoid some of the pitfalls of parenthood, he may attempt to replace certain suspect spontaneous responses of his own—anger at a misdeed, or the impulse to comfort a minor sorrow: things that he has sometimes seen work out disastrously in his clinical experience—with the carefully reasoned response of the trained therapist.

Within limits, there is nothing wrong or even unique about this. Every parent mistrusts his spontaneous responses from time to time, counts to ten before flying into a rage, asks a friend or a neighbor or his mother for advice, reads Dr. Spock, or simply stops to think about things before blundering into them. Every parent, therefore, occasionally substitutes an artificial and theoretical response for his natural impulse. Psychotherapeutic training, then, should be an advantage, since it is clearly preferable to have proper, useful knowledge than to be ignorant or less well informed, and unless one takes the extreme view that therapeutic concepts are wrong, one should assume, a priori, that a therapist parent would be better at dealing with problems. Alexandra Adler, Alfred Adler's daughter and a practicing psychiatrist herself, expressed some befuddlement when I mentioned that many therapists studiously tried to separate their work and home lives, saying she could not see why they should

_____

ments and to help Moreno's twelve-year-old son Jonathan overcome his trepidation about a date. Jonathan Moreno greatly resented the publication of this book, which he saw as an embarrassing invasion of his privacy. Later, as his version of adolescent rebellion, whenever his parents suggested working a problem out through role reversal, he said, "No, I don't want to do it that way, I want to talk about it." He has subsequently come to see the value of a more moderate use of psychodramatic techniques, and even uses them in his own family.[21]

deprive their own children of the benefit of knowledge and understanding that had proved valuable to their patients.[23]

Sometimes, however, the use of therapeutic concepts and techniques may become habitual and excessive, and rather than enhancing one's ability to act as a responsible and loving parent, may come to replace it, and not solely when there are problematic situations, but all the time. Parents can live by the book and neglect those spontaneous emotional responses that, although sometimes damaging, are also the foundation of parent-child relations. Quasi-therapeutic interventions may be intentional or may be reflexive carryovers from a life in the office that has not been fully left behind at the end of the day. Since a therapist's training changes the way he views himself and others, it is not altogether possible to tell where his acquired technique leaves off and his personality begins.

What are the effects and the good and bad consequences of parental therapy of their children? In a paper on the more general topic of doctors' medical treatment of their own children, Edward Levin states that it is a very complicated process that may have serious, long-lasting, and easily overlooked effects.[24] Whether or not the doctor himself can treat his child in identical fashion to the way he treats any other patient is only a small part of the question. The child's perception of the treatment and of the powerful parent's role is the real issue. Under any circumstance, children may be able to comprehend intellectually that painful medical treatments are for their own good, yet be unable to transform this into a meaningful realization, and secretly, more powerfully, perceive such treatment as a threatening assault. When the parents are allied with the doctor, they lose some of their role as protectors and side with the hostile forces.[25] It is alarming to a child when, after he hurts himself, his father or mother rushes him to the hospital and, in horrifying contrast to his or her normal role of knowing protector, stands impotently aside and defers to some stranger. When the parent *is* the doctor administering an unpleasant treatment, the confusion and distress are immeasurably greater.

Obviously there are common-sense limits to the caveat against treating one's children. A doctor faced with a first-aid emergency should feel glad that he knows what to do. The problem arises not from the knowledge itself, but when the roles of professional and parent are confused. Too often the physician parent *cannot* treat his child the same as any other patient, however much he may insist that he does: the situation provides an excuse and a justification for the emergence of other psychological ambitions that have nothing to do with the professional aim to cure.

When a parent-doctor goes beyond what any sensitive, educated lay parent is able or expected to do for his own children, one should presume that the doctor is acting out some remnant of his childhood "doctor game" fantasies. The use of procedures, techniques, instruments, or medications that require professional training for their proper application should be understood as an indication of such professional overinvolvement, which is unconsciously intended to allay the doctor's anxiety. This special treatment arrangement serves to transmit the parent's fantasy to the child. The doctor reassures himself of his power and knowledge as he cares for his child, who is now the sick victim of the parent's childhood "doctor game" fantasy.[26]

Ernst Simmel remarked in a 1926 paper that doctors often fall prey to the ailments of their specialty. Levin expands this to the next generation, commenting, based upon his own therapeutic practice, that "[a]t one time or another, every doctor in my experience entered into treatment realtionships with his children and every doctor's child developed symptoms and complaints that were dynamically related to their parent's professional interests. The ubiquity of these phenomena supported the hypothesis that they are psychologically significant, not fortuitous." Thus a pathologist's daughter became preoccupied with death, a pediatrician's son clung to infancy, a dentist's son was bashed in the teeth by a baseball bat, and "[a] therapist's son's speech hesitancy was relieved with the recovery of the childhood fantasy that his father could read his thoughts, making his own words superfluous. The boy was not paranoid; he was responding to incidental interpretations of his behavior that his father had made through the years."[27]

The therapist's situation is more complicated than that of the physician whose expertise is only occasionally and incidentally applied to the task of child rearing. All parents, whatever their profession, are constantly called upon to cope with their children's problems, questions, and developmental issues. The therapist's professional training therefore falls right in the midst of what it means to be a parent. A surgeon can send his child to a colleague for a tonsillectomy, but the therapist who wished to avoid dealing with emotional problems would have to send his child away from home permanently.

Moreover, the psychotherapist's learning may not be a useful addition to the knowledge and wisdom he has as a parent. Simply knowing things does not mean dealing with them well: knowledge can be used improperly, either purposely or inadvertently, or one can know things yet be quite unable to use that knowledge in a constructive way. Second, knowledge and techniques that are useful to a psychotherapist treating adults for one hour a week in an office may not be appropriate for the parent with a five, ten, or fifteen-year-old child who lives in the same house all day long. The objectivity of therapeutic tools, and the separation between parental and professional function, are infinitely more ambiguous than they are for a medical doctor—ambiguous for both the parent and the child.

One reason for inflicting therapeutic techniques and insights on one's child can be the simple and understandable one that the therapist is heavily invested in his work, and derives a large measure of his self-esteem from his success or failure in what he does. Raising a good and healthy child becomes an allied challenge, since the therapist feels he is also judged according to how well he constructs his own family life—how free of provincial bias he is, how delightful his marriage is, and how clever and mature his children are. There can be an insidious trap of feeling or wanting to feel that the child's healthy or unhealthy outcome is entirely one's own doing, and a temptation to strive for perfection, and an overestimation of one's own importance.

These issues came up in a startling way during an interview with a husband and wife, both psychiatrists. Owing to their schedules, I spoke with them separately: first the wife, later the husband. The wife told me:

> I find my therapeutic knowledge invaluable for myself as a preventative thing, for catching something right as it's developing, dealing with it right then and there before it becomes a problem or a symptom. In a little while my son will be home and you will meet him. We're prejudiced, but we think he's a fabulous kid, and really just about everyone who meets him, teachers, people, neighbors, friends, agree that he's a fabulous kid. He really is. And I think at least some of that is because he is the child of two bright, sensitive psychiatrists who have tried to use their therapeutic skills in understanding him and helping him along the developmental path.
>
> We are always watching the consequences of our interactions with our son. It's a very heavy responsibility, not that parenting isn't a heavy responsibility anyway, but *especially* knowing all

that we know and seeing all the catastrophes of bad parents in our offices all day long, and knowing the profound effects something that may seem very minor can have lifelong. There is something—I forget what—that some patient just told me, something he remembered from when he was very small, it must have been a very minor incident to his parents, but it had been with him for twenty years and he hadn't been able to get over it. And you just never know what's going to make that kind of impact. But *we* know, my husband and I, because that's our profession. It's a little scary to think about what our son is going to carry with him into his adult life, what he's going to be telling *his* analyst about us.

I asked for examples of instances when psychiatric knowledge might be a unique help or hindrance in raising their child. After saying that psychiatric knowledge was a double-edged sword, carrying the danger of overinterpretation or of believing one sees pathology where none in fact exists, she cited an instance where their training had been a marvelous help in dealing with problems. Their son had developed a phobia about riding on the school bus some months earlier. They had analyzed it and traced it back to a time when the family was on vacation and he was briefly lost. He had gotten lost in a very noisy place, not unlike a school bus, had been far from home and away from his parents, as he was in school, and they concluded that unconsciously he was afraid the school bus would get lost, take him away from them, and not bring him back.

We could really *see* the sequential development. We could plot it out and try to interpret it back to him. Well, he thought we were all wet with this; he didn't like our interpretation. But nevertheless we felt pretty sure we were on target, and we thought that most parents wouldn't have seen how all of these particular things were connected. We had the focus to see it, because we were both psychiatrists *and* his parents, and we had been there when the first trauma happened, when he got lost, and could see the resurgence of the phobic symptoms at particular times that recreated the original trauma. We could try to help him deal with his anxiety about it, whereas, I don't know, maybe another parent would have been exasperated with it, or overly sympathetic. They wouldn't have seen it as a symptom and understood its origins as we did. It was kind of neat that we felt really well equipped to handle it, just as we would help a patient try to deal with a symptom and see the onset and finally make an interpretation. The difficulty in this case is settling down, so I think that on some level he heard what we were saying even though he couldn't give us credit for it.

Soon afterward, this woman left the room and her husband came in to be interviewed. Also asked about the advantages and drawbacks of psychiatric knowledge in child rearing, he invoked precisely the same story, but for the opposite reason. He laughed at himself as he told how earnestly they had tried to persuade their son that his fear of the school bus stemmed from his earlier trauma on their vacation.

But then we found out that the school bus was incredibly noisy, that the older kids squeezed and crushed the younger kids, and that *none* of them liked it. The driver had already taken measures to have the little kids put on a separate bus that wasn't so crowded. So there was a certain amount of reality to his fear. We were trying interpretation on him, and he kept saying, "No, that's not it. That's *not* it." And he was right. It wasn't.

A disconcerting phenomenon is the fact that many therapists can be good with children in theory but not in reality. Psychiatrist Lawrence Hartmann, son of Heinz Hartmann, comments:

. . . having had a very famous analyst father and a well known child analyst mother, I don't think they were particularly smart, subtle, or sensitive, nor were some of my parents' colleagues. I knew the whole bunch of distinguished New York analysts of the 40s and 50s in their capacity as parents, because I knew their children, and I don't think, on the whole, that they were terribly attuned or interested or lively in focusing their greatest skills on their own children all the time. Ernst Kris was famous for his lovely descriptions of kids at the Yale Child Study Center. With his own children—first of all he didn't spend very much time with them, which was a widespread side of it: analysts of that generation simply didn't. But he also was not, to my mind, terribly penetrating, intrusive, or even *perceptive* about his own kids, although he learned to be about clinical kids. I think that's probably not such a rare finding. His wife, who was also a very well known child analyst, and my mother, who had been a pediatrician before becoming a child analyst, were pretty good intuitively at being close to children and friendly with children, but Ernst Kris and my father were not. My father was an ordinary, dignified, vaguely Edwardian upper class intellectual, who liked children theoretically but only got interested in them when they were teenagers and began being able to have more theoretical thoughts. Our parents were good at making theories about children. They were, in Kris's case, very good at demonstrating some things in children clinically, but that was a very separate category.[28]

Psychoanalyst Herbert Strean made an interesting observation based upon many summers of experience working in a camp for disturbed children. It had struck him how few psychiatrists, psychologists, and social workers were willing or, if they did come, able to function in the camp environment. They were fine at doing therapy with the children in the office, doing finger painting, talking, making interpretations, administering tests, all in neatly metered forty-five-minute doses where they were completely in control of themselves and the therapy. Yet these people, most of whom he says would be considered very fine child therapists, fell apart at camp, where there was no structured setting and things could not be made to progress in a way that could be easily reconciled with a theory.

"I used to encourage them to go out and get involved in a ball game, go on an overnight hike or whatever. If a kid wants to talk to you about his problems at camp, he's not going to make an appointment to see you in your office, he's going to see you as part of the setting, he's going to talk to you between innings, or while you're towelling off after your swim, or while you're walking through the woods. If you're going to relate to children easily, you must in some way enjoy the child in yourself, and these were people who were so self-conscious that they simply could not be spontaneous. I wondered to myself what happened to these people when they went on a hike with their own kids."[29]

The fact is, unfortunately, that many of them are precisely the same way with their children, though often it is less immediately apparent than when put on the spot by Herbert Strean at camp. They are people who, in all aspects of their lives, have found it easier to deal with people and situations that have been dehumanized and transformed into reductionistic theoretical entities. These therapists are people who tend to use, and to overuse, therapeutic principles and techniques, not from any malevolent wish, but to help themselves through an awkward and painful situation, to substitute for the vacancy that would otherwise be there: they simply do not, on the basis of their personal experience alone, know how to behave comfortably with other people. These are the people who fled into therapy to help with their own discomfort, who discovered there a refuge, a compensation, and a life, and who found it easier to immerse themselves in the gratifications of their work than to make the more difficult attempt to relate symmetrically with other people.

It is far simpler to tolerate discomfort in oneself if pain registers as a word on a display somewhere, to be taken into account and entered into the formulation, rather than as a sensation that burns inside. In the office, the objective theoretical manipulations of the scientist can perform very useful healing functions, whether the healer is healthy or not, but once past hurts have been undone it takes more to go further and create positive health. One PsyK remarked that his father had the best intentions in the world, and a psychological intuition that often let him zoom to the heart of his children's problems, but that once he had made an oracular pronouncement about what the true etiology of the problem was, he hadn't a clue what to do next. The natural sequel was for the loving parent to step in, but he didn't, because there was nobody there.

Quite a few therapists substitute intellectualization for true feeling, and view understanding a situation rather than some more immediate participation in it as the goal to be pursued. The son of one unusually reserved classical analyst told me he had envied his school friends who were spanked for their wrongdoings, because he had always gotten instead a long, exasperating talk. A suitable time after the misdeed, his father would enter his room and ask in a dispassionate, clinical way, "Tell me about it. What made you do this? Why did you do it?" When curious friends asked how his father punished him, he said, "We get hit with a Freudian whip." The most comical manifestation of this, which has now been enshrined in family lore, was the day when he made a mess on the tiled kitchen floor.

My mother had just come in from shopping, and I had taken a dozen eggs out of the bag and cracked one egg very neatly in the middle of each square tile on the kitchen floor. She hit the ceiling over that, and I was punished right away. But then later when my father came home she told him, and he came to talk to me about it. "Oh, no," I said to myself, "Not this again."

"*Why?*" he asked me.

He wasn't mad about what I had done, he didn't say "You damn fool kid, why'd you do such an idiotic thing?" He wanted to know *why* I did it, what *made* me do it, and above all why had I done it so *neatly*—one egg right in the center of each square? I don't think he really saw it as something wrong at all, the way my mother had, but just as an interesting bit of behavior whose motivation he wanted to figure out. I don't know what his conclusions were. I don't know what my explanation was. How *can* a little kid explain something like that, or at least in any way that's really going to satisfy a psychoanalyst?

It is distressing to realize that I have read articles on child rearing and proper parental attitudes by a number of psychoanalysts and psychiatrists whose children I have interviewed, and whose wise, compassionate, affectionate, theoretical pronouncements had no counterpart at all in their real family life. One woman who wrote very perceptively about ways in which parents should recognize and handle competitive and incestuous needs in their children was, in real life, emotionally remote from her children, highly competitive with them, and extremely intolerant of behavior on their part that did not fit quietly into the world scheme she had constructed for herself. Though she might have been a good therapist for her child patients, at least some of those children had substantial, emotional parents and robust down-to-earth lives to go home to once the session was over. Her own children did not.

Another woman, the stepdaughter of a prominent woman analyst, now herself a clinical psychologist, commented on the discrepancies in her stepmother's ability to help her or be close to her in various situations.

She wasn't wonderful at understanding what was wrong. Some things she was good at and some things she wasn't, and I'm not sure where the dividing line was. I got screwed up at college and came home, and she was just fabulous in going to bat for me, in not being judgmental, in seeing me through and helping me work it out. My father was furious, but she was just *there*. My sister had polio as a very young child, shortly after my parents got married, and she was *really* there then. So I know that she would have done anything, it's just that she was not good at it. She was not good at letting you know that *unless* you had a circumstance that demanded it. She couldn't possibly say "I love you" in any normal situation. She didn't know what the hell to talk to me about. I would sometimes go out in the living room where she had to pass in order to go to the bathroom in between her patients, sort of hang out hoping she would say 'Hi' or chat or something. But she didn't know what to say. She had no small-talk repertoire. She didn't know how to say, "Well, what did you do today?" or "What did you and Lynn talk about last night?" No graces about mother-daughter talks. If I had questions about sex or about a boy, I never brought them to her, and

I don't think she would have known how to talk to me on that sort of human level if I had. And yet, it's true that when I was *really* upset, or when I went through a stormy period with my father, she did know how to deal with it. Maybe in the larger situations she could be warm; I guess when I was in enough pain, or maybe where it was a pain that didn't involve her.

I remember once asking her something—I was upset about something concerning my mother's death, and I was trying to talk to her about it, and she said, "Well I don't know, I haven't had any patients like that." I've always remembered that as meaning that when she couldn't fall back on her own professional knowledge, she didn't have anything to offer. You can make what you want of that. I find it fascinating. She couldn't simply be a mother. Maybe I wasn't asking in a way that allowed that, but I think she could have done something, she could have provided some comfort or understanding.

It is striking that not only was the analyst-stepmother at sea when it came to crises outside her clinical experience, and not only was she inept at the warm, spontaneous aspect of motherhood, but even when her daughter described her as at her best, what she showed was "being there," "not being judgmental," seeing her through and helping work it out—all the neutral and facilitative qualities associated with a psychotherapist, not the passionate, loving help of a mother.

One might speculate about psychotherapists who have spent years of training and clinical experience willfully and abnormally working to transform themselves into an impartial participant and a transference object. They are taught that so much of what is directed at them in the consulting room, whether loving or hateful, really has nothing to do with them at all. They also learn that so much of what their spontaneous impulse would urge them to respond, whether throwing their arms around a crying patient or yelling back at an abusive one, would undermine the progress of therapy. Through an arduous process of professionalization, they acquire a knack for uncoupling themselves from the habit of taking things personally. This is called constructing a "therapeutic ego," and within limits it is essential, but when the therapist's ego was shaky to begin with, the therapeutic ego may move in and take up residence.

Many parents ponder the effects that they have on their children, and plan what they do in advance. Psychological notions have filtered down sufficiently that almost anyone will, for example, recognize that children sometimes act out in order to get attention, and that on occasion one should suppress one's natural impulse to go in and yell, because that's just what the kid wants, and doing so will only encourage such behavior in the future. It is mere common sense that a parent does not always act upon his or her first impulse. What is interesting, however, is the number of PsyKs who described a process in which their parents consciously disconnected themselves from situations and tried to manipulate those around them toward some supposed desirable end by positioning themselves, not as an active participant in the family dynamic, but as a passive force to be responded to.

Psychoanalyst Ralph Greenson relates the grotesque case of a young analyst in supervision whose zealous adhesion to analytic constructs completely blinded him to the realities before him. Faced with a weeping female patient who was upset over her son's serious illness, he remained steadfastly aloof. When the patient fell silent, the analyst interpreted it as guilt over her repressed death wish for her son. When the woman was subsequently silent and resentful, the analyst was indifferent to her emotional plight and never imagined that she might be justifiably disturbed by his hardhearted lack of concern. He had never even asked whether her child was better. Greenson remarks:

> I shook my head in disbelief. I asked the student whether he himself had no concern or curiosity about the baby's welfare. I added that perhaps the young woman's silent tears indicated the baby's condition had worsened. Or perhaps it indicated that she felt the analyst's behavior as a cold and hostile emotional uninvolvement with her. The student retorted that I might be right, but he felt I was overly emotional. I ended the session by telling the young man I felt his emotional unresponsiveness would prevent the formation of a working alliance. Unless he could feel some compassion for his patient and indicate this to her, within limits, he would not be able to analyze her.[30]

The patient subsequently announced that she was quitting treatment because she felt the analyst was sicker than she was.

A failure to respond to one's own child's needs is infinitely more damaging than the harm that a therapist can do to a patient. A child does not have the option of quitting, nor even the ability to perceive that he should, since this is the first and most important relationship he knows. Unlike the patient, who at best can perceive that a therapist is wrong, and at worst has some already formed notion of reality, the child who is raised amidst bizarre, distant, sometimes inappropriate responses has a very hard time establishing a workable sense of reality. Mercifully, few parents would take such an extreme attitude with their children as Greenson's analyst-in-training adopted with his patient, but the consequences still can be upsetting.

A successful real-estate developer and psychoanalyst's son told me:

If an issue came up, my father would try to be very rational about things and to view them within a psychoanalytic mode. He would try to posture himself as a father the same way analysts posture themselves as therapists. That was disastrous. I can't think of any really striking examples: they were all little things, but a lot of them, countless ones, all the time. When I was going through a rebellious phase in high school I didn't want to write any papers. My father said, "I don't care if you don't want to write any papers." He was afraid if he said that he cared, I'd rebel against his caring and abuse the care and refuse to write the paper. So he figured, "Well, if I just don't tell him that I care, he won't choose to act out on this issue, and he'll write the papers and he'll be fine." But he didn't see that there was an alternate interpretation, which was that I'd think: what the fuck's going on? Why doesn't my father care if I'm failing in high school?

If you spend fourteen hours a day, as Dad often did, positioning yourself so that people will react to you in a contrived fashion to help them grow, it's pretty hard to get out of that mode for the last two hours of the day when you're seeing your family. I don't think that he did. Another example of his posturing was when at the end of my first year in college I was pretty unhappy, moping around the campus, and I called Dad, pretty upset about things, and he said "We'll work it out." A week later I hadn't worked it out, and I decided to go home. We talked about it. I was pretty depressed, first romance broken up sort of disastrously, and various other problems. He said, "You know, I thought about coming up, but then I decided that your effort in working it out would be the best thing for you." Another case of the intellectual model riding herd over a basic emotional instinct, which I think he had, and which was the *right* instinct: to get his ass up there. That's what he should have done, and he would have if he had realized it, because he had a good heart, but he didn't do it, because that's not what a psychoanalyst would do.

If you're a father, unlike when you're a therapist, you have an unlimited impact, and you can't possibly fathom all the impacts you have. To return to the example of the paper in school, he didn't see that my reaction would be, rather, "He doesn't care about me. Boy, is my life *really* fucked up." In an analytic context you can figure those things out, you can figure out how the patient is perceiving you, you can calculate what to do in order to engender a given response. You cannot do that in your role as a father.

When there is active quasi-analytic intervention by the parent the child may have a very hard time trying to extricate himself. Not only is the parent an exceptionally powerful figure by sole virtue of being the child's parent, but his opinions are all the more penetrating when supported by a theoretical basis. A lay analyst I interviewed mentioned the case of a young man he was currently treating who was the son of a prominent psychologist. Part of the difficulty involved the father's intense fear of closeness and warmth, which had caused the son to feel depressed and angry:

> Now lots of fathers are afraid of warmth and affection, but I think there is a big difference between the psychologically unsophisticated man whose son wants a hug and who says, "Ah, don't be a fairy," or something to that effect, and this man, the psychologist, who won't hug his son and backs this up with profound interpretations about how it would have all sorts of effects on his virility, et cetera. Both men are frightened, in some way, of the possibility of homosexual contact, but the psychologist uses words to hide behind, and this, I think, can be more upsetting to the child, because the father sounds like such a brilliant authority. He *knows* the real truth, in the child's mind. He can prove it. It is not just some opinion he holds. The words and interpretations are being used to protect the parent, but the child doesn't see it as a protection, but almost as a law: I'd better stay away from my father.

This feeling of utter helplessness to resist or refute the parent's analysis was mentioned quite often in interviews. A PsyK woman in her forties expressed it most clearly:

> My [psychoanalyst] mother certainly *did* explain us to ourselves, and I remember feeling that I had no equipment to combat it. I already found her a rather austere, distant, somewhat cold person, and moreover she was using terms I wasn't master of, and which I assumed she knew, and therefore she had to be

right. I can remember her saying something like "I don't think your father likes women very much." Now, in the first place I have come to think that that's bullshit, but at the time, since she was saying it not as a person, but in her persona of analyst, and was saying it in a clinical sense, it was clear to me that it *must* be true. I remember her talking about my best friend and saying, à propos of something or other, "Well, she's going to have problems when she gets older." I gasped. Well, I guess she *was*. And certainly, when it came to me, I had the sense that she was privy to inside information that was not available to me. Even if I came up with an explanation of something in my own lay terms, she would come back with a clinical or quasi-clinical insight about it, and that would put the matter to rest. I didn't feel that the fact it was *me* talking about me gave me any authority. She knew better, because she was the psychoanalyst. I was very scared by the idea that she could know me better than I could know myself, and that this knowledge was not going to be used kindly, it was somehow going to hurt me. I carry this with me to this day: I am determined that nobody had better know me better than myself.

This woman, not surprisingly, has become a psychotherapist.

Another woman, the daughter of a psychiatrist and now a writer in her early fifties, says that she and her sister have spent much of their lives sorting themselves out from the influence of their late father. He was quite obviously a deeply troubled man, further embittered by a serious chronic physical ailment, who had spent much of his life suppressing his own emotions and trying to compensate for his feelings of misery and inadequacy by means of the intellect, through manipulation and authority. She believes, in a sense, that he was trying to help them in the sad sort of way that he had helped himself, but it was so inhuman and inappropriate that it came across as horrifying persecution.

We heard a lot of doctrine about how everything, in the end, was self-serving and self-centered, as a result of the id, I guess, and how in the end even the good samaritan was just getting his particular sort of kicks. It used to make me very angry, this kind of reduction of everything, although I had to agree at some point that it really was a kind of self-centered, solipsistic world and there's no way out of it. He talked about sublimation as a technique for living, there was a lot of discussion of people's hidden motivations, and great emphasis on being a clever detective—

his being a clever detective and knowing what so-and-so really meant or really wanted to do. An awful lot of analyzing my mother and her relatives, and looking down on them for their behavior. He told us that our mother was paranoid and that we should not take such-and-such thing she had said at face value, because what she really meant was something else. It kept me away from my mother for a long time; it was a miracle that I finally found my way back to her. And there was an awful lot of sneering at his patients. One of his favorite stories was about how when he got bored listening to people in his office he would fiddle with the curtain pull. He used to enjoy telling us about how various patients would misinterpret his doing that as his wanting to strangle them or wanting to caress them or whatever, whereas he, smart he, was just doing it because they were so damn boring.

He used to interpret everything we did. Everything had to have a reason behind it, and he was very insistent about nagging and trying to find out what it was. "Why did you leave your bicycle out on the lawn? What were you trying to prove? What were you trying to say about me or about Mother?" Well, sometimes I had just forgotten the damn bicycle. I used to feel sometimes that I was being pushed into making a statement about my behavior which wasn't true: if I was ingenious enough I would find an answer that would be psychologically satisfactory to him. It made me angry that I was subjected to this persistent questioning, and that I *always* had to have a reason. I wanted unreason, at the same time as I understood the power of reasoning. He got to the point that when I was in college I fell in love with a Jewish artist—we're not Jewish—and he sent me to a psychoanalyst to see if I was all right. He had nothing against Jewish artists, but he wanted to be sure that I wasn't just rebelling, in which case it wouldn't have been an acceptable decision. I don't remember exactly what the verdict was, I only saw the analyst once, but I think he told my father "Don't be an idiot! She doesn't need to come here for anything."

My father was not a person for small talk, and he was never spontaneously warm or friendly or admiring towards us. He was not interested in our lives except in terms of emotional understanding of feelings about things, or analyzing our feelings and explaining them away: "Don't feel shy, shyness is really self-consciousness." He wanted to know how we were doing in school, but more in terms of the dynamics of how we felt about

school and our teachers. Why we were angry. He examined us
constantly. I'm not very good at remembering the substance of
these talks, but they were analytical in the sense that they were
investigations of what was below the surface in terms of human
motivation. I was made to feel I should never take anything for
granted, should never believe in accidents: things were always
motivated, and you could figure out the cause if you only looked
at all the signs. The conversation was always of that—you see, he
really had few other outlets in life. He used to come up at night
and sit on the edge of the bed and talk with us, or have us into
his office, where he saw the occasional odd patient who came to
the house, and he would ask all these questions.

There was a big leather chair in the office and he would sit in
that chair and call us, "Come in and talk." We would go in and
he would be sitting in his analytic chair, and he would ask us
questions about how life was treating us. A lot of it had to do
with sex, which in itself may be interesting. He used to insist
that I could tell him *anything*. I should never be ashamed to tell
him anything that I did. That went on for quite a while, and I
used to think that maybe he meant masturbation. I never would
tell him, though. Around seventh or eighth grade my sister just
refused to cooperate anymore. She was establishing her independence and she wouldn't go in and talk. And then it devolved
upon *me* to tell her: he would tell me what he thought of her,
and I was supposed to talk to her and explain these things about
herself. It seems incredible to me now that I went along with it
for so long, but I wanted to make myself feel important and
loved by him, and I also *believed* what he was saying and
thought that she ought to listen to him. I really thought that he
could know everything, that if he had the right information he
could explain almost anything.

I suppose that he would have said he was trying to help us in
a psychiatric way by making us aware of who we were and of
what we might be, the terrors we might be encountering and
the guilt we might be raising up in ourselves. He told us often
that it was all right to hate your parents, they're the perfect people for it, of course you should hate them, and you shouldn't feel
guilty about it. And he wanted us to understand the way people
treated us in the world. When in grade school I became the butt
of the schoolground, and the kids used to make rings around me
and yell that I was fat and had glasses, my father instructed me
that the way to combat this was to laugh with them at myself. I

learned to do that. It worked, but it had the effect of making me the class clown, and then it took me quite a while to stop being the class clown and become serious. I complained to him another time that I didn't know how to look people in the eye, and that one had to be able to do that in order to show one was honest and sincere. He said, "You don't have to look at their eyes, just look at their mouths. They won't know the difference." He had an answer, a method, for everything.

Years later—one time when I spent a terrible night trying to keep an ex-student of his from committing suicide—I learned that he had talked to his students about us the same way he talked to us about everyone else. He delighted in telling our dreams and problems to the psychiatry students, and how he had come up with the right interpretation and we had instantaneously been relieved.

For myself, it took me a long time to get out of this frame of mind where everything was self-gratification and self-centeredness. Years later, when I first read Jung's *Memories, Dreams, and Reflections,* it was such a *pleasure* for me, having been brought up in this strictly Freudian world of reductionism. This seems very stupid, but I remember all of a sudden I said, "Goodness, there's more to sex than just sex!" I began to feel that it was legitimate to feel *upward* from an instinct as well as downward. There was a whole other realm out there that I had never discovered in my father's rendition of Freud.

Where the joy was in his life, I don't know. He *used* psychiatry as a weapon, as a defense, as a means of having power over people, and in the end it didn't get him very much. He used to say "Why, if you're an obstetrician, people bring you wonderful presents at Christmas, or if you heal someone they bring you all these presents, but *I* never got anything." In the last year of his life he was terribly lonely and terribly self-pitying, and when we went to visit him that's what he would beat us over the head with. He would analyze himself and present himself to you for your contemplation, what an unworthy, mean, and miserable person he was.

I've been wanting to ask you, in your interviews with the children of psychiatrists, have you found any happy experiences?

7

The Genuine Meaning of Things

I have *never* used analytic concepts in thinking about myself. Or, of course, maybe I did and I've just repressed all memory of it.

—A PSYCHOANALYST'S SON

The most conspicuous component of psychological analysis is the process of interpretation. What is specifically interesting about interpretation is that it provides a means not simply of understanding, but of redefining objects, thoughts, and feelings in mysterious, sometimes capricious ways. Things really may seem to mean whatever the therapist, like Humpty Dumpty, chooses them to mean. Interpretation can be silly, malicious, or profound, but it tends to be rampant in therapists' families.

The most obvious and often ludicrous example is the symbolic translation of objects according to the rules of Freudian dream interpretation. Martin Deutsch remembers his annoyance when he was around six years old and painted a picture of a soldier. The soldier, naturally enough at the time, was wearing a sword at his side, and his mother, analyst Helene Deutsch, promptly insisted that it was a penis. No, he said, it was a sword. "She insisted that it was a penis—this sort of thing happened all the time—and after a while I gave up. Obviously I was supposed to absorb this analytic concept, that when something hangs somewhere, one is supposed to say that it's a penis. Now I know that in some sense this is true, but why do you have to tell a kid that? What did it really have to do with me and my drawing?"[1]

The penis interpretation arises with laughable frequency. Another man remembers that after his father pointed out the phallic symbolism of an automobile stick shift, it made him think, every time he got into his Volkswagen, "I'm not going to shift. I'll have to sell this car and get an automatic." Another man took a different tactic than Martin Deutsch's resigned acceptance and, having been taught that anything higher than it was wide or longer than it was thick would represent a penis to his unconscious mind, for a time consciously trained himself to negate the thought of "penis" when confronted with a phallic object by reminding himself of the association before it could wreak its unconscious effect. He did not know what this unconscious effect would be, but he was determined to declare his independence from its insidious control through this curious and, one would imagine, rather distracting technique. What, if any, influence this superficial symbol interpretation has on the children it is difficult to say. It does seem odd, however, that children should be saddled at an early age with the weird dictum that there are underlying forbidden associations attached to all sorts of mundane objects, an idea justified by a theory that is widely accepted but which they cannot possibly comprehend.

Some therapists with whom I have discussed this phenomenon have wondered whether the unpleasant effects of relentless interpretation will not diminish as psychotherapy becomes more eclectic and the most rigid classical Freudians die off. The nature of the interpretations will certainly change—it already varies with the theoretical orientation of the individual therapist—but the ultimate effect is the consequence of the therapist himself rather than of the theory. Not all orthodox Freudians view everything in Freudian terms; conversely, even the most eclectic psychotherapist, if predisposed to flee from life into abstract theoretical considerations, will bring some unusual perspective to bear on all of his personal relationships.

More perfidious than symbol interpretation, which can often be little more than an extended parlor game, is the careless slinging of oversimplified reductionistic interpretations such as those used by the father of the woman in the last chapter. They teach a child an outlook on life that is terribly bleak and depressing. If all altruism is selfishness, if the woman who is afraid her child will suffocate in its crib secretly wants her child to die, if the father who worries about his daughter's sexuality is just somehow concealing his own incestuous lust, what faith can the child have in the simple facts of the real world, and how can he avoid the plague of creeping cynicism? Such statements, valid though they may be within the context of psychotherapy, require tremendous explanation before they make sense—and then their sense rests in a limited domain. Presented as revealed fact by a parent whose job it is to know such things, they are irresponsible and preposterous statements and, at face value, outside the consultation room, in the course of daily life, they are lies. The altruist *is* good; the mother *is* worried about her child, and it *is* a father's place in life to fret over his daughters.*

The specific effect of interpretations depends upon their nature, their accuracy, and the parent's intent. Minor incorrect interpretations may simply linger and confuse issues, as well as being an intrusive nuisance. More harmful are interpretations that are incorrect because, rather than portraying an accurate perception of the child's unconscious mind, they represent the parent's own unconscious difficulties—problems in self-image or in the parent's image of the child, which are then reified through interpretation and made credible through analysis's stamp of authenticity.

Therapists may use analysis to interpret reality falsely so that it better fits what they prefer to believe. A comical example of this is cited, again, by Martin Deutsch. At one stage in childhood he wanted to tell fibs, but he found that it was impossible because no matter what falsehood he told, it was not accepted as such. "My mother's thinking was that if you were in a state of grace, that is to say non-neurotic, you never had any need to lie. If a child did tell a lie, it would show that he was not in a non-neurotic state of grace, which would mean he had not been properly brought up according to proper psychoanalytic methods. Therefore *my* fibs were explained away. I was told, 'Oh, you misremembered.' 'Oh,' she would say, 'Isn't it interesting? He misinterpreted that.' And I was trying to tell a lie!"[3]

Many therapists go much further, and abuse their knowledge and position of authority to get their own way and control those around them. Any parent can abuse authority, of course, but the therapist is in an unusual position not only to enforce his rules and will, but to throw into question the child's motives, responses, and ability to

---

* If it were not true, it would be a bad joke that psychoanalysis did not formally recognize the "real relationship" until twenty years ago. Up to that time, everything that happened in the consulting room was viewed as part of the transference-countertransference relationship, and therefore was not to be taken at face value but as a distorted reflection of events that had taken place elsewhere. Then, at last, it was realized that some facets of the analytic relationship had mundane significance in the here-and-now: fees, scheduling, emergencies of various kinds and, on a more complex level, the fact that the patient's perceptions of the analyst were sometimes *accurate perceptions of the analyst* and not lingering remnants of someone elsewhere that had come to rest on the guy in the chair.[2]

defend himself.* An interpretation may be correct or incorrect, it may even sound downright silly, as analytic interpretations so often do to the uninitiated, but nonetheless it is presented as fact, and cannot be lightly dismissed. Saying to a child "You're projecting," as so many therapists have, is not merely a denial that the parent is doing whatever he has been accused of, but is a retaliatory accusation that the child is sick, the child is distorting, the child is either willfully or helplessly falsifying data.

Some ridiculous statements can be disbelieved: "At one point when I was nine months pregnant," one famous analyst's daughter said, "my father told me, 'You're pregnant because you want to be noticed.' Well, that's just plain crackers." In the best cases the child even knows precisely what is going on. One analyst laughingly mentioned the time he got his comeuppance from his fourteen-year-old son. "One day we were playing Ping-Pong, and he beat the shit out of me, and he was contemptuous and was making all kinds of remarks. But I knew that a fourteen-year-old has to struggle and rebel and that he was trying to take me on. He saw that I wasn't losing my cool, so he said, 'Let's play basketball.' So I huffed and I puffed, and he kept on telling me I was an old man and a jerk and a this and a that, and I finally got really annoyed and slammed the ball down. He looked at me and said, 'Just because I have an Oedipus complex there's no reason for you to act immaturely.' I'm sure that he was mirroring something about the way that I handled things, and it was enlightening."

With less dubious statements, however, and with younger or less self-assured children, even false interpretations cannot be dismissed completely. Interpretations have a different quality from other statements. There is a compulsion to hold onto such explanations, which makes it more difficult for the child to arrive at a real understanding of an incident or relationship. Saying that a child is "accident prone" or showing "sibling rivalry" are more potent statements than that he is clumsy or being nasty to his sister, since these masquerade as medical diagnoses, and the child can no more contradict such ostensible facts than he could contradict a medical doctor who says he has a strep throat.

* One analyst I interviewed mentioned a psychoanalyst, the head of the neuropsychiatry department at a major university, who parried all criticism from residents by means of interpretation, particularly Oedipal. The students, who were in the midst of that dreadful period of self-scrutiny and self-doubt that every psychiatry resident passes through, found it unusually difficult to hold their own. Finally they formed a sensitivity group and, working together, decided that he really was a bastard. Partly because of his amoral manipulations, he was eventually forced to resign from his post.

Interpreting the child to himself can be very confusing. Those therapist parents who believe they are bestowing the great benefits of their learned profession on their children by unlocking the hidden secrets of their behavior ignore the distinction between interpretation given in response to a patient's need and specific request, and that inflicted gratuitously upon a credulous and dependent child. In the first instance, it is a valuable therapeutic tool, while in the second, it may amount to a commandeering of the child's sense of self that is ultimately much more damaging than snooping through his diary and drawers, since it gives him the sense that there is nowhere to hide, not even in his head.

Correct interpretations can be far more frightening than incorrect ones, since they lead to an augmented impression of omniscience and omnipotence in the parent and a corresponding feeling of greater vulnerability in the child. All children's parents seem like godlike figures at the start. To psychotherapists suffering from a God complex it is inordinately important to cultivate and maintain this image, but even those who are not so inclined find the boundless adoration of their children a wonderful thing that it is difficult but necessary to surrender. It may be much harder for the child, however, to demote the parent to a mere mortal role when the parent's presumed omniscience is repeatedly confirmed by interpretations that are either correct or else so complex that they cannot be confidently disproved.[4] As a result, it is more difficult for the child to perceive the parent's limits and weaknesses and his own corresponding strengths.*

When the child is interpreted and understood, that bit of his self that needs to be kept secret if he is to construct a separate identity is invaded, and the child can feel helpless and at the mercy of the parents. Ultimately, the child may flee into a passion for secrecy, as Kohut has described, to protect the remaining nugget of inviolate self, or may rebel particularly forcefully against his parents during adolescence out of a greater than ordinary need to break away and establish his own free domain. It is inexcusable for a psychotherapist not to recognize these forces. It is unfortunately not a rarity for them to disregard them nonethless.

Sometimes, of course, the children succeed in penetrating the ulterior motives of the parents' analytic defense. One woman, a

---

* Sandor Ferenczi wrote a short article commenting upon the extraordinarily high number of male neurotics who had fathers in an "imposing" profession. It was harder for them than for most men to detach the Father-ideal from the real person of the father, which is a necessary step in the route toward independent adulthood. He also noted a monstrously exaggerated castration fear and consequent diminished potency in the children of men who worked with sharp objects: tailors, barbers, soldiers, butchers, and possibly doctors.[5]

lawyer in her forties and the daughter of a psychoanalyst, told of her emerging liberation from subjection to analytic interpretation, which she thought her father clearly used to protect himself and control others, since he was unable to set up a satisfying relationship on any other basis:

My father was terrible at dealing with problems. He would get angry at you and scream and yell, and then after he calmed down he would explain to you in psychological terms why he was right and why he had done what he did. When I was young it was very threatening, because, you know, you start doubting yourself. I would really believe him, and it would get me all the more upset, because I *thought* I knew that he was absolutely wrong, but then he would convince me that he was right. When I got a little older I realized it was simply that he was wrong after all, and that, moreover, he couldn't accept the fact that he was wrong.

The best instance of this was when I was in high school and I wrote a play. There was a class play that they did every year, and I wrote a basic plot outline, which was one of several that were submitted to a class committee. My father always insisted on knowing everything that was going on in my life, but I didn't tell him about this until very late, when my play wasn't the one that was accepted. And he just had a fit. A lot of it was that he wrote amateur plays himself, for the analytic society or something, and he would have insisted on helping me with it. So when I told him about the play he started screaming and yelling and ranting, basically saying that I had no right to write this play without telling him about it. He told me that it was a very *disturbing* play. It had a really disturbing message, but he wouldn't tell me what this message was. I wouldn't let him go on that one, and I kept after him until he finally told me what this tremendously emotionally disturbing message was. The message was: I want to be a boy. So what? That was a subject my girlfriends in high school discussed freely. I don't know whether he was just making that up when he needed some excuse for being so upset, or whether he actually believed it. If he really believed it, then that was really stupid.

There was another incident similar to that, but earlier, when I felt really horrible and stayed home from school one day. I rarely stayed home, but on this day my bones ached and I just felt lousy, and my mother decided I didn't have to go. Well, my father was furious. He accused me of playing hooky, and he criticized my mother for letting me stay home, and he ranted and raved. I was really sick, so this incensed me. I was so angry that I felt like throwing a shoe through the window. But of course with the sort of rational upbringing I had had, I had been thoroughly trained not to act so impulsively. So I waited, and I cooled off, and I thought it all over, and I decided that, all things considered, it was definitely a very appropriate response to the situation to throw a shoe through the window, which I did.

Of course he exploded. He screamed and yelled and blew the whole thing way out of proportion. And then, when he calmed down, instead of just saying, "I was really ticked off with you because you threw a shoe through the window," and leaving it at that, he had to explain *why* he had gotten angry, which was because of some deep significance about the way I was acting out in this manner. The whole premise of his argument was wrong, though, because he thought I had thrown the shoe through the window for a very different reason and in a very different manner than I had actually done. What's more, he claimed that his blowing up like that was therapeutic—not for him, but for me. It was just his duty to get angry in order to—I don't remember what his exact argument was, but it was something to the effect that he was carrying out some calculated therapeutic function by blowing his top. Rubbish. It was just anger.

Other PsyKs have a much harder time seeing through and jettisoning the parent's false view, because it has spilled over and been incorporated into so many aspects of family life. Two men I interviewed described strikingly similar situations in which their perception of themselves was permanently affected by their therapist parent's interpretation. One is a tree surgeon in his early forties. In first grade, this man had suffered from Legg-Perthes disease, a debilitating and painful hip joint deformity. He was on crutches for a year and for a long time afterward his coordination was poor and he often tripped over things. His father, a psychiatrist who frequently dealt with psychosomatic illness, maintained that the boy's persistent clumsiness was psychosomatic, though there appears to have been no clinical justification for his belief. Even if the boy's poor coordination had been psychosomatic, there was scarcely a therapeutic value in the father simply telling him so. "Now I have since then begun to believe that, having been crippled for a year, being on crutches and having my leg in a sling, it was understandable that I would occasionally trip over things and fall. But I missed out on that simple understanding at the time, and instead somehow got a psychological understanding that it was because of something I was or was not doing, that it was self-caused. There are five kids in my family, and my self-image was of the crippled, pitiful one of the family, and even more, the one who had wanted to bring this wretchedness on himself. It gave me a lifelong feeling that there was something wrong with me and that I had to come to the source of it. I have always had a kind of therapist's investigator overviewing my life as I went along, trying to figure everything out—a characteristic in my personality that I try to ignore more and more as time goes on." This man's choice of tree surgery as a profession was part of a quite conscious attempt to avoid intellectual and introspective pursuits. He wanted a very physical sort of work where problems and their solutions would be objective and clear.

A more puzzling and tragic case is that of a man, now a clinical psychologist, the son of a psychologist father and a clinical social worker mother. His father was a very unhappy person who committed suicide about four years before I interviewed the son, and whose identity was almost wholly wrapped up in his professional status: he had returned to school for a doctorate relatively late in life for the sole purpose of earning the title "doctor," which he insisted people call him. The father's behavior toward his family vacillated between the emotionally volatile and the coldly analytic and, as his son says, "he was too insecure to be a good parent, because he was afraid of the world and of letting people, including his children, see him as he really was." It was a relief to the son that his father worked so much that he did not have to see him more often.

This man's father interpreted a great deal, but the most significant event of his early years, the sequelae of which haunted him until very recently, was the fact that he was hospitalized for an extended period for a ruptured appendix at the age of three, and when he left the hospital he stopped eating normally. Foods tasted bad and smelled bad, and there were few things he would eat.

My father, and I suspect my mother, too, given her psychological training, assumed that this was a result of the hospitalization. Particularly since my younger brother had been born just four months before that, they figured there was all this accumulated trauma and I was doing it more or less to torture them, and that it was sheer perversity on my part. It wasn't until thirty years later that I came across an article in *The New Yorker* about a doctor in Washington who was doing research on taste disorders having to do with the salivary zinc level. A very abstruse sort of thing that nobody else in the country had recognized might be a medical problem, but the symptoms fit my case so perfectly that about six people I knew immediately called and told me about the article. I contacted this doctor and flew to Washington and had a battery of tests, and he found that even after all these years, at a time when my sense of taste had more or less returned to normal, my zinc level remained low enough for him to say that I fit this physiological pattern.

But for my whole life, until a year or two before I saw this doctor, my taste disorder was a major factor in my life. I would only eat a certain very limited number of comparatively bland things that weren't offensive to me. I couldn't go to somebody's house for a meal. I couldn't ask a girl out to dinner. If I needed to travel I had to worry whether I was going to find anything to eat at the other end. Obviously I found it very difficult to deal with, but my father made it even harder. He took it very personally. We fought about it at almost every meal when I was a youngster, because he saw it as a willful refusal to eat. I think at heart he was very embarrassed by me, because I was not normal, and I was so *obviously* not normal that I was a public reflection on his shortcomings as a psychologist and father. It's true that back in 1948 there was no counterbalancing evidence to suggest that this peculiar condition might be physiological, but his overexuberance about seeing everything as psychological made it impossible for him to consider any other kind of explanation even for a second. And, in fact, when I *told* him, in 1978, after coming back from Washington with pretty solid scientific proof that it was something real I had suffered from, he was singularly unimpressed. After thirty years I felt vindicated, but it just didn't have any impact on him at all. But meanwhile he had always made me feel as though I was crazy. I must be crazy. Who but a crazy person would eat like this, and persist in eating like this no matter what his parents did? He sent me to a therapist when I was six-and-a-half; again when I was nine, for four years; at fourteen, I was sent to a hypnotist. Nothing worked. I will be forty this month, and for most of my life I have felt like I was crazy.

One is entitled to ask why the fathers had made the interpretations they had, whether it was something they chose to believe for reasons based wholly on the relationship between themselves and their sons, or whether they would have reached the same conclusion had the person in question been a patient instead of a member of the family. It is impossible to say, but even had an objective therapist arrived at the same opinion, the effect would have been less intense and had a less durable influence on these children's self-image. However bizarre the latter man's taste problems may have been, and whether or not they were explicable physiologically or psychologically, there came a point when they had to be accepted as a fact and relegated, along with all the other facts of life, to the role of something that must be lived with. One would expect a good parent or therapist to help the child bear an obviously dreadful burden, rather than to superimpose the additional burden of insisting that the child was also fully, perversely, sickly responsible for inflicting such suffering on himself and everyone else. Clearly, it is easier for a therapist to do this than it is for the father, who is obliged to live with the situation and is not limited to weekly sessions. This is much of what makes the parental role infinitely more demanding, as well as potentially more gratifying, than that of the psychotherapist.

The professional and parental roles of the psychotherapist, similar though they may be in some respects, are in many ways diametrically opposed. In most types of therapy, therapists are to remain detached from their patients. There are distinct advantages to the therapists' studiously acquired ability to feel only impersonal concern for their patients. On the other hand, parents who regard their children with only impersonal interest are, by today's standards, bad parents. Patients purchase a service from a professional: the therapist is not their friend, and the ultimate aim is for patients to leave therapy and not need the therapist anymore. In psychoanalytically oriented psychotherapies, great emphasis is placed on the anonymity of the therapist, who serves as a blank screen for the patients' transference. In child rearing, on the other hand, one cannot remain disinterested, unemotional, and blank.

Patients in therapy are encouraged to relax their inhibitions in an effort to find the causes of particular bits of behavior, whereas, in a sense, parents must teach children the various types of inhibitions that transform them into respectable social creatures: giving them free license to express their drives openly would do them a great disservice.[6] Much of the therapist's value comes from being nonjudgmental, whereas parents must be judgmental, albeit in wisely administered doses, since only by doing so can they impart to the child a sense of values and a notion of acceptable social behavior.

Psychoanalyst Jules Glenn, who has criticized aspects of Freud's handling of the Little Hans case, mentions, among other objections, the fact that the interpretation and understanding of the child's drives may be experienced as a license to express those drives openly and may prevent the child from forming those defenses and inhibitions which, for better or for worse, endow one with a conscience that fits the rules of our society.[7] Freud himself recognized this drawback when he considered the possibility, much bandied about in the late 1920s, that through the wonders of psychoanalysis one could raise children who were free from suffocating and perverting parental repressions. Without first changing society itself, he said, this simply was not very practical:

> The child must learn to control his instincts. It is impossible to give him liberty to carry out all his impulses without restriction. To do so would be a very instructive experiment for child-psychologists; but life would be impossible for the parents and the children themselves would suffer grave damage, which would show itself partly at once and partly in later years. Accordingly, education must inhibit, forbid and suppress, and this it has abundantly seen to in all periods of history. But we have learnt from analysis that precisely this suppression of instincts involves the risk of neurotic illness. . . . Thus education has to find its way between the Scylla of non-interference and the Charybdis of frustration. Unless this problem is entirely insoluble, an optimum must be discovered which will enable education to achieve the most and damage the least. It will therefore be a matter of deciding how much to forbid, at what times and by what means.[8]

The rough-and-tumble humanity, even the pigheadedness, ignorance, repressiveness, and unfairness that down-to-earth parents sometimes display may be responsible for occasional problems in their children, but there is no escaping the fact that these very same real human features and foibles are also what give the child substance to begin with. One cannot use therapeutic corrective tools on a character that is not yet sufficiently formed, nor attempt to foresee and preemptively counter problems that have not yet occurred.

In *The Uses of Enchantment*, Bruno Bettelheim discusses the significant psychological function of fairy tales for children, and at the same time cautions parents against making these "real" interpretations of the stories known. The stories serve a purpose. If children grow attached to particular ones, then those stories may be helping them to work through some problem or conflict. Much of childhood is work of a sort, and the fact that it appears like play to us grownups who spend our days in more structured and tedious forms of labor does not diminish the serious and often painful nature of what children do. Children receive and assimilate feelings and facts, and at times it is more bearable to do so through the medium of a fantasy slightly removed from their lives.

Parents who offer a psychoanalytic explanation of a fairy tale strip it of much of its artistry and appeal. If a child's imaginary roles, beliefs, and games are a sublimated expression of something hostile or sexual, and the parent interprets them accordingly, the parent has not only ruined the fun and destroyed a harmless outlet for the impulses, but has turned what might otherwise have been a means of successfully resolving the issues into yet something else of which the child must feel ashamed:

> Explaining to a child why a fairy tale is so captivating to him destroys, moreover, the story's enchantment, which depends to a considerable degree on the child's not quite knowing why he is delighted by it. And with the forfeiture of this power to enchant goes also a loss of the story's potential for helping the child struggle on his own, and master all by himself the problem which has made the story meaningful to him in the first place. Adult interpretations, as correct as they may be, rob the child of the opportunity to feel that he, on his own, through repeated hearing and ruminating about the story, has coped successfully with a difficult situation. We grow, we find meaning in life, and security in ourselves by having understood and solved personal problems on our own, not by having them explained to us by others.[9]

What is true in fairy tales is true in childhood and adolescence generally. There are things that need to be worked out in one way or another in the child's own terms. Eventually, the healthy child will grow to perceive issues from an adult's point of view, but he should do so only as he begins to become an adult and is ready for that mature perspective. Forcing an adult interpretation on a child, in conflict with the child's own understanding, is to ram together two frames of reference that exist in different terminologies, almost different dimensions. It is pretty obvious whose is most likely to win out, but at what expense?

The therapist who is so taken with his ability to interpret and comprehend the concealed issues of childhood development that he cannot resist the temptation to use and to broadcast his knowledge, ignores the fact that sometimes it is better for the child not to know. The unconscious mind, after all, with its defense mechanisms of repression, sublimation, and the rest, did not come into being for the sole purpose of baffling and challenging psychoanalysts. Defense mechanisms are obstacles to be deciphered and overcome only when treating the pathological mind: in the normal person they are healthy functions that help in coping with life's inevitable problems. Just as one can defeat the purpose and value of a fairy tale, one can undermine the function of perfectly harmless play or fantasies by offering it to a child in the sordid form of repressed aggression or libidinal urges. The child has a right to be misunderstood. There is a place for therapeutic comprehension in therapy, but in the real world of people there is a genuine need to be a person and to respond with mere lay, which is to say human, understanding, and to accept one's role in playing out trite human dramas without trying to understand them. As PsyK and psychiatrist David Reiser says:

> The biggest hazard that an analyst has to avoid is his own narcissism and his own temptation not to react to the child as a real object, with warts, failings, and all. There are internal stages in the development of a child, among them the arousal of Oedipal and sexual impulses when a kid is three or four, and a need to begin to feel let down by the parent in late latency and early puberty. When a child reaches a certain age, he begins to de-idealize the parent, and begins to be disappointed and realize that his dad isn't the biggest, strongest, smartest person in the world. I think that a good case can be made that the best response a parent can have is to react with feelings and emotions, with disappointment that the child no longer idealizes him the way he did, with a certain defensiveness yet with a certain resignation. In other words, to react as flesh and blood.
>
> The developmental stages are in-built and unfold on their own, but their outcome—whether the stage is experienced as primarily traumatic and self-esteem defeating and neurotic, or whether it is experienced as growth promoting, consolidating and healthy—depends a great deal on the honest, undefensive, unguarded response of the environment to the child's behavior. I think that a "good-enough parent," to pirate Winnicott's phrase, whose kid is Oedipal, really can take pleasure in the child's vitality and robustness. He can probably discern at one level when the kid is banging into his groin and saying "Daddy I want you

to go away so I can have Mommy!" that there's hostility, but he also reacts to the kid with some sense of pride: "My son's growing up," or "He's a chip off the old block." Similar reactions can occur when a child begins to rebel in adolescence. I think a good-enough parent can be hurt and insulted and threatened by the child's increasing differentiation from him and his values, yet at the same time take a certain pride and pleasure in him: "Well, the kid has a mind of his own," "By God, no one's going to push my kid around; he's his own person." Along with the painful side of reaction to this child's unfolding stages, there can be pride, pleasure, and adaptation. All that is based on the assumption that there's some validity to what the kid is going through, and that the parent reacts with feelings, and that those feelings are known and authentically made available to the child, and are worked out.

The analyst who sees all these things and too quickly interprets them to somehow avoid the pain of his own involvement, and says "Well, you're just putting me down because you're at the age where you have to do that to be accepted by your peers" and so on, really robs the kid of a tremendous number of opportunities for self-definition and self-esteem. It would be as if you went to build up your biceps by using a Nautilus device, and when you went to push on the weights there was no resistance.[10]

Unfortunately, as we have seen, those who go into psychotherapy are often not the people best equipped to deal openly and honestly with their children and to roll aimiably with the punches. The ability to circumvent emotions and to harness and control situations intellectually is the crutch that has helped them get through life. Quite possibly, they themselves experienced difficulties with the developmental issues their children are going through. Perhaps they did not resolve them in a robust and satisfying way; and now to let themselves be apparently bested, for instance, in a transparently Oedipal contest may be beyond their emotional ability. They do not want the child to recognize that, after all, they are only human, because in their narcissistic belief this is not true, and they need the continuing adulation of the child to reinforce their belief in this cherished fallacy. Thus they may subtly, unconsciously on purpose, sabotage the child's efforts to grow. Reiser continues:

When their kids start pushing the right buttons and seeing that maybe the emperor doesn't have *no* clothes, but at least there are a few patches and holes here and there, the reaction is often defensive. This is aggravated by the fact that classical analytic theory teaches the analyst to blame everything on the patient, which makes for a convenient way of handling dysphoria in relating to the child. It's not that the interpretations the analyst makes aren't sometimes correct. If the analyst father says to the adolescent son, "You're putting me down and everything I stand for because you're feeling threatened and competitive and like you can never measure up to me in head-on competition," that's probably true. But such a reaction deprives the child of a chance to work it through. Not only is he stuck with his unconscious feelings, which have now been exposed, but he's also defeated once again—in this case defeated by the interpretation. I think analysts can protect themselves against being an object that's made of flesh and blood that when pushed by the child pushes back and gets things worked out in some kind of dialectic.

All of us, whether we're psychiatrists raising children or just parents in general, struggle with the question of whether we're doing a good enough job. I think it is important that the child know we are struggling, that it is an active issue that concerns us. When the parent is selfish and brings about a kind of closure at the child's expense in *either* of two directions, there is trouble. The borderline or abusive anti-psychological parent may say "This is all a lot of crap: my father used a strap on me and, by god, I'll use a strap on my kid." That kind of attitude can obviously be grossly non-empathic and distressful for the child. The other extreme might be the analyst parent or intellectual parent who has a book learned answer and an interpretation for everything, and conveys it with a certain smug sense of certainty that he has the answer: "Yes, dear, you're going through your Oedipal phase," or "Yes, dear, we know you're angry at daddy because he made you go to the potty." These two types of parents seem in some senses to be two opposite ends of the pole, but what the rigid fundamentalist spare-the-rod-and-spoil-the-child parent has in common with the rigid doctrinaire Freudian analyst parent is that both of them have an excessive sense of closure and smugness and lack of anxiety about the very fluid and often ambiguous and wrenching process of having to take stands with their children and *not* knowing whether they're right or wrong.[11]

Compliant PsyKs may accept the therapist parent's explanation of things and thus collaborate in the subversion of their own development, adopting the parent's terminology and perspectives and eventually incorporating his remote intellectual values at the expense of their own spontaneous feelings. These are the seemingly very mature children who get along well with their parents, since secretly they have supplied just what the parent wants. They are also, as a consequence, the PsyKs most likely to end up impaired in precisely the same way as their parent, and perhaps resort to the same means of handling their discomfort.

"It prematurely closed exploration for me," says one psychoanalyst and son of an analyst, a man in his fifties who has given much thought to the matter, "My father always had an explanation. He always knew the answer to everything. His explanations *may* have been true, may *not* have been true, but there was very little room to find out. In one sense it was very nice to have a father who always knew what the answer was, but I think that it prolonged my adolescence interminably."

This analyst himself was later alarmed when one of his own patients admiringly told him how comforting it was that he always knew everything, always had an answer for every one of her problems. He realized that he had inadvertently succumbed to the same temptation as his father, and that he was preempting his patients' enlightening and growth-giving explorations, just as his father had kept him from growing on his own by prematurely feeding him an answer that he could understand, accept, and repeat, but which ultimately had little meaning for him since he had not arrived at it himself.

From the child's point of view, one of the most insidious immediate effects of a parent's incessant interpretation is the invalidation of the child's feelings. This form of interpreting occurs with great frequency, and though it usually seems of little significance at the time, the cumulative effects can be quite distressing. The habit of interpretation and some skill at doing it enhance the parents' ability to reconstruct events to suit their own convenience and self-image.

A woman whose parents were both psychiatrists says:

My parents invalidated all of my memories. They still do that. They have a completely different childhood for me than I had. They have also reconstructed a completely different past for themselves. My father says now that he did this thing—I don't know if this is a defense or if it's true—but he says that he used to pretend that he was really opposed to things that I said that I wanted to do in order to test my commitment to them. Once I had a résumé lying on the table, and he saw it, and he said "This is so wonderful, you've done so many different things." And I said, "You were opposed to every one of those things." He said, "I was *never* opposed to them. I was only testing you. No, these are wonderful things." I really don't know if that's true, but I find it very hard to believe.

My mother, meanwhile, now seems to want complete valida-tion. She was really selfless when I was growing up, but it turns out it wasn't genuine selflessness, it was a kind of an ego prob-lem that she had. But now, through the wonders of analysis, she's really into being assertive. She wants me to keep telling her how great she is. She keeps asking me what I think of her, and I mostly think really good things about her, because she's a real wonderful person, but she wasn't always, and a lot of my memories of her aren't that wonderful. I began to tell her some of these memories a few weeks ago when I was visiting them at the holidays, because she kept after me to tell her, and she told me I was making it all up. She started bringing up all the nice things she had done, which are true also, but those are not what I . . . you know, things that all go well you don't have to dwell on, you dwell on the things that are not right.

One very simple form of interpreting and invalidating the child's emotional issues, no longer the sole prerogative of psychotherapists, consists of relegating everything to a phase.* This relieves the parent of any serious concern, since whatever it is, it is normal and transi-tory, and if one simply waits it will go away. It also promptly cuts off the child's act, which is drained of all significance and transformed from something meaningful into something inevitable and even rather cute that happens to everyone.

One young woman, who contacted me because her mother was a psychologist, she herself was going into psychology, and she was very worried that when she had her own children she might harm them as she felt her mother had harmed her, complained that her mother's favorite phrase, used in response to virtually everything, was "You're just going through a stage." "I wasn't a rebellious kid at all, in fact I

---

* Often the worst offenders are not psychotherapists but patients just beginning their therapy and still in the first flush of evangelical zeal over the miracles of interpretation. They tend to bore everyone silly, particularly their families, with enthusiastic amateur analyses untempered by firm knowledge or experience. Fortunately, this infatuation with therapeutic concepts usually dwindles with time.

was a goody two shoes, but if I ever did anything that in the least bit seemed like standing up for my own rights, she immediately belittled it by analytically picking it apart and passing the judgment that 'Well, it's because you're thirteen,' or because I was this or I was that. If I said something directly aimed at her, she would just turn it into something else and invalidate the statement. She still does this with my youngest brother, who is now twenty and a real problem. It's a bit harder with him—what's she going to say? 'Oh, this is the let's-get-arrested-five-times stage'? You'd suppose that sooner or later she'd have to admit that something was really going on."

Another woman, the daughter of a child psychiatrist, said:

My mother looked at everything and put it in patterns. At that time I think I was the only kid on the block who grew up in a house where people talked about "You're acting hostile towards me." I *hate* the word "hostile." I get *irate* at the word "hostile." "Why are you being so hostile?" my mother would ask, "Why is there so much hostility in your relationship with your father?" Whereas when I went to my friend Pat's house, her mother would say "Why are you being such a bitch?" There were no bitches at my house, just hostile people. What's more, bitches get sent to their rooms. I would go to my room of my own accord to escape from the conversation, but then my mother would follow me in to talk about my hostility. I just wanted her *out;* I didn't want to talk about it. I remember her saying "You have all this pent-up hostility. You have to deal with that. That is your biggest problem." I said to her, "If *that's* my biggest problem, then I'm in good shape."

My parents never said no to anything, but it really bugged me that anything I wanted to do, they would then sanitize and say "Oh, that's normal for someone your age." Once in seventh grade I was wracked with guilt, I couldn't eat, and I just lay in my bed and cried and cried. My mother finally came in and said "Whatever it is, you can tell me. I hear it all day." I had smoked a cigarette, and I was wracked with guilt. My mother laughed herself sick. She thought it was funny. So there was never anything I could do that would be so terrible, because it was normal, she had seen it in a patient. If I wanted to drink I could drink, though it was clear that they thought it was stupid. Stupid, not wrong, or at worst just something I was going through.

Invalidation of what the child is really feeling is a frustrating and infuriating experience. It is impossible to rebel, impossible to misbehave, impossible to try to get attention without the parent dismissing it as exactly that. When children act out, they are asking for something, and however circuitous and psychologically dishonest a means of communication acting out may be, these requests deserve some answer. Yet, therapist parents will often penetrate the subterfuge and then leave it at that, feeling that somehow the situation is solved. One man remembers the time when he was around eight that he was very upset about being punished for something. He deliberately broke one of his prized possessions, planning to tell his parents that they had done it by accident when they pushed him into his room, in hope of getting some much-needed sympathy. His therapist mother not only ridiculed the idea that anyone other than he had done it, but quite accurately explained to him his secret plan. Decades later he is still saddened by this memory. He had made an extraordinary sacrifice, admittedly a dishonest one, but in an utterly desperate cause, and he was not only denied the desired result but humiliated and made to believe that this heart-wrenching sacrifice was *nothing more* than a nasty trick he had tried to pull on his parents.

One young woman who remains extremely bitter over experiences with both her father and her psychotherapist is particularly upset about their invalidation of her feelings at times when she especially needed validation and recognition at face value. It is not clear to what extent her father's interpretations were accurate and how much they expressed something in himself that he had projected onto his daughter, nor is it really important, because the ultimate effect remained a usurping of her legitimate experience of her emotions and her perceptions of what took place in the course of her life, and of her resulting ability to work things out in whatever terms made sense to her.

My biggest gripe about psychiatry is that it disbelieves people. That was the essential crippling thing about my psychiatrist and my father, too: that there was not an a priori assumption of credibility. I'm not saying that you should blindly believe everything, but sometimes you should at least not *dis*believe unless you have a good reason to. But what's true in a court of law doesn't seem to be true in the world of psychiatry. My father called it "objectivity," which is one of his great linguistic tricks—he would always say that things were objective when they really were not. One manifestation of this, quote, objectivity, was his systematic refusal to believe people, who experience themselves subjectively and therefore don't know what they're talking about.

It was devastating to me that he denied my problems, or at least denied their extremity and thus the legitimacy of my extreme suffering. I was having a hellish time, but our family situation was perfectly normal, he said. "All families have problems." "Everybody" feels anger at their parents, and those who don't are suppressing it. My mother and I were fighting during my high-school years not because I had a legitimate gripe, but because "breaking away from your family is hard to do." Another good one was "adolescence is hell on everyone," and all teenagers are unhappy—my being anorexic was, I suppose, no worse than not making the cheerleading team. My favorite one was "nobody's perfect," speaking of my mother, and "she's doing her best." Fine. But this was the most painful of all, it was a total deflection of my feelings; it knifed me every time I heard it, because it implied I was wrong to be hurt and wrong to be unsatisfied and there was no validity to my complaints.

I was really delighted by the Jeffrey Masson book that said maybe these girls weren't making up the sexual molestation as some manifestation of their unconscious whatever, but that it was really true after all.[12] I *loved* that. Psychoanalysis seems to have this belief that you shouldn't believe anyone. *I* thought I was treated just as badly as I *said* I was treated, but my father, and later my psychiatrist, said "Why are you unconsciously provoking it? Are you unconsciously hostile? Do you need to like people who treat you like that?" Whatever it was, it was never "Gee, that must be really difficult," or "The world must be treating you badly." The helpful attitude to take with me would have been, "Well, you're really letting yourself be fucked over." That was it. If you want to point to me, don't ask how I'm provoking it, which doesn't get me anywhere, but how am I letting it happen, which gives me something to do. Say "Let's forget about your unconscious. We'll deal with that later, if you like. Let's start to be constructive and learn how to negotiate with people." Why not say that? Why disbelieve what I'm saying? Why not say "Well, it sounds true, it sounds believable." Why automatically believe that she's lying—just because everybody seems against her? Maybe they are.

This particular woman, fortunately, has seen through much of the interpretation and rationalization to which her father subjected her. Unfortunately, however, she continues to devote a great deal of her energy and considerable intelligence to replaying and refuting these unpleasant experiences. The lack of emotional validation remains; she is chronically uncertain about how she really feels, how others perceive her, and about what she wants to do and what is appropriate for her to do.

Quite a few PsyKs have pointed out the accusatory nature of the analytic inquiry implied in the preceding example. The first thing a therapist does is to ask what is going on within the patient, to try to figure out the patient's perception of something, the patient's feelings about it, the reason behind the patient's response. The job of a therapist does not require him to go out and verify the facts, though the job of a parent often does. The therapist is more concerned with psychic reality, whereas the parent is dealing with a child who is still in the process of determining what reality is and is not, what is fair in life, and what to expect from others. Asking a child always to look within himself appears very much like fault-finding—and in many cases it may genuinely be, when a parent is so concerned about his self-image that he wants the children to avoid at all costs anything that might damage it. Even when it is not, it is an unfair burden to imply that in virtually every circumstance this poor misused child must examine his own role in the affair.

"One day I was coming home on the bus," says one analyst's son, "and I bumped into a drunk, who yelled at me. I guess I was a bit upset about having a bum yell at me on the bus, and I mentioned the incident at dinner. My father's response—I guess I had said it was an accident—was to say: 'In psychoanalysis there are no accidents.' Which, of course, is true. It is true that, as long as you stay *on the couch,* there are no accidents. If you start driving cars, walking around, taking buses, trolleys, subways, and such, it is real hard to maintain quite the same control. The world just doesn't cooperate with the theory. I didn't find his response amusing in the least."

A psychiatrist's daughter says:

In my family I was never allowed to hate anybody. If I came home from school and said "I hate so and so," I'd always have to understand why this person did what he did. The bully was always the bully because he was really insecure. Everyone was allowed to do anything if they were only insecure. You had to be understanding when someone was mean or nasty to you or rejected you, because they were insecure, though of course you couldn't ever expect them to be understanding of *you,* also because they were insecure. If the boy you liked dumped you to go out with the prom queen, it was because he had to prove his virility by going out with someone society had accepted as the ideal, not "Well, he's just a shallow, vain asshole. He just wants to go out with pretty women."

A related issue to that of interpretation is the question of intrusiveness. When people think about psychotherapists intruding on their children's lives they imagine active attempts at analysis and interpretation and a meddlesome prying into the children's affairs. Though from the examples just cited it might seem that therapists do indeed leap at every opportunity to dissect their children's secret thoughts, this is generally not the case, at least not in such an overt manner, which would be obvious and relatively easy to resist. Most therapists could scarcely be described as intrusive in this blatant sense at all, since they are busy professionals whose schedules often keep them from spending very much time with their children. One woman began to call her analyst mother "intrusive" and then stopped herself, slightly puzzled and amused. "The reason I stopped is because it's funny to use a word like 'intrusive' when basically my sense of her is that she was not there. She was physically absent much of the time, and was not much there emotionally when she was physically present, and she was basically uncurious about me as a little girl, so you could hardly call her 'intrusive.' And yet she was. Intensely so."

The issue of intrusiveness arose very frequently in interviews, but it was rarely ever seen as pure nosiness. It assumed a more pervasive and intangible form, and one against which it is harder to defend oneself. On one level, psychotherapists may be seen by PsyKs as intruding on their lives simply because the therapists know and have seen so much and feel free to discuss it. One woman in her twenties, a journalist in New York, grew very annoyed even talking about her child psychiatrist mother's incursions into the domain of young people.

I get really angry when my mother talks about "the world of people my age" as if she knows what it is because she's heard about it from a few of her patients. Now she's into watching MTV so she will know what her patients are talking about. She went to see Bruce Springsteen because one of her patients gave her a ticket and said, "If you want to understand today's teenagers you'd better go see Bruce." It's sort of cute, but it makes me angry, because she doesn't have a *right* to be there. She doesn't have a right to talk about things that I like as if she knows anything about it. There's a part of a kid's life that their parents shouldn't know about. There's nothing I need to hide from her, but some things are simply mine. Music is very important to me, and she doesn't have a right to intrude. It's like the mother in *The Graduate*—why doesn't she pick on someone her own age?"

Psychotherapists can also be much more actively intrusive, though still without consciously meaning to intrude. Therapists spend their entire workdays speaking intimately and casually with relative strangers. In the consulting room, life's normal social boundaries evaporate and the patient may freely discuss even the secret personal habits and feelings that tacit agreement keeps him from mentioning to his spouse or most intimate friends. Reluctance and embarrassment give way to self-confession that is condoned and rewarded by the therapist. The therapist considers himself entitled to know these things, and he would be prevented from doing the best job he can if the patient resisted and refused to disclose them. The therapist may also come to enjoy them, since these secret facts give the texture and excitement of reality to the life stories he hears, and he is gratified by the patient's delight at finally being able to discuss them.

One young woman told me:

For a time my mother worked as a school psychologist at a girls' public school, and when I was in about tenth grade, when we were at the height of our period of mother-daughter conflict, she was after me all the time to open up. At school she had a loyal following among the girls, because here was a woman who would finally talk to them about sex and about femininity and about all of the things that were forbidden topics at school and at home. All of these other girls my age found her very approachable, so why, she said, wouldn't I open up to her? It was a constant tug of war between us. But I didn't want to talk to her, for god's sake, particularly since whenever this issue of talking came up she became very self-conscious, there was a particular sort of shift in the expression on her face, in the tone of her voice, the kind of concentratedness she brought to bear, that felt like a consciously analyzing posture.

Elements of the therapist's professional manner inevitably linger after the day is done. The boundaries may gradually erode between what is fair game for discussion and what ought not to be said.* The

---

* Conversely, I have been surprised and sometimes appalled at how willing psychotherapists often are to discuss their own personal lives and those of their families in embarrassingly open detail. Even when I was doing research for a book on the history and theory of the insanity defense, and my interviews had nothing whatsoever to do with the personalities and family lives of psychotherapists, psychiatrists sometimes treated me to the most extraordinary accounts of

community standards of the therapist's house, as it were, are shifted a few notches away from those that prevail everywhere else. Without intending to pry, and often despite an acknowledgment of and respect for people's right to their privacy, therapists have a certain expectation about what they should be entitled to know that creates a vacuum into which confidences are drawn. Since nothing is shameful, according to the therapeutic party line, there is no reason why the child should not feel free to discuss all aspects of his life. This passive intrusiveness is an even more pernicious invasion because, like a spy, it enters disguised as something else, and the child has a harder time in resisting.

A real-estate developer and son of a psychiatrist says:

My father was highly intrusive. No question. He was fascinated by our development, and he loved us, so he wanted to know what was going on. And because his way of looking at what was going on was more intimate than the way that most people look at what's going on, because he is used to looking at the intimacies of people's lives, he wanted to be pretty intimate. It was us, the children, who had to set the limits. "No, Dad, I'm not going to tell you what happened. The foreplay that went on is *my* life, not yours." That would happen. He wanted to know what was going on in our lives, and though, to be sure, he would always have a clever and benign way of phrasing it, he was very happy to know, at whatever level of detail any of us wanted to tell, what was going on in our lives. I don't think it was an accident that at least once or twice he walked in on things that he shouldn't have seen. He walked in on me a few times when I was masturbating. He walked in on my older brother once when he was with his girlfriend. There was a place for discretion, and he just didn't have it. All this contributed to my decision to leave home a little earlier, before high school was over. I was smart, and I went to college in the middle of eleventh grade. I wanted to get away from home.

A significant component of this not always so subtle intrusiveness is the fact that, while the parent feels entitled to know about the child,

---

their children's problems, their marital difficulties, or even their own health problems—confidences I had not solicited, which I could not be expected to want to know, and which were, by any normal standard, utterly inappropriate in the context of a relatively formal interview. They, on the other hand, seemed to find them fascinating topics of conversation, just as someone else would discuss a good book he was reading or an intriguing new problem at work. This happened several times with psychiatrists, though not once with lawyers or judges.

may even encourage the child to confide and assure him in tones of incredulity that there is no reason to feel ashamed or not to confide, at the same time the parent conspicuously does not return similar confidences. Not many parents do, of course, feel the need to discuss their problems and emotions with their children, but nor do they set up a situation where frank discussion is supposed to be expected and its absence will therefore be noticed. A great many PsyKs have spontaneously mentioned their parents' unwillingness to speak about themselves, which they saw as an unequal and unfair situation that placed them at a disadvantage. Worse, in the context of a family where open discussion is seen as so vital, the parent's withholding of reciprocal trust and openness may seem to the child like a withholding of love.

There are two different, not mutually exclusive avenues open to the PsyK whose parent insists upon intruding, interpreting, crossing the boundaries of the child's sense of self. One is to retreat into a passion for secrecy, which I have often encountered, and which Kohut mentions as the empathically assailed child's technique for preserving a healthy core of self. Paradoxically, this secrecy may sometimes be concealed beneath apparent frankness in discussing those things that his family demands be discussed, while the PsyK hoards up minor secrets the way a child may hoard a collection of scraps of paper and stones. The important point, after all, is less the defense of specific bits of personal data than a blanket need just to have something that belongs to oneself alone.

One prominent psychoanalyst proudly and repeatedly told her son that she knew everything about him and could see into his mind. The son, now seventy, says that this had lasting effects on him. "It is not really that I *hide* things from people, but I have always been careful to keep control over what people know of me. This has been true all my life, though perhaps it let up a bit after the age of forty or so. It was a question of defending my privacy, or of defending an area that was my own. This has had its problems in my marriage; my wife feels it and comments on it, but it is not that I don't want her to know things, it is just that by now I have an instinctive reaction to play things close to my chest."

Another man, a poet and painter, the son of two psychotherapists, said, when speaking of his adolescent romantic notion of love, that:

Something that always gave me trouble with my father was
that somehow it was all too sayable, and I found that intrusive. I

found it very intrusive, and trying to be cool or whatever and to make the appropriate response to parents who are so open about sexuality involved, I think, a lot of falsehood.

I knew the answers to questions I didn't want to answer. My parents are trained to meet a complete stranger and to very calmly discuss the most intimate facts of his life with him. I was just a person, a young poet, and highly secretive. I forget now, but there were a lot of fears about keeping secrets. To this day I think that there's a lot to be said for *what is not said*, particularly in the areas of nature, religion, and love.

If you *talk* about your girlfriend, it doesn't really correspond to the way you feel when you're with her, and it does your feelings for her a disservice to discuss them almost clinically with somebody else. What's nice about the feelings you have with someone is that they are not necessarily communicable. But I have the feeling to this day, with my parents, that I am somehow *accountable* for all my romantic life in terms of some kind of psychic economy. They expect me to give them a complete inventory of my emotions, and somehow to gauge how strong an attraction in any variety of departments I feel for somebody. And *they* feel like master detectives—that given a few tidbits of information, or having a glance at somebody I've met, that they can say A, B, or C is the motive for this relationship, and she is going to be good, bad, or indifferent for me.

They discuss me in psychodynamic terms like someone discussing current events. It's an interesting topic of conversation, and they don't see why they shouldn't chat about it with me. I don't think that they really have any picture of what my love life is like, of the extremity and the violence of my affairs. They picture it as me needing somebody, becoming dependent on somebody, somebody flattering me—you know, somebody tells me I'm a genius, and she's kind of cute and, wham, I get dependent on her. That's about their picture of it. And then she gets angry at me because I'm such an infant and won't hold a job. That's what they think happens. They don't know how close it all goes to murder. And they certainly don't know that wonderful transition between extreme emotional violence and creativity that is sometimes my day-in and day-out life, and which is a large part of my own self-image.

To tell you the honest truth, in all my life I never had a strong stomach, and all this openness made me a little sick. It would always come up at dinner conversations, and I couldn't digest my food. I wanted to get up and leave, but then they would say "You're getting up and leaving!" as though this were morally bad. It became, in fact, a moral point. It was bad not to be up-front about things, though of course when were they ever up-front about themselves?

I used to make attacks against honesty, or against being natural or open, simply because I was oppressed by it. That's why I have been accused of having a passion for obscurity and artifice. People say, "He reads all the difficult poets, and it's for snob appeal. He goes out of his way to be obscure in his writing, and either it's out of snobbery or self-aggrandizement or else he doesn't want to reveal what he really feels." Well the fact is that I *still* don't want to sit down and eat a meal that is going to be concluded with details about what influences people to attach themselves to other people. Sometimes it's better just to leave things alone. This has a lot to do with why I always liked to write, because writing gave the opportunity to quietly sit and without outside interference set down what you felt and, most important, to revise.

The alternative response to the parent's intrusion, which I have also encountered very often, sometimes in the same people, is to capitulate. If the parent insists upon knowing and discussing those interior thoughts that the child finds significant, and if it is only in this way that the parent relates to the child and lends credence and validity to those internal processes, then the child may go over to the parent's side, begin to divorce himself from the feeling of those things and come to know and discuss them intelligently and perceptively himself. He surrenders himself, in a sense, as a subjectively feeling self, and reifies himself instead as an object of scrutiny and mutual interest with his parents, a little hobby they all share.

PsyKs who take this approach and come to treat themselves with intellectual curiosity are very deceptive individuals. As children they seem bright, articulate, and mature. Their parents find in them everything they had hoped for. These PsyKs understand other people's motives as they understand their own, and they function quite well in the world of adults. Unfortunately for themselves, they function less well among other children, since they have ceded much of the spontaneity and emotionality that goes to make up childhood. Though they have the social graces of adults, they lack the social gaffes of the child.

As they continue through life, they always harbor this hole where the innocent delights of childhood should have been. It is harder for them to break away from their parents, since their enjoyment of their own lives is so wrapped up in their parents' enjoyment of it. In the absence of their parents they may feel very lost.

8

Contemplating Emotions

Cogito ergo sum.

—RENÉ DESCARTES

Cogito cogito ergo cogito sum.

—AMBROSE BIERCE

An academic in his early forties, the son of an enthusiastic and rigid psychoanalyst, says:

I think that probably the worst problem I encountered and one that I attribute definitely and directly to psychoanalysis—was an acute awareness of myself. I was incredibly self-conscious, and I always thought that everyone else knew what I was thinking and why I was doing whatever I was doing, and usually I felt that if they knew they probably thought that I was a fraud. It's interesting—I don't know how I got this impression, because my father never tried to *analyze* me in any way I was aware of, whether he would have been able to or not I don't know, but nonetheless I somehow acquired this sense, which I very definitely attribute to his having been a shrink: that people could tell what I was up to.

Probably the way that this came about was that I was so aware of all the little indications. I knew why I did certain things, or I thought I did, and I believed that other people must, too. It's like a kid who's afraid his face will give him away when he lies, and exactly because he's so worried about it, he turns bright red and looks so stiff and scared every time he lies that people can't help but notice. Whereas if he didn't worry about it in the first place, nobody would ever know the difference: they'd just say, "Oh, is that so?" and believe whatever he said.

So on the one hand I was always acutely aware of whether or not what I was doing would give away what I felt. On the other hand—and I'm really not sure how this fits together—I'm not sure that I felt much of anything at all, because I was so busy standing outside of myself and observing me, that I never just let it all drop and *was* me. In fact, just as I worried about how I seemed because I thought other people would figure out what was really going on inside of me, I daydreamed, not about how I would live things or how I would feel about them, but about how I would appear to others. I used to—I still do a lot—find myself in some situation that I thought was pretty neat, and rather than enjoying it for what it was, I would spend my time imagining: "If only So-and-So could see me now." I know that a lot of people do that, but I did it all the time. I did it to the point where I was living for external appearances alone, and if you had tried to pin me down on what I really wanted to do in a lot of circumstances, I honestly wouldn't have known. I'd never stopped to think about it. It had never occurred to me that I *should* do that.

The worst of it is that the kind of life you lead when you live in this self-conscious, daydreamy way, and try to construct your life so that it becomes something you imagine other people are impressed by, is a fairly remote, abstract sort of life. It's kind of lonely, and not very satisfying. It's also not very adventurous, which has depressed me since. I always thought I was pretty original in what I did, but it turns out I wasn't nearly as original as I could have been. I liked the image of being somewhat eccentric, and of just following my inclinations wherever they might lead. But you can only do so much of that when you are constantly monitoring and measuring your eccentricity, and worrying that your inclinations might lead you into an embarrassing spot. So you walk this kind of narrow line, and I think that's what makes you feel like a fraud.

What was it important for me to seem like? Actually I think I had a pretty good idea of what I would be like if I were a healthy person. It was important to be creative, to know a lot of things, to be respected. I wanted to have warm and easygoing friendships, where I could sit around with friends, lazily having fascinating discussions and not worrying about feeling foolish. When I was young I aspired to ruthlessly root out all of my problems and be pure and honest and really alive in some way. When I say I wanted to root out all of my problems, I think that I had this sense, from Freud, or maybe it came from King Arthur, that there was some tremendous value in shedding all personal fear or embarrassment and just trying to make oneself into all that one could be. It's not such a novel idea, but I carried it to extremes, at least theoretically, and even at times when I was taking drugs and having very bad experiences, I contrived to look on it as something of value, as a valuable ordeal or pilgrimage that was somehow going to take me someplace where I had to go—I may also have just been trying to make myself feel something that was strong enough to be genuine. But unfortunately I seem to have done it all wrong. I thought that this was what I should be doing, but in actual practice I was doing something very different. I don't seem ever to have confronted many of my problems. Once again I was creating an image of something I would like to have done rather than actually doing it, and I could just as well have daydreamed the whole thing, which would have given the same ultimate effect, and spared my body some of the abuse.

Embarrassment has inhibited me throughout my life and kept me from doing all sorts of things. Honesty has often gotten buried. I grew inward in such a complicated way that I didn't even know how to be honest in a relationship, for example. My motives and my notions of what I wanted in life were so far removed from the immediate concerns of the relationship that I wouldn't have been able to begin to discuss the sorts of problems that concerned the various women I was with.

A lot of these things have dwindled in importance over the years, partly through age, and partly through resignation and probably just by finding various ways to manage comfortably within the constraints I've grown to accept. It's depressing to think about them again, because I seem to have fucked up, and really not to have lived up to my early expectations. I look back and see so many failures and compromises and neglected opportunities that I can't really feel very confident about myself now. On the other hand, it's encouraging in a way to reopen the book on some of these issues, because I think I had just forgotten some of them, and perhaps now I should go back and think about them again from a new perspective.

One of the greatest feelings in life is the sensation of spontaneous action, where one acts, participates, loves, hates, and feels directly, with nothing separating oneself from the physical world and experience. One is master of oneself, has confidence, and engages others on common ground. But the psychotherapist's child, if raised with overt analytic understanding, may grow up in a world where nothing is quite as it seems to be. Actions are really reactions, if one only knows what to consider. A free choice is no more than ignorance of its determining factors. People cease to be *anthropomorphic humans*, masters of their fates, becoming instead psychological automata, the victims and products of whatever chain of circumstances has molded the trajectory of their lives. At worst, people are not even the product of the behaviorist's inhuman yet aseptic stimuli and responses, but are controlled by all that decent society holds most distasteful: by sexuality, excretion, perversion, and scarcely bridled envy and lust. The most altruistic sentiments dissolve under analytic scrutiny into sublimated selfishness. The world becomes a psychoanalytic "dystopia," a word the Oxford English Dictionary defines as an imaginary place where everything is as bad as it can possibly be. As Freud remarked in *The Interpretation of Dreams*, when one subjects oneself to analytic scrutiny, "One is bound to emerge as the only villain among the crowd of noble characters who share one's life."[1]

This attitude is scarcely the goal of psychoanalysis, an art dedicated to liberating people of the morbid preoccupations that deter them from the free living of their lives, yet it can be an unfortunate side effect, and usually, though only fleetingly, is. Candidates at analytic institutes and beginning analytic patients generally pass through an uncomfortable phase where everything is seen through the spectacles of psychoanalysis, every slip of the tongue or forgotten name makes one pause and attempt to reconstruct the underlying significance. Analysis becomes an obsession, and one in which the end point is not always clear. As one analyst's son remarked, "Analysis is very much like Plato. Except for the *Laws*, in the whole opera, there is not a single straight word. There is not *one* place where you can say 'Plato says that this is the answer.' It's all 'Socrates says this in response to that,' all the drama, the rhetoric, the irony, blah-blah. He never says 'What you ought to do is go out and X—': 'Take your mother out to dinner,' 'Call home.' It's all just a philosophical exercise, an arduous occupation. Then again, it may just be a vice. The same for psychoanalysis."

Adults can keep such theories and obsessions in perspective. Eventually some normal, if new, equilibrium returns to life, and their experience is enriched by a freshly available awareness of the hidden springs of consciousness. A child, on the other hand, can be permeated by such thoughts before he learns how to live. More than one psychoanalyst's child has told me that he felt his spontaneous emotions to be stunted by a tendency to intellectualize. The child who passed his early years being understood and interpreted by his parents may end up partly splintered himself, so that while the acting self tries to carry on its life, it is followed about by another ratiocinating self who draws attention to every fault, betrays the hidden greed behind an act of altruism or bravery, reveals the faulty decisions that led to a praiseworthy result, and torments the actor with the knowledge that he is just that, an actor, and not a very good one, either, since to a trained eye, he supposes, all his flaws and doubts and dirty little secrets betray themselves in every gesture, each innocuous turn of phrase, and in every self-conscious expression that crosses his face. The psychoanalyst's child may feel hunted down by an examining, evaluating eye that is ubiquitous and omniscient. One may come to believe, along with Jules Romains' unscrupulous Dr. Knock, that "healthy people are nothing but invalids who do not know that they are ill."[2]

What has been helpful for the psychologically naïve patient who, after blundering on impulse through decades of life finally benefits from a dose of insight and self-examination, here has proven to be a stumbling block. In any learning task one should first get to know the area, grow comfortable with it, gain some confidence, and only then commit oneself to the hard and humbling task of learning the precise rules. The analyst's son described at the beginning of this chapter was like a young musician pushed to practice like a concert soloist and polish his technique without ever having felt the initial personal satisfaction of the amateur making an interesting sound, and without having the opportunity to develop the passion that turns technical virtuosity into music.

A concept that comes up quite often with PsyKs is the capriciousness and fragility of experience. Geology, much like psychoanalysis, is the study of large patterns produced by the cumulative effect of small events. The position of one small pebble can divert the flow of a tiny rivulet that could grow to become a stream and the torrent that carves the shape of a region's landscape. This does not mean that there is critical importance to the precise position of every pebble.

In the trivialized, old movie version of psychoanalysis, one finds much the same type of process. The patient suffers from overwhelming, crippling, and totally baffling phobias or compulsions with no normal explanation or apparent solution. No amount of effort or courage can defeat the debilitating ailment, and it is terrifying to suppose that some fundamental flaw lies behind it all. Then the psychoanalyst, like a brilliant detective or master spy, prods here and there, follows the branching lines of stress back, nimbly eludes the defenses, and pinpoints one simple aberrant experience that has thrown the whole mental mechanism out of kilter. The patient is cured and lives happily ever after, curtains, lights.

For the child who comprehends the analytic notion of life in similarly simplified terms, the prospect can be far from consoling. In the condensed case history heard at the dinner table or gleaned from surreptitious reading of the texts in the study, cause and effect are so closely and directly related, with so few checks intervening even despite the passage of decades, that life appears as a very precarious business. When the adult with vast problems looks back, it may be consoling to find a small and simple cause. When the child looks forward, he may suppose that the slightest misstep now will lead inevitably to disastrous consequences later.

The son of one psychoanalyst said:

I picked up quite early that a lot of my father's patients needed help because their *parents* had been crazy, and that this had permanently affected their lives. And as a result I thought of my friends' parents from the standpoint of how they *should* be, or at least of how I supposed they ought to be. It was somewhat ominous at times to see the way my friends' parents treated their kids, because if it seemed bad to me, or weird in any way, it seemed as though I could almost see the germ of craziness being planted in my classmates. I guess in a way I kind of worried about my classmates' well-being due to their parents. I remember one kid in particular whose mother was an alcoholic and acted really freaky. One minute she was very nice—patronizing, actually—and the next minute all hell would break loose, she'd scream at him and get violent. It scared the shit out of me. And I always thought: god, this woman seems crazy, and therefore my friend is going to have to be crazy later on because of her. It was very sad. I was sure that he was doomed.

Another man, the son of a psychiatrist and a psychoanalyst, puts it even more bluntly:

One concept I heard from my father a lot—never in so many words, but quite succinctly nonetheless, and that repeats itself to me quite often, is this: Let's say I'm waiting in line, in a bank or somewhere, and I see somebody who keeps dropping his money, or who doesn't know where he is, or who looks completely nervously shot. I hear a voice inside my head which I recognize as partly my father's, saying, "This person has made some simple, rational mistake, some fundamental error in living." That is the way he always presented life to me. It's the System. And people's mental illness derived from falsely identifying some element of the System, which could be, for example, succumbing to mistaken impressions and falling in love with the wrong person. Somebody makes this error, and the next thing you know they're locked away on a ward somewhere. It's like the chess move where you're finally going to be mated because of this one little thing you did wrong.

I spent a lot of time in reflection: why is this happening? Always reevaluating, replaying every scene I've lived through. Going to bed at night and playing the day back again and wondering "Why did I behave the way that I did?" "Why did he behave the way that he did?" That was part of the attraction of drugs when I began experimenting with them, there was a great relief of finding that there was such a thing as intoxication, where you weren't standing looking over your own shoulder all the time and writing stage directions for yourself and then correcting the handwriting that you'd written the stage directions in. It got to be pretty crazy, but I don't regret it. I think that kind of introspection gives you certain advantages over people who are just downright sloppy in the way they lead their lives. But it is also a nuisance. You are always standing back. Any number of women have observed that about me and have been very frustrated by it.

Several PsyKs, in fact, have mentioned drug and alcohol use as a method of combating their tendency toward endless speculation. One said he had learned to use them to "cloud the intellectual aspect" of things and allow himself to function in a simplified world. His father actually helped him in this endeavor by giving him Miltowns when he was upset or confused. Another man phrased it slightly differently, saying he used barbiturates and liquor to "discolor" situations; by reducing the subtle hues of experience into blacks and whites and a couple of grays, the logic of relationships, ambitions, and problems became narrower and at least seemed more clear.

The chess analogy is a particularly accurate one in light of the function psychotherapy serves in the lives of many psychotherapists and comes, therefore, to serve in the minds and lives of their children. Children of therapists are, by and large, the children of unhappy people, people whose unhappiness often came from their own difficult dealings with their parents and experiences as a child, and who have learned to cope with their discomfort through an intellectual understanding and emotional distancing of themselves from their problems.

Allen Wheelis, in "The Vocational Hazards of Psycho-analysis," beautifully relates a clinical vignette of a young man whose problems finally led him to become a psychoanalyst. At some stage in this man's struggle against his own loneliness and misery, he recognized the value of insight. Having learned the power of insight to solve problems and to stave off his personal pain, this man came to idealize insight, to think it the answer to everything:

> Larry's insight occurred at the time of bad trouble. Such an experience, if it proves repeatable, will have far-reaching effects. One will come to rely on insight as on nothing else. So far as personal security is concerned, he will value it above friends, fame, love, or money. It is something of which no chance can deprive him. It is utterly reliable.[3]

This led him to psychoanalysis as a profession and as a method of continuing his life. Unfortunately, however, such a flight into reason is not a very satisfying way to lead one's life, and it is not aways even a very good way to conduct psychotherapy.

A paper by psychologist Stephen Appelbaum tells a sad yet funny example of a therapist's blind faith in insight. A long-term alcoholic and drug addict entered into therapy with a psychoanalytic candidate. In the course of treatment, this woman, who had not previously been very psychological minded, gained considerable insight into her own behavior and became quite good at psychological understanding. Both the therapist and the training analyst who was supervising his work, in their enthusiasm over this technical triumph, overlooked the fact that the patient had fallen behind in payments for her treatment. As it turned out, despite her gratifying proficiency in intellectually grasping elements of her problem, the patient had, unbeknownst to the analysts, reverted to drinking and drug abuse, and was spending what she should have paid in therapeutic fees on drugs and alcohol. As far as cultivating insight was concerned, treatment was very impressive: as a therapy to solve a problem, it was a ludicrous failure.[4]

The therapist parents who have taken the route of the encapsulated wound remain on the defensive in all their relationships, including, at times, those with their children. Life at some stage ceased to be an easy give-and-take with others, and turned into an adversarial intellectual contest in which one wins through dialectical gambits, propaganda, and psychological warfare. These parents regard their children sometimes as additional opponents, more often as fellow defenders of the besieged fortress, on whose faith and dependence they particularly rely. They also, of course, as fundamentally benevolent people, try to impart some of their acquired wisdom to their children, but unfortunately for the child the parent's wisdom may be a sickly variety of self-defense and a flight into intellectual dissection of emotions and distancing of oneself from things.

The PsyK is given an implicit or explicit paranoid world view and supplied with an arsenal of tricks that oblige him to evade and defend himself against situations he has never had the chance to evaluate on his own. The defensive gestures of the parent have been transformed into a philosophical system that masquerades as objective science, and since the parent rewards the child's belief in this system, one that truly does have certain convenient advantages, PsyKs are often tempted to accept it, and start to become cynical, defensive, and artificial even before knowing whether or not they ought to feel genuinely disillusioned. One analyst's son, when describing what passed in his house for father-son chats, said that they would go into his father's office and "he would sit in his chair, which he sat in all his life, and I would sit in the adjacent chair, and without very much eye contact he would go on, and after a while he would really get on a roll, explaining the world to me, picking apart other people, psychoanalyzing the family, dissecting himself and myself." He had warm recollections of these really rather nasty-sounding talks because these were among the few times he passed alone with his father.

Even the genuinely valuable aspects of psychotherapeutic thought are not helpful unless the child is ready for them and knows how to use them properly. The man who has been saved through religion may want to pass religion on to his son. But merely furnishing a child with a point of view, a few rules, and a faith, is not sufficient to insure his salvation. Neither faith nor insight can simply be given. Faith, to have meaning, must be acquired on one's own. Insight, by its very nature, demands a questioning of superficial appearances and rejection of ready-made answers. Providing tools someone does not know that he needs and does not know how to use burdens him rather than helps. False insight can very easily be a defense against change; one covets and works hard to achieve valued and praiseworthy discoveries, but without integrating them into any program that leads toward improvement.[5]

A prominent analyst and son of an analyst reports that:

The net effect of it for me was a certain kind of withdrawal and a sense of abandonment, a certain grandiosity and—well, a lot of bad judgment. You really have this identification with your father going on in adolescence, you are identified with this kind of magic, with this smug understanding of all the events in the world, when in fact you don't have it, in fact you're no better off than anybody else, *in fact* you're probably much worse off, since you can't delineate a simple cause and effect. You have never been trained to look at cause and effect, because instead you were being trained to look at the effect and the hidden *hidden* cause; you're never to look at what you really see, because there's always another explanation for it that doesn't meet the eye. I don't know quite how to say it, but your simple explanation for why you feel the way you do is constantly obscured, and you end up in a quagmire of interpretation and confusion. It affected my experience of reality.

I had a very smug feeling that I understood a lot more than other people did about life in the world. What it did was to help push me into a premature maturity, or rather a premature *false* sense of maturity that fed into my feeling of grandiosity. You feel that you are in possession of information about the world and about yourself and other people which gives you some great advantage. In reality it doesn't, and as a matter of fact you are covering up the fact that you're not a simple bread-and-butter person, you're not a simple cause-and-effect person, you're really much more confused about simple causes and effects than most people. That is how I experienced it: it was a complication that ultimately made things more confusing and difficult.

In practical terms, it encouraged me to take on more than I should have at a much earlier age, including marriage, children, and medical school. Since I had this sense of pseudomaturity, and an intellectual grasp that obscured my ability to come to grips with things, I denied the reality of the situation and denied the fact that I really couldn't handle it. In relationships, I found that I was not starting from the surface down, but taking the analytic approach and going from the bottom up. In doing analysis, the traditional school of thought since ego psychology has been that when you work with a patient you work from the surface down, in contrast to the Kleinians, who work from the depths up. I was acting like an analyst of the old school treating myself as a patient, ignoring the simple and obvious experience and plunging straight for the depths. If somebody hurt me in a relationship, my tendency was to look at their motives, not to stop for a moment and recognize that I'd been hurt, and take whatever the appropriate action might be.

Thank God I eventually came to see the trap I had fallen into, or followed my father into. If I had continued, I would have become more and more constricted, more and more anesthetized, more and more a zombie, more and more impervious to reality, more and more living in my own world. You can talk to other analysts' children and you can talk to other analysts, but you're not going to have much luck with the guy who puts gas in your car, or with anyone else who sees things in terms of the simple causes and effects that govern daily experience in the real world.

One paradoxical feature about PsyKs that conceals a treacherous trap into which they have fallen is that they tend to be bright, charming, and charismatic. They do seem terribly mature. One model of their cousin, the minister's child, is that of the "little adult." Preachers' kids grow up in a household where the ideal is to exercise control over one's base emotions and passions, to sacrifice oneself for the good of others, to be self-effacing and self-denying, to rise above petty temptations and desires—in short, to act like an adult, not like a child. Or rather, to act like some hypothetical version of an adult, and to do so at a time when one is really and most emphatically still a child. Such children have repressed their impulses, they have not honestly come to grips with them and gotten them under real control.

PsyKs fall prey to a similar syndrome, though in a less conspicuous way. Their lives are not publicly on display in a church, their parents do not represent such a rigid and possibly artificial way of living, their values are not so overtly at odds with those of their peers. PsyKs are not told what they should do—far from it: nondirectiveness is common—rather they are told *how* to do it, which is responsibly and with full awareness of their motivations and of the consequences of their acts.

The PsyK's own notion of self-worth and sense of values can be painfully weak. Narcissistically disturbed parents may stress the importance of having a strong ethical sense, and they appear to have their own set of moral principles, but often this is little more than a theatrical decor concealing an ethically impoverished interior.[6] They suspect others of being fundamentally dishonest, fraudulent, and opportunistic, while they themselves, with no genuine internal ethical sense, may change their position to suit the circumstances or even entertain mutually exclusive ethical attitudes. It is a very fluid sort of hypocrisy that may masquerade as enlightened liberality and which may even be rationalized by the dialectic tricks of psychotherapy. Whether the children consciously recognize this or not, it is the sort of influence that does not fail to be absorbed. Where, then, are they left when the decision of right and wrong is entirely up to them?

The painful troubles of living from the surface in can be made much worse for the PsyK who has not only been manipulated into gratifying the narcissistic parent, but who has been taught a doctrine of self-abnegation and perpetual catering to the other person—like the girl whose mother excused anyone who was insecure—that legitimizes if not sanctifies this approach. There is little of the robust satisfaction in life that supports real growth of the person in the child, for the family's gratification is based on prestige, appearances, insight, understanding, and the translation of common sense into uncommon knowledge. Looking right and having proper manners are recurring themes among PsyKs. Therapists themselves spend a great deal of time thinking about what should or should not show or be known, and how actions, intended one way, may strike someone else in another. This can easily come to mean that to truly seem the way that one is, one should act in the way that creates that impression.

The son of a psychiatrist and a child analyst says:

I don't know anyone's parents who were as artificial as mine. I always envied my friends' households, which seemed more relaxed, natural, with the possibility of enjoying ordinary activities, of people enjoying one another's company and being affectionate to one another. I didn't see very much of that at home. I didn't see much feeling between my parents, as though they were together because they wanted to be. It was based more on criticism of other people or on an agreement about standards: "Your bed should be made. We both agree." "Your shoes should be tied. We both agree." On the other hand, I didn't see the real perils of neurotic, fearful attitudes or confusion that I sometimes saw in other families. My family represented a certain kind of order. There was orderliness in going home, and that I liked in a precious sort of way. Up to the age of twelve or thirteen I suppose I seemed like a model child. I was very polite, probably obedient, shy. I could impress people socially; if you could get me over my shyness I could say things that would make people feel either impressed with my intelligence or charmed by my sensitivity. I don't think that at the time this dawned on me as being any kind of vanity, it was just this thing that happened repeatedly, it was the texture of the world, and it was the only texture I knew.

I can't say that there was much joy in my childhood. I used to lie in bed as a child, and I would think: Is there any reason to keep living? And I would try to think of something that I was going to do, like go to an amusement park, or some other thing that was still in the future that was probably going to be fun. But otherwise, I'm not sure why, I found it very painful going on from day to day. I don't know what, if anything, my parents thought. They probably tried to nudge me along to get me more involved with other people. But by the same token they were themselves very reserved and relatively isolated. There were never a lot of people in the house, and it all had this kind of almost solemn aura, a very low-key fatality about the whole thing. There was never a hint that life in the world was a lot of fun. There was not a lot of élan.

My sister had a bit of a hard time growing up, she's a little bit lost, but I don't think she has the sense of being completely at odds with the world. I think it was harder to grow up being a boy in the family. There was no sustenance, there wasn't really any sustenance for the project of being a man. I think—if I were to have a family, I think that in some sense my life would have to have come together by then. I might say that I had spent all these years coming up with some method by which to solidify myself and feel whole as a man, and I may have used this or that rationalization or prop or so forth, but when I had a child I would have to feel somehow that all of that past had somehow fused, and that I had some intuitive sense of myself. With my father I felt, and still feel, that he's so busy still proving *himself*. . . . The way an adolescent will get a car or get a different pair of trousers, something that identifies him, or works on this or that job, or adopts a certain slightly condescending way of talking about women just to prove that he's cool. It *never stopped* with him. It didn't stop when I was born or when I was a child or while I was growing up. And of course I took some pride in him, but it was pride in his *invention:* he gave ostensive definitions to things, he said 'This is wonderful, and you certainly ought to be proud of me because I did it.' He made it his business to enforce the idea of his competence, he enjoys doing something and making everyone acknowledge that he did it just right. I didn't get an example from him, and then when I began to grow up he would complain that I was incompetent and couldn't do anything. My sister has mentioned this, too, so it is not just subjective, it's not just the judgment by a boy of his father. All I got was practical advice on how to keep up appearances: how to dress, how to talk, how to appear well-bred. I didn't realize that the public was so simple-minded, but what my father was telling me was, "It's a lot of sham, and here's how it's played." Well, to a certain extent he is right, but there's no nourishment in that attitude.

I was completely privileged in what I got. If I wanted a book, or a musical instrument, or something that had a particular fascination for me, then suddenly it appeared in my life. It was mine, it was in my room, the guys at school couldn't destroy it and weren't interested in it. Mine was a pretty specialized, self-involved kind of world. I could mostly enjoy things that were quiet and subtle, like poetry and certain paintings. And I had the sense that all of that was agreeable to my family. There was a space in which there were these objects that either spoke to me about the world or about *a* world that I was interested in, or they were poems describing that life. They were artifacts that were a little bit fragile, that were considered precious, and that were somehow guarded from the invasion of brute force. And I did feel as though, yes, my parents endorsed my interest in those things. It kept me in an enclosed world. Perhaps in some way I was going to fulfill the creative project of my father's that had been curtailed so that he could make a living and get married and raise a family. Because he did tell us that, that he could have created this great work if only he hadn't needed to see patients and support us kids. I know. I spent years theorizing in bars about extraordinary works that I might do, and going to bed at night actually believing that I was somehow going to embark on this tremendous project, starting first thing next morning.

I was living in this darkness, always dealing with something to do with death. I was trying to do something representational about my most secret pathos, and I didn't tell anyone that. I didn't tell people that I didn't want to be alive, or that this world was so frightfully drab and unromantic that I wanted to escape into whatever I could create. But then I began to meet people from another world. I met people through school who lived in a neighborhood where everybody played guitars and ate pizza, and sat on porches in the evening and talked, and went to the beach, and talked to these girls they knew who walked around in bathing suits and drank sodas, and things were relaxed and real. I would stay at a friend's house and he would ask all these questions about people's bodies and bodily functions and so forth, and suddenly it was like, Yeah, shit, you can talk about all this, and here's somebody who's curious about this stuff and you can talk to them about it. So I had a glimpse of that world, but for some reason it didn't become open yet. I was always on the fringe of it, my clothes were always a little too clean, I was a little too stiff, and I always wanted to back out of this or that.

Then I met a girl, and I decided that I was going to make her a conquest, and I was going to invite her into my world. We slept together—I was real young—and later through her I met these people who went to the public high school and were intellectuals, but there was a rough-and-tumble aspect to them, they were intellectuals with a ragged edge, rebels, troublemakers. I finally felt like maybe I had found a world that I could live in.

So in my early teens I found things to do. Instead of just being negative I could drive off to the ends of the earth in the middle of the night, stay up all night, smoke grass, or lie in bed with a girl smoking cigarettes and feeling like I was in one of those grainy movies. There were actually things you could do with other people that had a little bit of the quality that I was looking for. I felt like I could almost get my feet into the world a little bit, almost touch it. Maybe if I watched the people I was around, how they went places and got things done, maybe I would find my own way of being a human being or being a man or whatever it was that I was after.

But I knew during all that time, I still knew that I was really different, and it would still come to a point where everything would be a little too vulgar, and I would move back to the fringe, and the fringe bordered right on the family again, which was whitewashed walls, clean carpets, no dust, everything very hygienic, clothes that were neatly ironed, everything proper and in place. I guess I couldn't decide what I wanted. My family represented a kind of orderliness with no blood, no life, and then my contemporaries represented a world with some life in it but which entailed giving up a certain amount of that privileged feeling of having all your needs met. At that point I knew that my parents began to disapprove of what I was doing.

I think, at heart, my parents had some of the same problems as I had, and that that played into our relationship somehow, though we never talked about it. I bet on some level they were terribly sensitive to things. They are probably people who hurt a lot over the years, and they have invented this sub-paradise that they can inhabit where things will be all right, and they won't be bothered by it at all.

If psychotherapists often have a God complex, then their children suffer from being the children of God. This is true in several confluent ways. First is the basic problem of the child of any narcissistically impaired parent, who becomes that parent's crutch or flattering mirror, who is good at empathizing, good at understanding others, but not very solid in his or her own sense of self, which is defined largely in terms of the parent's approval. One woman I interviewed was unusually charming, witty, brilliant, and articulate. People had told her throughout her life that she was destined to be a politician because she seemed so charismatic and independent. She discussed herself and her family openly and honestly, and it was hard to imagine anyone better adjusted than she: in fact she herself said that she was the best-adjusted person she knew. Soon afterward she admitted that she was not very good at expressing her feelings, but was better at identifying and rationalizing her feelings than experiencing them, which was an advantage in that it helped her to deal with them, and a disadvantage in that they did not seem to be really her own. She adores her mother, a child psychiatrist, and though she resents much of her mother's intrusiveness, and discussed this resentment quite openly, the overall picture was exceptionally rosy. When I asked whether her closeness to her mother ever posed any problems, a curious change came into her story.

Yes, there is a very definite problem with that. The first thing that pops into my head as you're talking is, maybe this is all just my perception, and it's not all this rosy and I'm not this well adjusted: I've just been brought up as the center of her universe to believe that I'm wonderful but it's entirely her creation. That's a very definite possibility. I panic at the thought that, God forbid—my mother is just never going to die. She just isn't. She can't do that to me. But I panic at that thought. The thought of not having my mommy just flips me out. I can't deal with it. I know that if anything ever happened—*which it won't,* it never will—but if, God forbid, it does, I'm going to be a mess, a basket case.

I define myself—it's not a conscious thing, I don't say to myself, Gee, how would Mom react? but I inevitably react the way she would. Sometimes it scares me, because I see myself playing shrink with my friends or whatever, and I don't like it. I don't want to have the same kind of life she did, including being a psychiatrist, spending twelve hours a day being understanding and "supportive but nondirective." It is hard for me to act like a grownup around her, even though I'm almost thirty years old. We will walk into a restaurant and she will read to me from the menu, or as soon as the food is put down and before she takes a bite she'll say "Here, have some." She needs to give. That's what gives her life: giving and giving life to other people.

I just keep promising myself that she will always be there. Yes, maybe all those other people who aren't well adjusted and don't get along with their parents will have the advantage over me in the end. I'm going to have a *real* tough time. When my mom was late picking me up at the airport last Christmas, I freaked out. It was raining that day and I was sure she had had an accident and died, and here I was sitting in the lobby of the airport, crying, wondering what I was going to do. She was fine. My father had gotten lost driving around the airport.

This form of closeness to the parent, of parental dependence on the child that results in the child's dependence on the parent, makes it more imperative for the child to play the parent's game, to see things in the same way, maintain intact the fragile intellectual world, and makes it far more difficult for the child to abandon it all and strike out independently. Curiously, it is not always clear that the child is being compliant and good. Some are very rebellious and get into trouble. By most people's standards, they look like a terrible burden to their parents. But when one looks more closely, one may find that in truth this rebelliousness itself is in utter conformity with what the parent wishes to see.

There is another more conspicuous form of the children-of-God influence that pushes from the outside to keep the child in. Many psychotherapists have an exceptionally high opinion of themselves. They have studied human behavior, they know the ultimate source of all human creation and endeavor, and they are qualified to pontificate on anything. Some of them express disdain for their patients. But even when psychotherapist parents are humility incarnate and would not dream of claiming superiority by virtue of greater knowledge, there is much in the therapist's position in life that, to the child, implies this superiority. One son of two analysts, now an analyst himself, remembers that as a child he always felt thankful that his parents had both been analyzed. He did not know precisely what it meant or what the effects had been, but there was the vague sense that something dreadful had been avoided. Another had simply been raised to believe that psychiatry was in some sense the ultimate profession: "Early in my life, every adult I knew who was not a relative was a psychiatrist, and I was fairly old before I ever realized seriously that there were interesting adults in other professions. I didn't know any of them, except for my extended family, who were in the button business in New York, and that was always looked upon as most definitely not interesting."

At the dinner table, PsyKs hear stories of patients' problems and the therapist-parent's simple explanation and solution. It's so obvious; why couldn't the patient see that for himself? The children themselves absorb the fundamentals of therapeutic understanding quite readily, and it seems surprising that other adults should be so blind. Patients are known to adore their therapist, to want to be their friends and participate in their lives, but the therapist will not permit it, and restricts them instead to an hour at a time—an hour for which they must pay. Within the family, unfortunately but quite naturally, patients may be viewed as a nuisance. They call at all hours, they make unreasonable demands. Says the son of two psychotherapists:

One of the very odd things about the whole field is that to most people it's pretty dramatic when somebody they have a close involvement with threatens to commit suicide, or has a nervous breakdown, or gets a divorce, or somebody dies. You go out of your way to be sympathetic, and it starts you to thinking about things. Whereas that's absolutely quotidian for psychiatrists. They wouldn't *see* anybody who wasn't having nervous breakdowns or wasn't psychotic, neurotic, or didn't have relatives dying on every side. So it's perfectly natural, unnatural though it may seem, that they gradually get accustomed to things that no one should ever get accustomed to.

I remember a family story about somebody who called my father to say that he was going to commit suicide. Somehow he had gotten my father's home number and called late at night wanting to talk, and my father allegedly told him, "Well, I'm sorry, I'm not working now and I can't talk to you, but my office is right on your way to the river, so instead of drowning yourself tonight, why don't you wait until morning and stop by on your way there? I have a free hour at eight." I appreciated later that this was the way you were supposed to deal with certain types of suicidal patients, and that if you know what you're doing and you know the patient, maybe that's an appropriate and helpful response, but at the time it seemed like a pretty horrible, careless thing to say. Well, no, wait: it may have seemed horrible in some sense, but not careless, because it never occurred to me that my father might have misjudged the situation. It wasn't conceivable that my father would take that attitude and then the patient *would* jump in the river. I think what came across as condescending, in my mind, was the fact that here was someone so emotionally worked up that he was going to kill himself, and who probably *believed* that he was going to kill himself, while my father didn't take it seriously at all, because through years of training and experience with patients like this, he knew what was going on in this guy better than the guy did himself, and he knew that he *wouldn't* kill himself, and that therefore, in the great scheme of things, the doctor's sleep or the chance to see the concluding minutes of "Perry Mason" was a more important consideration than this patient's false belief that he was in the last hour of his life.

The PsyK himself, on the other hand, is in a very different and more privileged position. He lives in the therapist parents' house, sees his parents in their bathrobes, eats with them, argues with them, can see all their human failings and weaknesses that are invisible to the patients. He is much more important in his parents' eyes: the suicidal patient can easily wait until morning, but the PsyK's scraped knee demands immediate attention. The therapist's child is partially immune to the ostensibly objective and faintly demeaning dissections that are performed on other people through analysis of their behavior and motives. By living within the privileged domain and being included on the parent's side in discussions of what "we" know and what other people do not, there is an unspoken assumption, if the child chooses to adopt it, that he is somehow entitled, by some sort of birthright, to a position above everyone else. This feeling of belonging to the priest class is sometimes explicit and is quite often detected as an underlying current. The psychotherapist's family is special.

This sense of privilege tends to be reinforced by the outside world, since the general public believes most emphatically in the curious powers of psychotherapists and, to some degree, the extension of those powers to the rest of the family. PsyKs find that their friends' parents expect them not only to be better adjusted, but also to share some of their parents' professional knowledge and insights, which indeed, bright and perceptive young people that they are, they often do. A surprising number of PsyKs relate tales of friends and friends' parents consulting with them on psychological or ethical issues in ways that required not factual knowledge but clinical expertise. PsyKs often become miniature therapists who attract troubled friends, and they may take pride in the fact that they are the only ones who can understand them. "I didn't have friendships, I had a clientèle," is a phrase which, in more or less identical terms, I have heard any number of times. In the words of one psychiatrist's child:

I seem to be sort of like my father. I have the kind of knack where people always ask me for advice and for help. And I think I am good at it. I'm not easily shocked, I can sympathize with almost anything. At the same time I am not very tolerant of weakness in myself. I am a perfectionist. It doesn't altogether make sense that when I'm alone I rip myself to shreds, but when I'm out in the world, then everyone loves me. And I love everybody, too; I'm a real humanist, whatever that means. But there are some problems with that way of living. It's a very self-effacing way to be, which is not altogether good. So recently, I have been trying to be selfish, I try my *damnedest* to be selfish, and it's not natural to me, but maybe if I was a little more selfish it would be easier for other people, because we could interact more as equals. I went to a psychiatrist once, but she wouldn't believe that I had problems of my own: I was too clever and articulate and wonderful, and I understood myself so well, that she wouldn't believe there was anything really wrong with me.

The net effect of the tendency to intellectualize, the approval that the family and society give to the results of this personally draining technique, and the internal and external sense that one somehow belongs to a privileged class, is to make it more difficult for the PsyK to change. Alice Miller, writing of narcissism, remarks:

A patient once spoke of the feeling of always having to walk on stilts. Is somebody who always has to walk on stilts not bound to be constantly envious of those who can walk on their own legs, even if they seem to him to be smaller and more "ordinary" than he is himself? And is he not bound to carry pent-up rage within himself, against those who have made him afraid to walk without stilts? Thus envy of other things can come about as the result of the defense mechanism of displacement. Basically, he is envious of healthy people because they do not have to make a constant effort to earn admiration, and because they do not have to do something in order to impress, one way or the other, but are free to be "'average."[7]

Yet even though the intellectualizing PsyK may feel uncomfortable and envious of mere mortals, having succeeded so well thus far, to go back and undo the damage that has been done, to try to rejoin one's emotional self would entail a significant degree of regression—and it is not clear what one would find. They may not altogether like what they have become, but they have so arduously and cleverly constructed such a seemingly clever life that it would be difficult to abandon this cherished edifice. This is particularly true since they do not know what they would become, like the girl who was afraid that if she did what she wanted to do she would end up going insane. She had no familiarity with the potential person within her.

To undo the PsyK's work of a lifetime is a difficult task, one that can often not be done through routine psychotherapy. It was therapy and insight and intellectualization, after all, that produced much of the difficulty to begin with. The therapist's child is immune to that startling burst of insight that is so effective with many patients, and self-scrutiny is the last thing he needs. What is called for, difficult though it may be, is a more arduous and painful process that involves cutting down some of the proud artifice and allowing this child of God to join the rest of the human race, to feel, to rebel, to sacrifice being ever-popular in exchange for a meaningful quality to the affection of people who do like him.

9

Sex,
Drugs,
and Other
Problems

> My parents raised me to believe
> that they would never say no to
> anything I asked because I would
> never want to do anything they
> would want to say no to.
> —A CHILD PSYCHIATRIST'S DAUGHTER

A writer in her thirties, the daughter of two psychiatrists, told me:

The first time I realized that I was the child of a psychiatrist was when somebody told me her parents didn't like her coming to my house because my family only talked about sex. Which really surprised me, because they didn't, hardly ever.

I read a lot of psychoanalytic literature when I was very young. I remember reading Reich when I was in junior high school, and I read a lot of pornography, because it was around, partly because of my brother, who belonged to the Evergreen Book Club. I read a lot about abnormal sexuality before I ever experienced anything you could consider normal, and as a result I was afraid of certain kinds of perversions which I thought were really rampant. I was scared because I thought there was much more S & M (sado-masochism) than there really is. There is S & M, but not everybody's into whips and shit like that, and I think I thought that they were, and that this was what I would have to expect in life because you just couldn't altogether avoid it—just another rough part of growing up, getting chained to a bedpost and flogged.

My father was very pro-sex. He had a utilitarian attitude toward sex which he taught me long before I thought about having sex myself. He took the attitude that there was a function of the orgasm, there really was this *function,* and you had to make sure that you had sex often enough, or else you'd be unhealthy. It gave it a kind of medicinal quality. I worried because I wasn't having sex yet—I was young at the time, and there was no reason why I should have—but I worried that I must be unbalanced.

Asked whether her parents ever sat her down and explained the facts of life to her, and whether she supposed their approach was more enlightened or enlightening than that of her peers' parents, this young woman replied:

The facts of life? Now this is strange: I remember my mother talking about homosexuality before I had ever learned about heterosexuality. They were in their room with my older sister, explaining the facts of life to her, and I caught the tail end of it and said, "Teach *me* something." And then, being a kid and not wanting to share or to get hand-me-down information, I said, "Teach me something that you *didn't* teach her." So if they taught my sister heterosexuality, then I wanted to learn some other kind, and I remember my mother telling me that sometimes people from the same sex fell in love with each other. That made a strong impression on me. I've had a lot of homosexual friends in my life. I think that somehow homosexuality was sweet to me, somehow I felt that it had been condoned.

My parents were very weird about sex, actually. It was easy to discuss, but in a detached kind of way. I remember that long after I'd started having sex, I mentioned it to my mother for some reason, and later she just forgot. Completely slipped her mind. She didn't want to remember. Even when she was forced to acknowledge it, she didn't altogether comprehend the fact. I don't think my mother really hooked up sex with what it was that I did. I did something else. There was some more wholesome thing that her daughter did, which wasn't the same thing as the stuff in the books. I don't know how I did it or what it was. I remember her going with me to get birth-control pills, and it was completely *abstract,* it wasn't related to sex or related to men, it was some mother-daughter ritual, something just between women.*

* Another woman, a designer in her fifties whose father was a psychoanalyst, said that when she was about to get married her parents sat her down and asked "Don't you think you should

She was generally very uncomfortable with sexuality, and some of it was justified on psychiatric grounds, rightly or wrongly. We weren't allowed to wear nightgowns. I wasn't allowed to walk around in a nightgown, which I've come to believe is a perfectly acceptable thing to do. But not in my house. My mother wouldn't permit it because she was really into unconscious sexual responses, and she thought that by doing that I would really disturb my father and brother, even if they didn't know it. She gave a lot of power to sexuality. Sexuality was this *really* powerful force that was always active somehow.

So I guess those kids' parents were right after all: my household *was* obsessed with sex. There were books on sex in the *living room*. If a kid came over to my house, there were big books that said "SEX" in huge letters on their book jackets. So I guess kids used to love to come to our house. They always loved to come because there was sex and there were drugs. It's true.

When I was in high school, my father had all these drug samples around. They were in his office drawer, and we could just go in and take them by the handful. There were Dexedrines and things like that, and at one point in high school I would take them and write papers like crazy, which probably had something to do with my being such an over-achieving student.

My parents never really faced up to my drug use in any serious way. They seem to have decided that drugs were a prevalent problem and that they would have to live with it, and then they forgot about it as a real concern, though interestingly enough they did use it as a convenient explanation for everything. They attributed a lot to drugs. If we were angry with them, it was because we were taking drugs. If we were upset or quiet or depressed, it was because we were taking drugs. We were constantly accused of taking drugs when we weren't, but whether they really believed that we were, or whether this was just some polite fiction, I don't know. They had all these drugs in their drawers, and it *certainly* never occurred to them that I might be taking those, except perhaps to give to my friends, which indeed I did. I gave drugs to my friends all the time, be-

go see a doctor?" "I asked why. I didn't know what they were talking about; I thought maybe it was my brain or something. My mother said, 'Ahem, well, to have your body examined.' I said 'What's the matter with my body?' They said, 'Well, you know, people do that before they get married.' Here I had *lived* with this guy for three years or so. Where had they been? What did they think I had been doing?"

cause I had them by the ton, and it just seemed right to share the wealth.

The funny thing was that at the high school I went to in Chicago my father was the disciplinarian or whatever they called him. If you had trouble in school, you were sent to my father. Everyone except me, of course; when I got in trouble for wearing short skirts, or when I got caught reading *Naked Lunch*, I was sent to the religion teacher and I got to discuss philosophy. But the other kids would have to go to my father and discuss their drug taking, which was really pretty funny since all the drugs had come from me, or ultimately from him."

One would expect psychotherapists to do better at dealing with the various childhood and adolescent problems that all parents eventually face. Indeed, with some types of problems their training and experience do give them an edge over their less well-informed nontherapist peers. When there are major traumas such as deaths of close relatives and family uprootings—circumstances that call mostly for patient understanding and for an awareness of potential problems and implications—they find themselves better prepared. Therapists know the protocols for dealing with the catastrophic and the unforeseen, and when in doubt they have highly competent colleagues whom they can call on for advice.

When it comes to developmental issues such as early sexuality, toilet training, and the changing affections and rivalries within the family, the therapist's training can be a help or a hindrance. In most instances described to me where training was seen as an advantage, it was so in a relatively passive way: it did not help do something, but rather reassured the parent that nothing need be done, that there was no cause for concern. It kept the parents from overreacting and occasionally helped them to arrive at a particularly apt way of explaining something to the child. These parents, in a sense, inadvertently put into practice Freud's idea that preventive analysis for children would be difficult or impossible and that one ought better to analyze the parents.

On the other hand, therapeutic knowledge can be misleading when dealing with such issues. It can foster a smug and undeserved sense of confidence, can incite the parent to intervene and short-circuit a perfectly normal developmental process, or it can lure the parent into perceiving significance where none is to be found. One analyst recounted the story of a colleague whose response when her four-year-old son got a small cut was, "The cut is going to get better, don't worry, *nothing will fall off your body*. Your ear is on, and your wee-wee is on. . . ." In her well-meaning efforts to soothe the castration anxiety she imagined he would go through, she made her son worry about something that had never occurred to him.

Another psychiatrist reported with embarrassment his own overly zealous efforts to be helpful. His family had recently moved across the country, and his seven-year-old son was separated from his grandmother. The grandmother came for a visit, and when she left the boy began moping around. "Then he developed a recrudescence of a sleep disturbance and started coming into our bedroom and was afraid of being alone in his room. I said to my wife, 'This is understandable. The child's had a lot of losses, and now having his grammy back and then losing her again must have stirred all kinds of things up.' I do think that's true, and I conveyed all this to my son in a way that he perceived as empathic and not intrusive. But my wife, who's not a psychiatrist, said, 'Well that's all fine and good, but you forget that in spite of our agreement, it was a week ago that you brought home *Alien,* and his nightmares and coming into our room also began when he peeked when he wasn't supposed to and saw that creature popping out of the spaceman's thorax.' "

Most of the crises and chronic problems that plague parents as their children grow up—sex, drugs, delinquency, smoking, drinking, popularity, and academic and athletic performance—less clearly involve therapeutic knowledge. Therapist parents are not being asked to undo something that has already been done wrong, to add the voice of reason or act as objective moderator. They are there as parents, to do the damage or the good in the first place, and they are dealing with the fluidity of day-to-day life rather than large and distinctive clinical problems. And as parents, psychotherapists are notorious for being exceptionally liberal and permissive with their children. By now this reputation has been significantly embellished in the interests of humor, but it unquestionably has firm foundations in fact.

Psychiatrist A. Wilmot Jacobsen relates a wonderful anecdote about Adolf Meyer, a famous early psychiatrist and a founder of the mental hygiene movement:

When I was in medical school after the first world war, the late great Adolf Meyer was my teacher. He was an awe inspiring person, and when five of my classmates were invited with me to dine at his home, we were on our very best behavior. As we sat stiffly in the living room before dinner, we could see through the open door into the dining room. There we beheld a table gleaming with rare crystal, finger bowls, priceless candelabra, flowers—quite a contrast to what we were accustomed to in our cheap boarding houses.

Suddenly the front door burst open and the daughter, about five years old, came running through the room. She was obviously angry, and ignored her father's suggestion to stop and meet the guests. As she passed into the dining room, the magnificent table setting must have affected her like a red rag to a bull. She grabbed the nearest end of the table cloth and kept on going. I still shudder as I recall the crash of glass and silver!

When the crash occurred complete silence fell over our small group. Then, as if nothing had happened, Dr. Meyer continued with the subject under discussion. There was never any mention of the episode. Mrs. Meyer, who was supervising arrangements in the kitchen, had restored the dining table to its pristine state by the time we walked in to the dining room.

I am sure the young lady received no punishment. Her father disapproved of this, and also of giving orders to children. Probably some time later there was a family discussion and it was pointed out that such behavior was ill advised.[1]

This ludicrously exaggerated form of genteel hands-off child rearing has gone somewhat out of fashion in recent years, as psychotherapists have come to recognize the drawbacks of setting no limits at all. Still, therapists do have a strong and widely acknowledged tendency to abstain from action, to examine things, to think and talk about things, to let each individual make his own responsible decision as best it might suit him rather than to impose arbitrary rules. "If I have any generalization about analysts' children," says psychoanalyst Henriette Klein, "it is that they are overindulged. Theoretically analysts should know better. They have had more advantages and a longer period of training than anyone else. When you consider the discipline that analysts go through in their own formation, it is ironic that they have so little in their families."[2]

Everett Dulit, a child psychiatrist who believes that in general there is no more than a stylistic coloration to life as the child of a psychiatrist, agrees nonetheless that in the area of discipline there may be meaningful differences. Therapist parents tend not to be very decisive or clear about the consequences of the child's acts, something which has both positive and negative aspects. Up to a point, it is constructive not to take everything purely at face value, to consider all the complex issues that may be involved, and to reach a more profound resolution of problems:

> It is for the better that they recognize that the spirit of what the child did wrong counts more than the letter, and that they sometimes get involved in psychological discussions about the child's missteps rather than simply saying "That's wrong. You're punished." But it is also for the worse, because these conversations often end up being *just* talk, endless discussions with a curious floaty quality, with no action, no reaction, no consequences. There is a lack of the productive clash of strong emotions between parent and child, which can be especially problematic in the years around five to eight, and again around thirteen to sixteen. While sometimes discussion is very useful, there really are times when you can't just keep backing off into endless, endless talk, and you have to say "That's wrong, you're punished, that's it."[3]

Most often, psychotherapists are not simply amoral libertines whose permissiveness toward their children reflects the wild abandon of their own lives.* Their permissiveness rarely takes the form of an active philosophy that no standards *ought* to exist. Rather they question the forcible imposition of arbitrary values and emphasize, or overemphasize, the child's own sense of responsibility. So large a part of adults' problems stems from the distorted values and worries forced upon them as children that it seems preferable to give their children gentle guidance and lead them to learn the reasons rather than to blindly obey meaningless rules. The parents may or may not have encountered the particular problem at issue in the course of their therapeutic practice, but their job has given them a way of dealing with things and approaching new issues, and they try to pass on this rational approach to their children as well: think about it, consider the consequences, it's ultimately your life and you're not going to have parents watching over you forever. We trust you, go ahead and decide for yourself.

---

* There are, of course, exceptions. One businessman in his thirties, who does not drink and has never used drugs, had a psychiatrist father who used every kind of drug, drank too much and kept a flask in his office, and who had immersed himself in the counterculture of the sixties: "One of my father's most disingenuous arguments was: What a great sacrifice he had made to *feign* radicalism for all those years, at great personal sacrifice to his naturally conservative self, so that his sons could rebel against this and all be successful, straight professionals. Perhaps it worked."

This is, at any rate, the rationalization that is provided for the therapist-parent's policy of noninterference, though in reality, within the context of the whole of their lives, it often rings false. Psychotherapists, for example, tend to be very enlightened about sex—they are more or less forced to be by the nature of their jobs—but in their personal lives they may be quite inhibited.* Many PsyKs envy the earthy world of their friends' families, where people take pleasure in one another's company, even pleasure in quarreling, and can demonstrate real affection. In contrast, their own family lives are often stilted and dry. A PsyK in her fifties commented that sex was really a funny topic. "My parents were as liberal as anyone could be: 'Sleep with anyone you want, at any age,' they said, as a result of which I didn't lose my virginity until I was twenty-one.† They were always very open, but there was some sense in which the subject was a fraud. I think that kids just seeing their parents put their arms around each other or kiss each other gives a message about sexuality, but my parents never touched one another."

Somewhat similarly, from the son of a psychoanalyst:

In the field of sex, there's no doubt that my father's point of view was very enlightened. I mean, he would actually tell me things like, "Go out and have some sex." "Why don't you go in the car and lay someone?" I would tell this to my friends, because I was rather proud of this point of view. Most parents— well, I don't know what most parents did, but my father would say, "No, sex is great." From that point of view he was very enlightened. He would try and bring knowledge from the office into our discussions of my problems, and would couch things in terms that were familiar to him from the way that he dealt with those things all day long. But I don't think I perceived any greater perception or ability to deal with me. I don't think he was any more successful at it than anyone else. Somehow I thought he was a bit less successful, and that is largely a function of him as a person. It is not that analysis made him that way, but

---

* Freud thought that sexual enlightenment was preferable to ignorance, and that many problems of people's later lives stemmed from misapprehensions of sexuality or from early notions that tainted the idea of sexuality not with feelings of tenderness and love but of secretiveness, wrongdoing, and the forbidden. According to Edward Hitschmann, Freud lightly remarked that the chief problem with masturbation is "that one must know how to do it well," though Freud's son Oliver told an interviewer that his father had counseled him against masturbation, and that he had found their discussion of the subject upsetting.[4]

† Another woman remarked that it was very hard on her not to have a curfew, and she used to lie and tell boyfriends her parents were very rigid and insisted that she be in by 10 P.M., just so she would have an excuse to go home.

just that analysis didn't make him any other way. My father was unhappy. He had an unhappy childhood, and he remained an unhappy person all his life. He is a rather secretive, noncommunicative person. I grew up very much on my own. And the fact that I was *never* told what time to be home, and that he was very open in his attitudes about sex, about marijuana, about all sorts of things that drive other parents crazy—that enlightenment was not really enlightenment due to the fact that he was an analyst who had a greater, more worldly perception of things, it was more a function of who he was. And who he was was a hands-off person; hands-off with his son, hands-off everyone. His unhappiness made it difficult for him to deal with his own problems or anyone else's problems, or to deal with people, period. I love him, I still do, he's a wonderful father in many respects. He is someone you can easily respect; that kind of distance creates an aura of respectability. But he is not someone I was ever very close to.

He once told me, "Well, if we were to do things over again we might do it differently, we might not have let you go on your own so much." And I remember thinking at the time—I didn't say it to him, but I thought to myself, "Gee, I can't imagine that that was a conscious decision. I can't imagine him saying to my mother, 'Hey, why don't we just let him go off as he wants to? Push him every now and then when we think he should be pushed, but generally let him find his own way in the world.' " I can't *imagine* that was a conscious decision. I think that remark betrayed an apology of some sort, but one that was false at the base.

A number of PsyKs have complained that their therapist-parent simply never wanted to hear about their problems and insisted that they should work things out for themselves. It was not simply, as is sometimes suggested, that after a hard day at the office listening to real catastrophes the parents had little interest in paltry domestic concerns, though it is true that this plays a small part. They might wish to know a great deal about what was going on with the child, and might like to discuss problems to excess in a detached intellectual manner, but when the child was feeling hurt and uncomfortable, the parent was uncomfortable as well, and shied away.

Says the daughter of a psychiatrist and social worker:

My parents only dealt with things when they really came up and confronted them directly. The sense that I've gotten, now that I have some distance from it, is that they really didn't want to know what we were doing, and that as long as we were functioning okay, and keeping up a respectable image, and not drawing attention to ourselves, that we could do whatever we wanted to do. All of us did a lot of drugs, and they *really* made it clear that they didn't want to know about it; it was okay if we were going to do it, as long as they didn't know, as long as they didn't *have to* disapprove. Once someone told my parents that I was doing drugs, and then they were forced to sit down with me and say that it was not the thing to be doing, but when I tried to say "Be realistic, I am going to do this, and it doesn't seem to be hurting me any," they couldn't bring themselves to give enough to discuss it. They wanted me to say "Okay, I won't do it anymore," and then keep it from them. Which is what I ended up doing a lot. Their whole attitude just begged us not to tell them things and to spare them the harsh realities of dealing with their kids' problems.

Much of the psychotherapists' liberality is in fact a convenient and attractive masquerade disguising an abdication of parental responsibility. Through their professional habits they have come to regard the emotions, sexuality, and questions of identity and self-worth that make them personally uncomfortable with clinical interest and dispassionate ease. They become observers rather than participants, in both their practice and their family lives, and are placed in the attractive position of exercising authority without having to accept full responsibility.

One of the rewarding aspects of psychotherapy for some people is the fact that patients are independent adults who lead and accept responsibility for their own lives and come to therapists only about relatively specific problems. Like back-seat drivers, the therapists who are so inclined have the gratification of giving gratuitous advice without the personal consequences. In their own lives, they do not want to make decisions and face painful emotional realities, and they shy away from making decisions for their children. Instead they relegate their children to a position very similar to that of a patient or to that of another adult. Through a curious psychological reverse logic they say to themselves that if they treat their children like adults, then they are adults, and if they are adults, they do not need parental guidance.

Analyst Herbert Strean describes this phenomenon in a form more easily tied to the narcissistic parent-child relationship. Strean, who has had many therapists and PsyKs as patients, observes that "a person who becomes a therapist, I think, is very hungry to be parented himself or herself. Maybe unconsciously he turns his son or daughter into a bit of a parent, and he or she becomes the child." It is difficult to effect quite this transformation in practice, so the form that it takes instead is for the parent to be unusually friendly with the child. They tend to be pals and get along as equals in a seemingly mature relationship where neither is asked to assume responsibility for the other. "I think this often shows a certain reluctance to being a full parent. If you are my father, I expect you to be different from my pal. I expect certain things from you as a father. I expect to rely on you in ways that I do not expect to rely on a friend or pal. And I have a feeling, at least with the parents I've worked with who are therapists, that there was a subtle abdication of the role."[5]

In some circumstances it is very difficult to maintain this pretense and to abdicate all responsibility. If the children continue to demand attention or help, or get into trouble too glaring to ignore, many therapist parents almost visibly transform themselves into different people, into psychotherapists who can discuss the problem clinically. I have heard of many cases where, when there was a home office, the parent would say, "All right, let's go into my office and talk about it." They adjourned to the office, behind a soundproofed, closed door, away from the normal life of the family, and the parent slipped into the accustomed, comfortable role of the psychotherapist, insulated by his professionalism, dealing with someone else's problem.

Often this trait manifests itself in terms of the types of problems the therapist parent can deal with. Curiously, small problems may be unbearable, whereas larger ones cross the threshold into something within the clinical domain. One analyst's son who had running feuds with his father says:

He was not a warm person as a father, and we were never close or comfortable with each other. When I was seventeen or eighteen, I got to the point where I could admit to him that I was doing things that were wrong, but it was not because I had come to have faith and trust in my father, but rather that I recognized it was an effective way of bothering him. "Oh, I'm going out to get drunk tonight. So long." And I would go out and get drunk, come back and get sick, and get thrown out of the house.

He had a terrible temper, and sometimes he would completely lose control. I think I almost hit him once. He would yell and scream and become kind of inarticulate. Later, when I was seventeen or eighteen—I was back from college, having been thrown out for malfeasance—our fights would occasionally spill over into the street, which was unusual for our dignified neighborhood. The neighbors, happily, were discreet; people didn't open the windows and hang out to watch. I sound flippant about it now, but I remember being shocked at my father *not* having control. That was the scary part of it: that whatever I was doing wrong must be *terribly* important, because one doesn't like to get like this. Maintaining control was extremely important to him, and if he could avoid flipping out he would. But he couldn't control it, and he would get this way over minor things, like a D in algebra, coming home drunk, or losing a baseball glove. He simply could not handle my problems, because he couldn't handle himself.

With major problems he was better. I got into trouble one time with the police. I had some friends who were trying hard to get into trouble and who finally managed to do it. I think one of my father's fixed ideas was that other people had some strange desire to get me in trouble, and that there were all of these people lurking around who wanted to lead me astray. He didn't say why. Perhaps there was a bounty? So these friends of mine stole a safe from a supermarket and brought it down to our house at the seashore. When that hit the papers it was a source of real embarrassment: "Young X, son of prominent analyst . . ." You'd think that that would have floored my father, but I don't remember catching any serious shit about it. This was a different situation. It was "Here we have a major problem, let's deal with it." It was not like failing algebra or something, it was a problem on a level he knew how to handle.

What are the effects on the child of having a parent who is very permissive and who abdicates responsibility and pushes it off on the child? Often these PsyKs seem just fine from the outside. Their classmates envy them for having such an easygoing and friendly relationship with their wonderful, enlightened parents. Adults find them responsible and mature and able to discuss the reasons for things, which is, of course, precisely the way they have been bred to be. They themselves may feel privileged for a time to enjoy such personal freedom and the admiration of others, but ultimately they often do not feel so fortunate.

PsyKs are encouraged to accept responsibility, but as it turns out, they may in many ways be particularly ill-equipped to do so. They are

asked to make decisions at the same time that they learn the therapeutic caveat that decisions are often suspect because guided by
unknown unconscious motives. Their parents furnish them with few
external standards by which to gauge whether or not a decision was
correct, because psychotherapists so often eschew any absolute definition of morality; there is no fixed right and wrong with which one
can comply or against which one can rebel. Discussing the problems
of permissiveness, psychoanalyst Jules Glenn comments that one of
the things a relatively strict upbringing accomplishes is to give the
child a conscience:

> If, on the other hand, the child thinks that his parents are saying
> you can do any old thing you want, then his conscience becomes
> weaker. The conscience is what tells you you *shouldn't* do any-
> thing you want, and in fact you shouldn't even *think* anything
> you want. But psychologically enlightened parents sometimes try
> to make overly subtle distinctions. They say, "It's okay for you to
> be angry, but you're not allowed to hit anybody." That makes a
> certain sense, and it is good to be aware of it, and if a parent
> says it in moderation it is not going to have any ill effect, but if
> that is a persistent way of dealing with the child, then you are
> trying to fine tune the degree of aggression and the expression of
> aggression in a way that is simply beyond the abilities of a
> child.[6]

The PsyK who has been taught the various intellectual and psychological considerations, and the correct way to manipulate and
discuss them, must make up his own mind, then try to decide whether
he has come to the right decision. It has more the quality of an
abstract debate than of a conviction hard-won through personal experience. Often what they really learn is merely a method of making
a good show of responsibility: how to rationalize, how to use their
considerable intellectual and linguistic skills to persuade others—and
to some extent, at some times, themselves—that they have made a
mature and self-motivated decision.

Freedom and responsibility can be tremendous burdens at an early
age, a complaint that comes up with great frequency during interviews.

Says the schoolteacher son of an orthodox analyst:

> My father never gave us opinions on anything. He was always
> listening, never participating, and he never spoke unless he was
> spoken to. My brother and I learned very early that we had to

decide for ourselves. We had to make our own choices. We had a lot of responsibilities that our friends didn't have, and in that sense I think we had to grow up too soon. If our friends didn't know what to do, they would ask their parents. Every time we asked our mother, she said, "Well, see what your father says." *She* didn't give opinions, because if she said, "I think you should do this," and we did it, and my father found out, then he would get on her back: "Well why did you tell them to do that?" She would get analyzed before we would get analyzed, and we would get analyzed for doing the wrong things. If we asked him, "What should we do?" he would say, "Well what do you think you should do?"—you know, the standard analytic thing: always answer questions with questions. It was only if we decided to do the *wrong* thing that he would step in and try to find out what had motivated us to do it.

The thirty-year-old son of a psychoanalyst and a clinical social worker is more explicit and emphatic about the unpleasant effects of his parents' insistence on treating their children like adults:

My parents incorporated a lot of their psychological professional beliefs into bringing us kids up, such as having us make as many decisions on our own as possible at as early an age as possible. I think they thought this would make us into sturdier people. I believe they were trying to strengthen the ego, to encourage us to develop as strongly and independently of parental guidance as possible, emphasizing—or overemphasizing—the ego above the superego. But in the end it led to a great deal of guilt and anxiety. A lot of it was wrong. They should not have done it. I think that it was too much for us to make those kinds of decisions, and I blame them for it. I would never raise my kids that way, and my sister has not, she's gone very far towards the other extreme.

An example? Well, the ones that come to mind are all very small, which is part of the point. A simple one is something like smoking cigarettes. If I was caught smoking cigarettes, it would be, "Well, what do you think about whether you should be smoking?" I had to think about it maturely, in the big context, over years, with all its implications, when I was really just a ten-year-old sneaking a smoke in the alley. It wasn't a severe reprimand and just leave it at that, which I think might have been very effective. If there had been just external guilt applied to me as a child, I think I would have reacted and would have felt it externally, and that would have been it. I would have gone on and decided for myself whether it was worth it to go through that kind of reprimand or whack on the butt in exchange for the benefits that I got from smoking. But instead, there wasn't a reprimand. It was: you decide for yourself. They kind of loaded all this information about what might happen onto me and then backed down and left me up there to decide for myself. The decision became very different, and it became a much *larger* issue than it should have been.

The effect of all that was and still is excessive guilt and anxiety related to minor things. I think I tend to dwell on things more than I should. I think it takes away a lot of spontaneity and lightheartedness. I tend to say "What if this?" "What if that?" It causes vacillation.

I think, really, that I was robbed of a childhood, because by the time I became aware of the difference between myself and external surroundings, it very quickly became obvious to me that I had to make the decisions, and it was a very lonely, awesome task, as opposed to having parents who protected me, who made decisions for me so that I could just frolic around in a Garden of Eden free from responsibilities for the first part of my life.

Another effect of the parent's permissiveness and reliance on the child's own sense of responsibility can be, paradoxically, to hold the child in tighter check and undermine his independence. Kohut very precisely if somewhat cryptically describes the case of certain narcissistic parents who cannot say no to their children's demands. He dismisses the most obvious psychological explanation, that these are people who cannot stand frustration themselves and therefore do not dare to frustrate their children, and says, on the basis of his own clinical experience with such cases, that there is a very different cause:

[T]here are . . . parents who cannot say "no" because they are afraid of the frustrated child's anger as the manifestation of the fact that the child's self is beginning, phase-appropriately, to become separated from the self of the adult, to become an independent center of initiative. The predicament of such parents, in other words, does not concern conflicts about frustrating the child's drive-wishes; nor are they avoiding the frustrated child's anger as the feared expression of a dangerous drive—they are reluctant to give up the merger-enmeshment with the child whom they, phase-inappropriately, because of the defective condition of their own self, still need to retain as part of their own self.[7]

In other words the parents' permissiveness is another unconscious manipulative method to keep the children within the parents' domain, where they will continue to provide the mirroring and adoration and vicarious sustenance that the parent requires. If the children are given nothing to rebel against, then they will not rebel and consequently will not become independent and abandon the parent. It is almost a bribe—not quite so overt, and not tendered in expectation of very clear-cut returns, but part and parcel of the pattern of intrusiveness and usurpation by which the parents have always shared more of the children's lives than is strictly advisable. They have intruded, like a virus, more of their own way of thinking and acting into their children's own way of living.

The children often respond to this without knowing it. To them, as to everyone else, it may seem that they enjoy unlimited freedom and have a wonderfully mature relationship with their parents. Nonetheless, when looked at more closely, they do not take extraordinary license. At heart most of them are good kids, since at the same time that the parents have given complete liberty and trust, they have made known their expectation that this trust will be upheld, and the children internalize this daunting expectation even more than they might the dictates of a fixed law. It is an effective means that coaxes rather than coerces into line. The children may live in a permissive atmosphere, but they conduct themselves responsibly, and not wholly from their own freely exercised recognition of the personal rewards of responsibility.

In extreme cases, the PsyK's obedience in order to protect the vulnerable parent can be clear. "I *dreaded* hurting my father," says the son of an analyst whose disappointment was very close to the surface. "That was the thing that could always bring me up short. I hope to God I never do that with my kids. If I withheld anything or did anything that didn't meet his expectations, he didn't yell at me, he didn't scold me, but it was as though I was withholding my love from him, as though I was hurting him. And his being hurt scared me. It was too heavy a thing for me as a kid. Between adults, that's one thing, you can deal with it, but a *kid*, how does a kid deal with hurting his father?"

More often the operative factors keeping the child in line are better obscured within the delightful, close, mature relationships that prevail within the family. The issues of responsibility and control may not become clear until much later, if ever.

Says the daughter of a psychiatrist:

My parents are the most liberal of any parents I've ever heard about. And I think, for me, it worked out very well, because I happen to be a very self-disciplined person. But the down side of them being so unbelievably liberal was that they did want to know a lot about what was happening, they wanted us to be able to tell them if we were thinking of doing something that was probably going to be outside the boundaries. They wanted us to be able to tell them as though they were our analysts, so we *should* be able to tell them, not as though they were our parents and we ought to feel uncomfortable. An example of this overly analytic approach to something was that they sat me down when I was about fourteen and had a serious discussion about sex. They told me that if I was ever interested in "sexual intercourse" —which was the only word my father ever used, because he always used the proper clinical term for such things—if I was ever interested in sexual intercourse I should tell them first, and they would take me to a gynecologist to make sure that I had appropriate birth control.

When you think about it now, fourteen seems a little young. It certainly was for me, at any rate; I hadn't given them any indication that sex was on my mind, and it wasn't. They were very detached about it: the issue was not moral, although he did say "If you ever should fall in love with somebody and want to have sexual intercourse with this person . . ." It was clearly just that they didn't want me to get pregnant. It was very practical. There weren't any moral overtones about it at all. And then if we were ever going to smoke dope, too—to smoke marijuana, I mean—if we ever thought of smoking marijuana then we should tell him first, and he would discuss with us whether or not it was a good idea and what the possible consequences could be.

It was always presented as though the eventual choice was your own, whether to indulge or not in whatever it was, but that you had to tell him—well, you didn't *have* to, you were strongly encouraged and expected to tell him—first. It made everything unbelievably sanitized and analytical and documented. That was very strange, and when I tell people they think that it's very bizarre. I think the real down side of that candidness and rational discussion is that it takes away any kind of spontaneity or the ability to rebel. You *couldn't* really rebel: the things available to rebel against were quite minimal. It's hard for me even now to be much more spontaneous about things, because, growing up, from the time when we were very young, I was told: "If you think of doing this, tell me and I'll discuss the consequences with you." Smoking dope wasn't just, geez, go have a fun time, but there were *serious* consequences. Screwing around with somebody, the consequence was becoming pregnant, and that was bad. All of that is true, of course, and I'm sure lots of parents tell their kids not to do them or to be careful, but with me the issue was *planning ahead*. The whole notion of planning ahead has made it very difficult to be spontaneous. My father is very rigid in his thinking, and being in control is a real big number, as I think it is with most psychiatrists. He certainly made it very clear to us how important it was to be in control at all times. Once you were out of control it was a very bad thing. And knowing and understanding and thinking things through was the way to stay in control.

Things really did work out according to plan, too. It's pretty amazing, but the first time I was going to sleep with a boy, when I was about seventeen, I went to my father and told him. The boy was somebody my family knew, a nice kid, good student, and I said, "Well, we've decided it's about time, and you said I should come talk to you and here I am." He asked whether I was sure that I wanted to do it and I said I was, and it was okay. He said, "You and your mother go and make an appointment with the doctor," and that was it. There was no confession, there was no discussion after that. The same when I wanted to smoke dope for the first time. I said "You asked me to tell you, so I'll tell you." It was no big deal.

Amidst the permissiveness and apparent unbounded trust there was a cold, hard, scarcely perceptible but extremely powerful set of expectations and rules. This woman felt free as a child and adolescent, but she subsequently grew disillusioned and embittered, because she gradually recognized that she had been manipulated into doing what was expected, and retrospectively feels that the liberty she enjoyed was not the liberty that really mattered, and that all along she had been kept well under control. Amidst her mature freedom she was always accountable for her actions. Knowing that she could talk of anything she did made it somehow essential that she never do or think of things that she would not be able to talk about.

This form of manipulation is particularly debilitating in the long run. To be given responsibility without genuine authority undermines a person's sense of self-confidence and removes precisely those feelings of power and of being in control that ultimately make responsibility bearable and rewarding. A child may be oppressed by a domineering parent who allows him no authority at all, but this child, at least, is not deceived, and will later be in a fine position to rebel and to establish himself in opposition to his parent. The PsyK who is assured that he has complete responsibility but who secretly lacks any meaningful authority, since expectation hovers above him and draws him to it, is crippled in his sense of self. He has a harder time rebelling, because there is nothing one can put one's finger on that incites one to rebellion.

In many ways the worst aspect of being given responsibility by a friendly but abdicating parent is the simple feeling of abandonment and betrayal that some PsyKs may feel later in life. It can be lonely and frightening for a child to be told that he has responsibility for himself. Yet having been given credit for maturity and responsibility by the parent, it is personally demeaning, and not always even possible, to then go to the parent saying, no, I am not mature, I'm upset and need help. Instead, one bravely tries to work things out on one's own, bluffing one's way through and then rationalizing the bluff, feeling somewhat puzzled and neglected by the parent's inactivity. As David Reiser remarked, it is not good that the parent seem all-knowing and all-understanding, or even all-trusting. It is important for the child to see that some things are not known and that the parent is trying. It even sets an encouraging example to show the child that one really can try and fail, and need not make the perfectly correct decision every time. Whether the parent does the right thing or not is certainly important, but in a significant way right and wrong are secondary to whether or not one cares. At times PsyKs are obliged to act out excessively to get an honest response. One analyst's son says:

My father was against corporal punishment. He hit me only once, and I deserved it, I provoked it, I *begged* him to do it, I told him that he wouldn't do it and that he was afraid to do it and that he was a pussy—I called him every name in the book, and finally he hauled off and smacked me. Of course I ran upstairs completely humiliated and crying in quite a dramatic way.

But then I made him feel so guilty that he later apologized. Looking back, I deserved it, and he should never, ever have apologized. He should have told me I deserved it.

A thirty-five-year-old musician and child of two therapists, who is now bitter about the lack of guidance and discipline he received, says:

I started smoking grass when I was about sixteen and got really heavily into it. I was dealing for a while in high school. My father had died by then, but my mother knew about it, yet she didn't say a word. She just tried to pretend, to me, that she didn't know it was going on, even though I knew that she knew, and she must have known that I knew. She found a whole lot of my grass in the house once and never mentioned it. Later she told me she had flushed it down the toilet. Even later I learned that she had really kept some and tried a bit with her friends.

A while after I started doing grass somebody offered to sell me some pills—Seconals or some other kind of downers. It had never occurred to me before that, but immediately I thought, "Shit, I don't have to buy this stuff, there's a whole cabinet full of it in my house." That's how I got started on stronger stuff. I never bought drugs in my life, ever. Either people gave them to me or I got them from my father's office. My father used to buy drugs by the truckload, and of course there were all those samples, and after he died they just stayed in his office. I would swipe the keys and go down and take them whenever I wanted. I remember there was a bottle of a thousand Methedrine pills. They all went. There were dozens of smaller bottles of Dexedrine and Benzedrine. I took them, too. I didn't like downers, so I gave them all away, which made me a lot of friends who in turn gave me drugs that I did like. And there were hundreds and hundreds of those little sample packs of amphetamines—six in a pack, with one pill showing through a little cellophane window. I'd take five and just leave the one in the window, but then after a few months, when nobody said anything, I would go back and take those as well. It should have been impossible not to notice all those pills disappearing, but I never heard a word. In retrospect I really hold that against my mother. I came damn near killing myself, and she scarcely said a word, even though she had to know something was going on. I looked like hell, lost twenty pounds, stayed out for days on end, didn't eat, rarely went to school, and at one point I was so strung out that I was hallucinating and could barely make sense. She maintained that she always trusted my judgment, and as it turned out she was right, I was very strong, and ultimately very sensible, and I probably came out of it a better person in some ways, but I will never believe that she really *knew* that she could trust me. I think she just said that as a way to cover up the fact that she didn't know what to do and so she was going to hide and do nothing at all, and keep telling me that she trusted me as some way to beg me to be careful.

One time, narcotics agents came to my house because a relative of a person who was supplying some of the grass I was dealing tipped off the police. They arrived at this huge impressive house with a search warrant for every kind of drug under the sun and I think they were a little overawed. They didn't know what to do. They certainly weren't going to search the entire house, which would have taken weeks, so they contented themselves with trashing my bedroom and insulting me and looking like they dearly wanted to knock me around a little bit. The grass was hidden down in the basement, so the only thing they found was a hash pipe belt buckle I used to wear all the time and which reeked of hash. They confiscated that. The funny thing was that when they were leaving they had the secretary call my mother out of her office, where she was seeing a patient, and they gave her some simple-minded cop crap like, "We want you to know, Dr. R., that we're here to help people. If you ever have any trouble with your son, don't hesitate to call us and we'll come right over and give you a hand. People think all we do is arrest people, but we really are here to help." It was pretty extraordinary stuff. My mother listened very politely and thanked them, but I could tell that she could scarcely keep from laughing. The fact that they were such ludicrous morons probably saved me from getting in more trouble with her—it appeared as a farce rather than as what it really was, namely two narcotics agents arriving at her house with a search warrant. Oh, the last shot was that I was really upset about them taking my belt buckle. I had taken good care of it and it was full of good resins and I didn't want to lose it. So I said, "But that's the only belt buckle I have. My pants will fall down!" And the narcs said, "Well, let that be a lesson to you." That was actually probably the sternest lesson I did get about drugs while I was growing up.

10

Therapists'
Kids
in Therapy

> You know, the New Testament
> would have you believe that it's
> the continuation of the Old
> Testament, but in reality the
> *Introductory Lectures on
> Psychoanalysis* is the continuation
> of the Old Testament.
>
> —AN ANALYST'S SON

In the early days of psychoanalysis, many analysts believed in prophylactic analyses, whose purpose was not to unravel existing neurotic entanglements, but to handle preemptively the potentially
traumatic events that dot the landscape of childhood, thus ensuring
that development would proceed with a hitherto inconceivable lack of
conflict, letting problems be solved before they arise.

Karen Horney was among the first to seek prophylactic analyses for
her children. Her eldest daughter refused to go, but her second
daughter, Marianne, was sent to Melanie Klein for analysis at the age
of eleven or twelve. The child analysis she went through at this very
early phase of Melanie Klein's professional development consisted
essentially of lying down and relating the events of the day. Occasionally Melanie Klein would make an interpretation, or equate some
mundane object or act with a sexual object or act, then she would
send the girl on her way with a few parting words of analytic wisdom.

At that time they didn't know anything about interpersonal
relationships, which hadn't been discovered yet; it all had to do
with the libido, which you were supposed to get straightened
out. It had nothing to do with real problems I may have had.

216

My parents didn't talk to Melanie. Melanie wasn't interested in talking to my parents. It really had very much nothing to do with anything. I was put on the couch and went through this meaningless procedure, which doesn't seem to have hurt, and which couldn't possibly help. Certainly there was no psycho*ana-lyzing* or psychologizing—none of what one finds nowadays: now anybody who has anything to do with psychiatry, psychoanalysis, or psychology tends to over-psychologize. But personally, I don't see where our lives were affected by analytic concepts.[1]

Horney's youngest daughter, Renate, was slightly affected, though not quite in the anticipated or hoped-for direction. She had experienced some difficulties at school and later with tutors, and in an attempt to resolve these problems she, too, was sent to Melanie Klein. She spent much of her time in analysis hiding under the couch with her hands over her ears so that she would not have to listen to Melanie Klein's interpretations. She did hear enough, however, to learn a few sexual words and phrases that she had not known before, and by way of sharing her new-found analytic knowledge she took to writing these words everywhere and sending obscene letters to some of the neighbors. This was the end of Renate's analysis.[2]

Ernest Jones, in a somewhat similar way, sent his eldest son Mervyn to Melanie Klein for analysis, though with almost imperceptible results. As Mervyn Jones records in his autobiography:

> I suspect that my father, who was championing Mrs. Klein against the opposition of others in the profession, seized the opportunity to demonstrate his faith in her by sending his son for treatment.* He recorded that the analysis was a success, but I have my doubts; I'm sure that I retained many neurotic traits, and any analyst who might have tackled me in later life would have had to start from scratch. Anyway, I have forgotten—or, I ought presumably to say, repressed—everything about my sessions with Mrs. Klein except the journey to her house and the look of her room. The analysts whom I know react to this confession with bewilderment, with disapproval, or sometimes with amusement.[3]

---

* The chief "other" when one speaks of Melanie Klein at this stage was, interestingly, Anna Freud. Sigmund Freud wrote a stern letter to Ernest Jones in 1927 objecting to his apparent support of Klein against Anna. "You are building up a campaign against Anna . . . claiming that she has not been deeply enough analysed. I have to call your attention to the fact that this kind of criticism is dangerous and [either "illegitimate" or "not allowed"]. Who can be analysed enough? I can re-assure you that Anna has been analysed much longer and deeper than you." Freud, of course, had analyzed Anna himself, though Ernest Jones may well not have known this.[4]

Sigmund Freud's view on the value of prophylactic analyses was less optimistic than that of his followers. As early as 1916 he expressed doubts about the practice on grounds that the causes of neuroses were too complex to permit their avoidance by simple means, and that if, for example, one took care to protect the child from supposedly pathogenic sexual experiences (meant in the broadest sense of the word) one ran the risk that, on the other hand, one's protectiveness might be too successful and might inculcate excessive sexual repression in the child, or that, conversely, through overprotection one might send the child into the world defenseless against the sexual demands encountered at puberty.[5] He reiterated and expanded his reservations in 1933, saying that psychoanalytic inoculation against childhood neuroses, which would necessitate a certain openness about sexuality and lack of repression, was simply impossible amidst life as we know it. As far as he was concerned, the best way to obtain the optimal balance between love for the child and appropriate authority without the intrusion of pathogenic factors was simply to do all that one reasonably could to make sure that the parents, teachers, and other important adults surrounding the child were free of pathology themselves.

The passion for prophylactic analyses rapidly died of its own accord as the early analysts' zeal was tempered by time and experience. No one, to my knowledge, would now think of sending a child deemed perfectly healthy and well balanced into psychotherapy for preventive purposes, and most people would consider it unethical of a therapist to accept into treatment someone who clearly did not need any. Nonetheless the vast majority of PsyKs do go into psychotherapy at one time or another—proof to some that they truly are screwy, but more plausibly merely an indication that in their families psychotherapy is perceived as something available to be used. It is the way that one deals with one's problems, and there is no stigma attached. Says one psychotherapist and PsyK, "I remember talking to [a famous analyst's daughter] when we were both over in London studying at Anna Freud's clinic, about having fathers who were analysts. We were laughing, because to us it was never 'Are you going into analysis?' it was just a question of 'When are you going into analysis?' It was understood all your life that you would go into analysis, either for personal growth or because you were crazy. Early on, you didn't know which it was."*

Another PsyK, the daughter of an analyst, says:

* A New York training analyst remarked that Anna Freud's clinic in Hampstead used to be jokingly regarded as "the finishing school for analysts' children."

My father was from the generation of Jews that did not believe in either religion or Judaism, so Freud was the religion. His picture hung in the front hall and he was God. All his theories were the basic tenets. One did not question them. I did not question them. My brother and I were sent, from birth onwards, for any problem at all—fear of the dark, wetting our beds—I feel I was in nonstop analysis. I think it was done with a perfectly good motive, too. My father believed in it. He thought no adult should be unanalyzed, he felt that it was part of one's education. It didn't occur to me at any point that there was another way to live, and in fact when I got married I thought "I have to start saving for my kids' analyses"—the way other people save for their kids' college educations.*

Psychotherapists, not surprisingly, paint a very rosy picture of their children's mental health. One could probably not find any other population that so proudly and insistently boasts of such pleasant, mature relationships with its children. They readily admit that some or all members of their families have been in therapy, and they do so with such disarming forthrightness as to convince anyone that they feel no shame at all, and that they have reached an enviable degree of confidence stemming from perfect clarity of perception and a selfless ambition to do what is best. If there are problems, they say, then one should seek help. This is what they would recommend to potential patients, and they will do no less for themselves and their families.

Some studies of PsyKs in therapy reach conclusions at variance with this cheerful self-image. One, by analyst Herbert Strean, offers a disturbing and rather grotesque collective portrait. From a review of only twelve children of analysts, psychologists, and social workers who had entered psychotherapy with him, Strean found surprising similarities in the nature of the problems and the patients' responses to treatment.† His description of a typical case is as follows:

The spouse who was the therapist made the first contact [by] phone, requesting a "special favor" or "a very personal request"

---

* Not all PsyKs follow the parental faith so piously. Says one man, "My father sometimes called himself Lutheran, but he was really anti-God, and properly speaking he was Freudian. My mother came from a Presbyterian background, and she became a Sullivanian. I don't know what that makes me—ambivalent, I suppose."

† The problems that Strean generally found in the children when they did come to therapy were obsessive character disorders or obsessive compulsive neuroses. The parents, he says, had been too much "friends" or "pals" with their children, indulged them too much and held them too close, and through this subtle psychological hold made the children feel guilty and depressed when they attempted to assert their independence.

which "could not be discussed over the phone." Frequently, the parent considered an office discussion as undesirable and preferred a luncheon meeting or social visit. In most cases, the parent only knew the therapist superficially but over the phone he was told that he, the therapist, "knew something about children" and that was why he was being consulted. When the therapist's office . . . was suggested as the locus for discussion of the "personal request," most parents balked and either wished to continue the discussion further over the phone or stated that the professional office was "inappropriate." When their preference for the place of the discussion was even superficially explored, in a couple of cases the therapist was told "to forget it" or "never mind, then."[6]

When most people consult a professional they expect and agree, of course, to do so in the professional's office. But even in subsequent meetings between therapist-parent and therapist, the parent continued to avoid the therapist's office, preferring to meet in his own house, his own office, or in a restaurant—in other words, in a place that was neutral, or where the parent had a certain advantage. When the parent broached the subject of his child, it was in an embarrassed, roundabout sort of way. While explaining the problem that called for psychotherapy, the tendency was to depersonalize the situation by lapsing into jargon: "he has a lot of repressed hostility and a powerful superego," "his Oedipal problem has never been resolved and his phobias certainly tell us that," or "his peer relations are impoverished but his object relations towards adults seem less narcissistic." The parent characteristically said that the child related well to him or her, but had problems with the spouse. In many cases the parent omitted altogether any mention of his or her own relationship with the child. In initial and any subsequent meetings, it proved peculiarly difficult to obtain much family history from the therapist parent, which severely hampered the treatment process.

Another researcher examining psychotherapy for the psychiatrist's family, based on experiences with six wives and five children of psychiatrists, mentions similar problems that therapists may have when family members need help, such as shame at having failed, and fear of revealing their secret shortcomings, such as alcoholism, to colleagues.[7] Undoubtedly these factors do enter into the picture; it is inconceivable that they would not. Among people I have interviewed, some therapists who feel guilty or embarrassed about exposure of their family secrets solve this problem simply by going out of their way to recommend, or to have a colleague recommend, someone whom they do not know and are unlikely ever to meet. Sometimes they appear intentionally to select someone to whom they feel superior—a psychiatrist or medical analyst, for instance, might choose a psychologist or clinical social worker—so that if necessary he can belittle and contradict the therapist's opinions when they seem in the least bit threatening.*

Others, however, purposely select close colleagues, particularly if their children are young, and then try to meddle in the therapy and monitor its progress with conspiratorial quasi-professional concern, something a good psychotherapist will staunchly resist. One PsyK never trusted his therapist because he believed, rightly or wrongly, that the therapist was in collusion with his father. He refused to discuss anything of importance, and spent endless long hours without uttering a word. "There were many sessions where we both sat silent the whole time. Of course, this was 1954, and he was a strict, old-school Freudian, so he never said anything anyway." When he was old enough to make the decision, he quit therapy. "Later on, when I chose a therapist on my own, the first thing I established was that he did not and would not ever have anything to do with my father."

When the parent is uncomfortable about therapy for the child, the ultimate danger seems to arise less from the fact that the parent delays seeking therapy or tries to undermine it, than from the fact that the child is consciously or unconsciously aware of this reluctance, which then keeps him from participating in treatment as unreservedly as he might. The child does not want to do anything that might hurt or upset his parent. For a PsyK raised in a house where confidentiality is highly regarded, where the anonymity and good name of the therapist-parent is of crucial importance, and where the parents often have such a strong overt or covert interest in their children behaving maturely and well, it can be difficult then to air all of the family's dirty laundry, even though it is not infrequently related to the cause of the problem.

One analyst's son, whose father was prominent in the regional analytic community, remembers precisely this problem:

> I was afraid at the time that my analyst would have a certain opinion of my father. I think I was probably very defensive

---

* Conversely, one psychoanalyst I interviewed had once treated the daughter of his own training analyst, who came to him some time after her father's death. This analyst found it upsetting to learn what an unstable person and horrible father his still-idealized analyst had been, and in retrospect he saw it had been a gross error on his part to accept this young woman into therapy, in large part because he would have preferred to maintain the untarnished image of his mentor.

about that. My father was considered a sort of a maverick, a little strange, not one of the gang. He had tried to develop some ideas that were not consistent with a very straight and narrow interpretation of analytic dogma as it was, and often he perceived hostility toward him on the part of his colleagues, which bugged him. Every time he gave a talk he would be bitter afterwards, and would say something to the effect that "Well, a lot of these guys, they just don't like me." Therefore I was afraid that the analyst I was seeing was going to be biased in his interpretations, biased because he thought my father was a nut because of his contributions to the professional literature, or eager to come up with an interpretation that would confirm, on psychological grounds, the low opinion I supposed he must have of my father's analytic concepts. Looking back, I think this guy must have been in a bit of a bind himself, and he handled it pretty well, because I would bring all that up, I would say "Do you think that my father is a nut?" and he would say, "No." I would say, "Well, what do you think of his work?" And he would either say, "I don't think that is really to the point," or else, "I think you are asking me that because you think I will be biased, but I am not." He would never answer the question; he would answer what was behind the question. I don't know what it meant in the context of the transference, but this was an issue that preoccupied me during much of therapy.

Despite these initial conflicts and reservations, however, I have found that by and large, no matter how uncomfortable the parents may feel, their tendency is not to shy away from therapy, at least not for very long, but to err in the opposite direction. They do just what they claim to do: they very willingly send their children—as well as their spouses—into therapy. If anything, they do so much too willingly. Faced with a minor problem, their immediate response is to seek objective professional help, often in circumstances where most less psychologically sophisticated people would confront the problem within the family or leave it to resolve itself with time.

As with so many therapeutic issues, it is difficult to say what is true and what is only rationalization. In the absence of any objective standards, amidst widely differing class and cultural views, one cannot really say with much confidence at what point it is an enlightened choice to seek therapy and when it is merely blind faith. True, there are problems one cannot resolve on one's own and, true, one should not feel ashamed of seeking help for them. Some of those others who do not resort to therapy have made a mistake. But when is help useful and when does it preempt a useful and ultimately fruitful struggle?

One psychiatrist's child, who is now an outspoken adversary of psychiatry, states:

My father banked psychologically on the integrity of the institution of which he was a member. When I did the usual little-boy things and later on the usual adolescent things, he sent me to a psychologist instead of handling the problem himself, and that, itself, was part of the problem. Instead of saying "Don't do it again," and then walloping me if I did do it again, he unravelled and analyzed and pulled it apart, and then tried to reassemble it in front of my mind so that, behold, I could marvel at this masterful construction and see the error of my ways revealed. That sort of thing, in reality, made you wonder where his authority was, because he would never really take a stand, and when things got bad enough he would just farm you out to somebody else. It took me a while to realize that he really loved us and cared about us, as well. He didn't get directly involved in anything with the family, because he had this barrier.

So I went to therapy for a couple of years, and the whole thing was rather a joke. This therapist had lots of toys, and I could never understand why I was going to this lady's house to play with all these shiny cars and blocks and things and to listen to her lecture me on my impulses. I really didn't get anything out of it. She wasn't the brightest lady in the world, I don't think, and she certainly was wedded to whatever it was that she was trained on, so she brought no flexibility or receptivity or creativity or humanity at all to the process. If anything, if I hadn't been as strong as I was it might have done me some harm, because she actually told me at one point that I had been very sick when I first came to see her, and that just was not true. Basically she had the same problem my father did. She also, by the way, had the most unruly son you ever met, and he would sometimes just barge in during a session and start making trouble. She couldn't get him to behave. Well, the proof of the pudding is in the eating.

Occasionally a therapist will use therapy as a way to push his child into line, as other parents might send theirs to a very tough summer camp. One man in his fifties, the son of an atypically harsh, quite well-known early analyst, was sent to a psychoanalyst to be hammered into shape.

My father always said, when I was younger, that I had to be disciplined. Not that I had to develop some discipline, but that I had to *be disciplined*. He said "If there were some way that I could put you in jail . . ." I'm not making this up, he probably thought about it, but decided there were too many legal obstacles for that, even with all his connections. He also diagnosed me at various times as insane, schizophrenic, homosexual, and he predicted that I would end up in prison or the electric chair. It's nice to be loved. When I was around twelve he sent me to a child analyst, because he had some theory that I went crazy on weekends. Don't ask. So he sent me to her to have me analytically straightened out, and his underlying assumption, of course, which was perfectly clear, was that he was right and I was wrong, and since analysis was his game I would come out of it disciplined just the way that he wanted. I actually lived with this woman, if you can believe it. She didn't have a very big apartment, but I lived in the maid's room for a while, and he paid her some immense fortune for her work. I don't know how long this went on, but this woman, this analyst, bless her, finally gave my father her official report, which was in essence: "This kid is in real trouble, but he is in no more trouble on the weekends than he is during the week. And the only thing I can figure out that is different on the weekends is that *you* are around." I could have told her that, but nobody asked me.

Many psychotherapists, under the benevolent guise of seeking help when it is needed, use psychotherapy as yet another way of abdicating their parental responsibility and avoiding the painful confrontation of problems. Unfortunately, this means that many problems are not resolved where they lie, which is within a context, quite probably the family. Instead the parent excuses himself, saying the problem is the child's to deal with in isolation. The decision to seek objective professional help, camouflaged as a recognition that families often get caught in patterns they cannot break out of themselves, comes instead from the parent's distrust of his own response and of his ability to handle the situation. Ultimately, though, the flight to therapy deprives both child and parent of a valuable opportunity to learn and grow. The parent misses the chance to learn from mistakes. For the child it may turn into a very ethereal experience that has little to do with anything.

Therapist parents are generally very reluctant to join their children in family therapy, even though most of them, if asked in their professional capacity, would readily say that there is often a need to treat everyone involved. It is one thing to send an adult into treatment to reconcile himself with childhood problems that lie irretrievably in the past; it is quite different to send a child into the same sort of therapy when the problems are still right there in the present, waiting for him when he goes home. Nor does psychotherapy necessarily help in these circumstances, because, unlike the reconciliation that takes place within the family, where someone wins and someone loses and the end result is there for better or worse, the therapeutic rumination does not lead to a change in the family. It is nondirective, and leads to a change in the child's perception of the situation of the family, but not to something that can always be taken back and applied. At times the child ends up almost as an intermediary carrying on an attenuated debate between psychotherapist and parent.

"Take a kid who's living with his parents and he's having some friction with them," says the son of two therapists, discussing the long and unpleasant experiences with therapy he has endured:

I don't think even the healthiest person will get along with his or her parents all the time. But this person who is having some kind of conflict is going to a psychiatrist, and the psychiatrist says of this conflict, in a supportive sort of way, "Your mom and dad are wrong. Don't think you're crazy, you're basically right." Fine. But then what's he supposed to do? He comes back home and says "Doctor So-and-So says you're wrong." And they say, "Ah, well, is *that* what he said?" or "Oh, no, you're only distorting what he said," and they browbeat the kid, who goes back to the therapist and says, "I told my parents that I disagreed with them about A, B, and C. That's what you told me, isn't it?" At which point the psychiatrist will say, "Shouldn't you have been a little more understanding of their point of view?" So the kid goes back to the parents and listens—all the while feeling smaller and smaller—to their point of view, and tries to do what they want or expect of him. This makes him highly uncomfortable, so he goes back to the psychiatrist, who says, "Can't you *assert* yourself more? You have to find your own value system." So the kid wanders out and looks at the stars, and is probably still circling around to this day. Ideally, what you want is to have a person *in* society. There's a lot of shit coming down, and he agrees with some of it, disagrees with some of it, and at night—this is what happens to most of us—you go home and replay it all and decide where you were right and where you were wrong. There's an end to it. It may or may not be the correct one, but it is an end.

Being sent into therapy can be alarming to a PsyK. For those who have been raised with the sense of belonging to an implied priest class that understands others and is somehow above them, it is an upsetting form of betrayal. They, like their parents, feel sympathy for other people's problems, are always delighted to listen and help, and can easily voice reassurances that there is no reason to be ashamed to seek help when one needs it. But they do not feel that way about themselves. Part of what was gratifying about being benevolent and helpful is that it buttressed their sense of self-esteem and made them feel superior in comparison. To be helped oneself is to lose this advantage. Many PsyKs have always been determined to solve their own problems on their own; several have commented on how alarming and deeply humiliating it was when their parents suddenly began treating *their* problem as something to be approached with the confidentiality and nonjudgmental compassion heretofore reserved for the parents' patients. Abruptly, the children feel expelled from their privileged position and turned into stigmatized mortals like the rest. Before, it was they who peered through the shrubbery or sneaked looks at the patients met in the elevator. Now they are the ones who need solicitous protection. Their parents hide their therapy from siblings and friends, and in sheer contrast with their loudly proclaimed sentiments, the parents now give the child every reason to feel that it is shameful.

"My brother was in analysis for three or four years before I ever heard about it," says the son of one analyst. "My parents were very secretive about it, and when it came out by accident, they told me never to mention it to him. Twenty years later, he still hasn't mentioned it to me, though we talk about all sorts of intimate things. When I went into analysis I felt very humiliated. I experienced it as a real abandonment, too. All of a sudden my father was saying, 'Well, you're one of them now; get along with you, boy.' "

It is also, in a very practical way, disconcerting for a PsyK to find his difficulties elevated to the level of needing help. One analyst's son first went into analysis at the age of six. His parents were separating and he was having bad dreams, was depressed, antisocial, and generally unhappy. Whether or not analysis was truly necessary, neither he nor anyone else can ascertain now. "I was unhappy, but I wasn't really that serious, I don't believe. I was never unmanageable. I never failed school. I was never paralyzed by depression. I think it really was that my father could afford it, and that he believed in it and thought that it could help me become more vigorous." Going to therapy, however, had an unfortunate side effect. He went to his analyst—"his analyst": at such an early age this had become an attribute of his life—two or three times a week for nine years. His family lived in the suburbs. His analyst's office was in the city. When he had an appointment, his mother picked him up after school, drove forty-five minutes into town, sat in the waiting room during his hour, then drove him home again. Later he took the train by himself, a roughly three-hour round-trip. His social life suffered from all this lost time. His self-image suffered even more from the fact that, though he didn't think there was really much wrong with him, his parents, in their infinite wisdom, seemed to find him so mentally unhealthy that these extraordinary measures were called for.

The method of using therapy in place of honest interaction can be merely an effective extension of techniques some therapist parents have always used in the family, employing their analytic knowledge and their dialectic skill to direct blame and criticism away from themselves and onto the other person. For the child who has suffered from that form of manipulation, therapy can serve, under the guise of truly objective intervention, to confirm the therapist-parent's position and further erode the child's sense of confidence and ability to assert himself. It is no longer just an argument between parent and child. The parents, by choosing a supposedly objective outsider who nonetheless shares the parents' own philosophical views, have brought in an ally who further contributes to some of their less fortunate effects on the child.

An analyst's daughter who works at a publishing house says:

My father used therapy as an excuse for not being a father. He would say "Go talk about it with your psychiatrist," and that was a cop-out. It also gave me the impression that I was boring and he simply had no interest in dealing with things that concerned me. It was a constant theme that therapy was supposed to fix your problems, not talking to your father. Confrontation with the person who fucked you up in the the first place was discouraged. You weren't allowed to say, "Dad, I'm really pissed at you," you had to work it out in a weird intellectual way with somebody else. But why? Why not stop what your parents were doing to you instead of going somewhere else to work it out in your head?

My psychiatrist, rather than helping with things, compounded the problem by her attitude. She invalidated my feelings; if I said I felt something she would say, "Oh, no you don't," or "You can't," because in her world construct what I thought was real did not correspond to her analytic notion of reality. She created these weird intellectual scenarios, and then made me feel that I had to hunt for them all the time, which was an incredibly inhibiting thing. If I was angry at someone, the question was "What am I feeling?" or "What's wrong with me?" If some guy didn't like me, I wasn't supposed to think, "Boy, this guy's a real jerk," or "Gee, you really led me on, you creep," it was always "I must like guys who don't like me back—that's my problem, it's my fault, and I'm really stupid." I felt like shit. The strange thing was that she would come up with a concept, and use the words, but it wouldn't correspond to what was really going on in my body. But who was I to know? I was biased, while she, and therapy, were objective.

When I was having bad problems with my father, instead of saying, "Boy, you must be really furious at him," she asked, "Do you have any sadistic impulses toward him?" as though there was something *wrong* with it. "Do you want to punish him?" implying that something was *wrong* with wanting to punish him. Hell, yes, of course I wanted to punish him; I wanted to throw him out the window! But there isn't anything wrong with that, as long as I didn't actually go ahead and do it. My psychiatrist would always invent these little scenarios for me, of what I was unconsciously doing. Why did I get home late? "You're trying to punish your mother. It's hostile." What was the hostile import of that? Or why was I seven minutes late getting to her office? "Because you don't want to be here." She was right about that one. She never wondered why I might not want to be there, or why I wouldn't want to go home, or why I should feel hostile toward my mother or father. The construction went: "You don't want to go home, which means you're hostile towards your mother. If you stop being hostile then she will like you better." I had to adapt. That was always it. Of course, I was the patient and they weren't, therefore it was I who had to get better.

Later I asserted myself and went to a different psychiatrist who was totally unlike my father. My father interpreted this egocentrically, as a rebellion against him, rather than as an autonomous move of desperation to escape from a doctrine that threatened my very existence. He called my action "the weapons of the weak," an incomparable phrase which both totally interprets my actions in terms of himself, and also implies that the weak need no weapons—he has the idea that emotional black-mail is something the weak perform unjustly all the time, passive-aggressive behavior, and so on, and automatically de-fends himself against such weapons rather than trying to distin-guish right from wrong and see clearly when a person is reacting against him rather than from some sort of neurotic need.

I began getting more and more enraged at my father because of the way he was reacting to my crisis, not understanding it in the least, denying it, using all kinds of amoral verbal acrobatics to justify his position, all the while he denied that he had any position but a purely objective one. I wanted confrontation. His only responses were to tell me that "I only wanted to apportion blame" (crime of crimes), "confrontation doesn't do anyone any good," or, of course, "work it out with your psychiatrist." I fi-nally realized that I was not really trying to win, but to achieve mutual understanding, and to the extent that I sought victory it was the victory of balance, of retribution through acknowledge-ment by another person that they have done you wrong. There was no spite or malice. My father couldn't perceive this simple human need; he called me controlling and provocative, not to mention narrow-minded (I could only see what I needed, and not how I made other people feel). But I finally stopped listen-ing and started looking. He was the one being narrow, he was driving me to desperation and then denying it, he was fighting through rigidity rather than raising his voice, he was not enter-ing into my feelings, and by God I *knew* it! I realized that this was a tack my parents had taken with me all my life, which was to fit unfair, manipulative words to a situation they could seem to describe, or blame me for not entering into his feelings when the person who was having the crisis was *me*, and the onus was on *him* to enter into my feelings.

I realized I would have to sever relations with him completely unless he would listen to me. I'm sure he saw this as an ultima-tum, another "weapon of the weak," I suppose, which of course it wasn't, it wasn't a punishment, but simply an unpleasant real-ity, and moreover a reality I would have done anything to avoid. I began to fight to get him into family therapy. This was somewhat like tugging a very large mule with spikes on his hooves—and an articulate mule, at that. I was provocative, "stubborn" (implying that I had no reason to be), narrow, etcetera. Luckily I got a friend of his to push from behind, a psychiatrist colleague who started recommending joint therapy as one way to go. So we went for a while, and it worked a little.

Some PsyKs readily accept the idea of personal therapy, some in a healthy, dispassionate way, others through a lingering childhood faith that psychotherapy is the answer to everything. They have internalized the parent-therapist's world view of analysis as a religion, of insight as the cure to all ills, and of therapy as the thing that finds the real meaning of life that lies under, or beyond, superficial impressions. In a paper on the problems of terminating analysis, Melitta Schmideberg, an English psychoanalyst and the daughter of Melanie Klein, includes an interesting description of what many narcissistic patients may imagine they will attain through analysis. Some PsyKs carry this idealization even farther.

> The patient's assumption that perfect bliss characterizes the condition of a fully analyzed person really expresses his longing for past happiness; an idealized memory of his babyhood is projected into the future. As a baby he was happy, had no need to work or to make decisions and was in fact all important, judging at least from the love and admiration his parents gave him. Analysis is for some patients an escape from life, a return to childhood. This type of patient lives almost literally only through and for the analysis. He would feel guilty if he were to deal with a difficulty or get over an emotional crisis without first having it analyzed. He prefers analysis to ordinary everyday methods just as, from guilt over his wish for independence, he had to prefer his parents to ordinary people or other children. He would like analysis to protect him against reality as his parents kept him from life; he wants to remain a baby and puts off any effort or unpleasant decision until the situation "has been fully analyzed," with the expectation that in the life after analysis work will never be an effort, there will be no need for renunciation and no decision will ever cost pain. To justify these absurd demands he proceeds to exaggerate his real difficulties in order to prove that they are neurotic and therefore curable. Everybody has to make a certain effort when learning something new or reacts with pain to frustration, but for such patients as these it is a narcissistic insult to be like others; it is so much more flattering to suffer from inhibitions and bizarre pathological reactions.[8]

When there is a sweet parental endorsement of therapy and problems that the PsyK carries throughout his life, it can easily lead the child to cultivate problems and treasure them: it may have reflected an element of reality when one analyst's son facetiously commented that of course shrinks' kids are crazy, but that "unlike other crazy people, we're proud of it." Jules Glenn relates his experience with a clinical psychologist who may inadvertently have encouraged symptoms in his son. The child was having nightmares, and the father was very interested in them. Every time the son had another nightmare, his father would sit down and ask him about it. "He would not make interpretations, but he was inordinately interested, and the result was that what would have been an ordinary series of nightmares became much more for the child. He seemed to develop the nightmares in order to please the father. My treatment consisted of advising the father not to get into these discussions, and soon after he stopped the nightmares went away."[9]

One woman whose parents were both psychotherapists was in therapy herself quite often through her life, and went into analysis when she left home for college. She found that she had intense and mixed feelings toward the process. It was difficult to form a proper transference because there was such a strong association between the analyst and her analyst father and because she already had so many fantasies about what took place in the consulting room. At the same time it was a very seductive situation. "A lot of my own therapy had to do with the fantasy of wanting to be a patient and wanting to be treated by my father, to gain some of the attention I felt I had not gotten as a child. I guess some of my fantasies were sexual: he spent all day in that room, one hour with each person who lay down the whole time, and nobody else could go in while they were there. I fantasized about what secrets he must have heard, and what power he had in terms of being able to help them when they were sick. Illness has always been a thing in my family, taking care of people, so I wanted to be a patient, and particularly a patient complicated by an illness. In my family there were certain benefits to being ill, you got attention, you could be dependent."

There is a great deal of truth in the old joke that the psychiatrist's child, when asked what he wanted to be when he grew up answered "a patient." This idea arises repeatedly in interviews in one form or another, not always as an overt wish to go into therapy. "My father was so intimately involved with other people's lives, and I wanted him to extend that awareness to mine," says a thirty-year-old musician. "And so, while I was grateful that he did not come home and interpret me, at the same time I wished that he would apply that intimate knowledge he talked about vis-à-vis someone else, to me."

Similarly a writer in his fifties, the son of two psychiatrists, says "I am very interested in secrecy, and I think that I am very interested in being a secret, though not in the sense of obscuring myself from view. To the contrary, I may be secretive precisely because I want attention. As far as I have figured it out without benefit of analysis, my parents shared a profession that investigated secrecy, and therefore, perhaps, there was some kind of Oedipal configuration that made me want either to become their secret, to become as interesting to them as their patients were, or to become like them in their secret profession."

Even without any apparent emotional attachment to therapy, the idealization of the therapeutic process can turn itself into an intellectual addiction. The son of an analyst reports:

> I've been in and out of therapy for many years, and it didn't occur to me until rather recently that you could get better. I had always thought of therapy as *what happens* when things are really going to shit, when you're getting down toward the bottom and you don't want to go down any further, and how to keep from sliding. But it had never occurred to me that it's possible to enter into psychotherapy, of one sort of another, to start, go through a course of treatment, and stop: "I'm better!" I only know of one person who said that he finished, and he was sent into therapy by the court after he killed someone in a car accident while driving a stolen car. He was obliged to go to a psychiatrist weekly for a couple of years, and when the stipulated term was up he didn't have to go anymore so he was done. That's the only case I know of nice, clean termination.
>
> This notion that therapy never ended must somehow have come from my father. In fact there's only one of his patients I have a clear impression of, and that was a patient he had forever. I think he had opened his practice with her. She would call frequently, first thing in the morning. Her code name in the family was "Whiney." I think at some point he discharged her, but his view of her was that no one could have cured this person. It was just not a possible task. But he had been working at it for ten years before he realized that, and finally, about another ten years afterwards, here he still was not knowing quite what to do.
>
> The first time I was sent to therapy was when I was sixteen or sixteen-and-a-half. I was going to college early, and before I went off my father sent me over to a colleague of his, I think just

to get a second opinion that I was all right. Something like an auto inspection. Unfortunately I didn't turn out quite right and got kicked out of school, and I guess there was a warranty on me so this fellow took me back. I think my father took the idea of me seeing a therapist as in a way removing responsibility from him. As long as I was seeing someone else, it was not necessary for him to try to straighten me out. Someone else was going to straighten me out for him. But I think that outside of the analytic community, getting thrown out of school is not normally considered psychopathology. It's normally considered a sign of being eighteen. Everybody gets thrown out of school. The college that I went to was particularly tough; it had an entering class of 130 and a graduating class of 30. People would make mistakes and get shot. But my father considered that this was pathology—and it is, it is psychopathology in the sense that being eighteen is a pathological state.

So let's see, college difficulties were the first thing that sent me into therapy. I think I was just *sent off* at those points when college was not working out. Then when I was in medical school and not enjoying it, not doing well. "Not well" equals "time to go and find someone to see." So I started myself at that time, and went to see another analyst. If I had been interested in staying in medical school, it was the wrong thing to do, I think. You don't get a behavioral response from a classical analyst. You know, if what you need is, "I got a big exam coming up in a month and I don't know any biochemistry," you're not going to learn any biochemistry from any four, eight, or twelve hours in a chair. I don't remember how long it lasted.

Then a few years later I started again. My business was not particularly prosperous, though I enjoyed it. We had a baby, and suddenly there wasn't *any* money coming in, my wife wasn't working, and there wasn't any food for months and months. I pretty much abandoned the business and went into the school-teaching trade, and a little while later, my wife said, "There's something wrong here. This is not going well. It's time for you to go back and get readjusted," because I suppose I had indoctrinated her as well with the idea that psychoanalysis was what I did when I was not right. We still didn't have any money. I was making maybe $9,000 a year and trying to pay off accumulated debts, but it still seemed worthwhile. A large part of that is not rational; part of it is that I've got the religion. I don't understand the religion, I don't *really* know what it's about, but I've got it. Very strange. The college that I went to, St. John's, in Annapolis, is a principally Platonic enterprise. What it's about is examination, is inquiry. All there are is questions: there aren't necessarily answers. It's a peculiarly powerful institution, whether it's good or bad. It warps people permanently. And the analytic notion is very similar. At least in my understanding of it, which is to question, examine, look at, turn it around, ask what's going on, how does this happen? It is terribly important. Somehow much more important than the answer. There really *isn't* an answer; there's no end to it. And if you accept that notion, you're stuck. You do examine all the time.

I don't know what the point of analysis is. Being *happy* is not the point. That is, the sixties notion of feeling good, of sex and drugs and rock and roll and New Mexico and the hog farm and all. Analysis *doesn't* feel good. It's not pleasant, not pleasant in the least. It's horrible. It's lovely sitting around talking to anybody: anybody *except* an analyst. And it's even OK talking to an analyst, if the meter's not running. But if the meter is running, and it's forty cents a word, it's really hard, it's a bad job. The point is not feeling good. The point is not being happy. I don't know what the point is, except that they are the last Platonists: the unexamined life is just not fuckin' worthwhile. And examining *life* is all it's about. Those people who go into the office are not—in the view I've always had—sick people. Maybe some of them are sick, but going into the office, by itself, does not indicate being sick. They're going for insight.

A great many PsyKs take the opposite approach, and though they may find the concepts of psychology and psychoanalysis intellectually stimulating, they either do not believe they could derive any benefits from therapy or they positively rebel against the infliction of something they have grown to find distasteful.

A filmmaker in his forties says:

I'm the son of an analyst and I never went to an analyst. There are various reasons, but number one among them is simply, Why should I pay *all that money*, over *all those years*, for a process that may yield results which are so intangible, so undefined. Absolutely not. I would obsess more about the process I was undergoing and the money I was spending on it than on any benefit I might derive.* And then my personality simply is not one

---

* Many PsyKs ridicule the easily self-serving analytic justification for charging high fees and refusing pro bono analytic patients on grounds that therapy is of no value to the patient unless

that can tolerate the idea of someone going deeply into my mind and motives in the classical sense. I need more feedback than that. I really do not like to talk about myself a great deal, and I certainly wasn't prepared to sit down for hours in a week and talk about myself and hope that I could come to some sort of conclusions with a little prodding from some disembodied voice behind me.

The other thing about it all is that, after all, I could never divorce my father from analysis. Behind every analyst I would see what I saw as the same workings my father went through. Growing up, I knew that my father was wrong a lot of the time. He didn't understand me a lot of the time, he didn't understand my mother, and he had a difficult relationship with her. He was a psychoanalyst, but I was under no illusion that this made him infallible. It didn't even give him a reliably *greater* expertise in dealing with things. Even when I saw my father on infrequent occasions acting in his role of analyst, delivering a paper or something of that sort, it still seemed to me largely a profession of perceptions and insights, which is to say *not* a profession. It was not as if a biophysicist was talking some esoteric language you knew nothing about, and all you could tell was that this was another world to you, that everything in this other world was labelled differently from what you knew it to be, and behind simple mechanisms of life as we knew it, someone was perceiving another process you had no idea of. When I thought of analysis, that was *clearly* not the case. Their perceptions, their language, the way they looked at things, were largely the same as mine. Perhaps directed toward different avenues, somehow, but essentially largely the same. They would frequently refer to writers; my father delivered papers on novels at times. That was his source. His source was not Einstein's theory of relativity, some explanation that would take an entire blackboard of inexplicable formulae to explain; it was a source that was as open to me as it was to him. All I had to do was to look at that source and perceive it in my own language and my own way, just as analysts did. The way they translated that source might be couched in a few odd terms here and there, but essentially it was the same way I would translate it into my own terms.

So their perceptions were basically the same as mine, and I

---

he pays for it. One man suggested that if analysts really believe this—that it is not for themselves, but for the patients' own good—they should donate the money to charity or, better, hold it in trust for the patient until he is better and can spend it more wisely.

could never figure, I'm just *talking* to some *guy*. Maybe an intelligent guy, maybe a nice guy, but why should I be paying this guy fifty, seventy, eighty, a hundred dollars an hour just because he's nice and intelligent? It's not as though I'm paying a dentist who's going to drill my teeth. That I can accept, because I haven't the faintest idea how to drill my own teeth and I can't ask my friends to drill my teeth and fill a cavity. But some of my friends certainly could function in the same way this analyst is functioning. I don't understand what it is about his training and his perceptions that would lead him to be exclusively capable of doing this, and in fact, based upon my knowledge of my father, and my contact with a lot of his colleagues, I have wondered at times whether many analysts might not be uniquely *un*qualified to do it.

Many PsyKs find it hard to consider going into psychotherapy because they doubt that it could have any genuine effect upon them. Their unconscious minds have been inoculated against the element of surprise or seeming magic that is so valuable with most other patients. If anything, their problem stems from an overawareness of motivations, an overabundance of self-accusation, and a cutting off from the original emotions that a lifetime of narcissistic intrusion and intellectualization have wrought. Their ratiocinating self needs no further encouragement, and indeed some of them, if engaged on dialectic grounds by the therapist, can out-argue and antagonize him and transform the intended therapy into a battle of wits. "We grew up with these skills, while they just learned them," says one with pride and belligerence. A number of therapists who have treated PsyKs agree that they can be difficult patients, in part because they have already incorporated so many therapeutic colloquialisms and tricks of the trade into their array of defense mechanisms. For a great many, the preferable therapy is one that does not try to outmaneuver them but that is closer to the down-to-earth approach which the parents had not used: therapy without jargon, without abstruse concepts, that is aimed at enticing out and strengthening the spontaneous self within them that had been so laden down with intellect.

One child of two therapists complained of a brief and repugnant contact with analysis, during which he spent all his time trying to outguess the analyst, anticipate the interpretations, and educate his defensive mechanisms against these more polished forms of assault. He was furious on those few occasions when he let something significant slip and it was picked up by the analyst. Finally he left alto-gether, and fortunately wound up with a more humanistically inclined therapist, who used no visible analytic technique but simply allowed him to grow comfortable with himself for the first time. To many PsyKs, no type of therapy is acceptable, and they fly to alternate forms of treatment, such as self-knowledge through drugs or through self-expression in the arts.

"I found it difficult to think of going to an orthodox psychiatrist," says one woman. "Because I thought the two gestures—my parents and the therapist—would cancel each other out. I felt that there would never really be privacy for me in a psychoanalytic office, because I'd be so aware of my parents being present, which I think would be enough to make it not be valuable. When I finally did go into therapy I sought out different kinds, really unusual forms. One of the people I went to said that he thought I'd made a very wise decision, because he thought I would be very slippery, a very slippery patient."

An unfortunate number of therapists who deal with PsyKs, how-ever, do not have the presence of mind to abandon their typical methods of practice, and they fall into a drawn-out intellectual strug-gle that may be informative and even entertaining but which does not ultimately do the patient much good. An artist and the son of two psychiatrists, who takes a bleak view of psychotherapy, says:

> I went into therapy when I was mentally and physically broken
> by drugs, and didn't have any other choice. It's like going to a
> bad surgeon when your heart's malfunctioning. I didn't think
> about it: I just went. I was desperate. I was desperate enough to
> overcome my dislike for psychiatry, like somebody who has an
> aversion to certain foods: if he's starving enough he'll see some
> allure in the stuff. I didn't expect much from it, though, and I
> didn't get anything from it.
>
> I have a horror of handing my life over to someone. Even as I
> was doing it—I look back at notebooks I kept at the times when
> I first saw a psychiatrist, and there are constant references to
> letting someone put his hands in your life and that kind of thing,
> a real sense that something which had an almost sacred bond
> with your being, with your self, the whole project of your
> living—it suddenly wasn't quite all yours anymore. You had sold
> your soul, you were in the hands of the receivers. I still think,
> today, that somehow bound up in the terror of actually being
> responsible for our own lives, is our dignity, and when we give

up that little edge of fear by getting solace from somebody else, I think we sacrifice some of the beauty and the physical pleasure of living. We numb it a little.

Addiction to drugs and to alcohol were really my biggest problems, and none of the various psychiatrists I saw ever did anything significant about it, nor did I really expect them to. What I expected from psychiatrists when I went was tranquilizers. It was just like when you want to borrow money from someone and you have this half-hour conversation with him before you get around to it. I never pictured a psychiatrist as somebody who was going to answer the phone to me in the morning. You know, he was somebody with an answering service. People in AA will do that. They'll hop out of bed in the middle of the morning and run over and get you. They'll actually put themselves out, physically, mentally, not for any tangible reward. Whereas psychiatry bases itself on tangible rewards.

I don't know what use psychiatrists are. Psychiatrists never gave me any practical help. You know, the way sometimes you have a problem with a pipe, or with a garbage disposal, or a carburetor. You know, the kinds of things you get from friends— every once in a while they just tell you something you need to know: the right kind of tape to use, or the right kind of glue, or you need a chisel this wide. They never gave me that kind of stuff. I don't know if I just didn't have the right kind of problems. Maybe they had these vast funds of household hints and I just never tapped them.

They weren't much help with personal problems, either, though I didn't really think I had them that much. I had a lot of these meaningless sort of sexual flings. They weren't really anything that I had any problems with: I had no scruples about that. Sometimes I would walk in and I would say, "Ah, it's amazing how a mixed-up slob like me knows so many pretty girls who want to go to bed with him." And the doctor would say, "Well, you know, you're such a romantic. They're suckers for that kind of stuff." But I would never say, "Well, I don't know, I can't really get it up for Mary Lou after the first . . ." You know, we didn't really have that kind of relationship—I mean, if that had ever happened to me, I wouldn't have told him. I was too cool. And sometimes I talked about the kind of sadomasochistic stuff I did. It didn't strike me that they were real clever on that score, either. Any problems or clues just went right past them. It was like those little incidents in grade school, like not doing your work for a long time and the teacher doesn't check you, and then one day she found the book that you hadn't done any of the work in for six months. These little secrets, these little bad secrets and these little traumas you get into, hiding things. None of it ever really seemed to get unpieced. If somebody doesn't tap right into your fantasies, if they don't pick up the thread of it so that you're talking the same language . . . We never got onto the real link between love and others, you know, my concept of myself and other people.

Possibly I was just immune to the effects of psychotherapy. Psychotherapy, like a placebo, operates by indirection, and there's the rub as regards my getting help from a psychiatrist. There is no feeling of indirection, no surprise in terminology, no surprise in the approach. Five minutes after I was ever even mildly touched by the originality of a psychiatrist's statement, I could identify his source: book, chapter, page, and paragraph, and it was rather disheartening, because here you had thought the guy was getting some kind of intuitive feel for the situation and someone could understand you at last. I would read things on narcissistic disorders that my parents had gotten the week before, and then I would notice it on my psychiatrist's writing table. I would say, "How do you like it? In chapter four, doesn't the case of Mr. M. bear some resemblance to me?"

As for clearing up the unconscious by discussing it, my own belief is that there is something inherently mysterious in life, and that you can't clear it up. What you're doing is you're tampering with something I'm tempted to call divine, and you're going to make trouble. Psychiatry is *probably* nonsense. It is probably a refined form of nonsense in the technical sense that you find in Wittgenstein, meaning assertions that can neither be validated or invalidated. In other words it doesn't submit to the kind of verification that is necessary before you can say whether something is true or false. Therefore it is neither, and therefore it is nonsensical. It is also arbitrary and devoid of values.

The psychiatrist is the perfect guy to get a little bookworm who doesn't want anything but some peanut butter and the latest publication of some obscure university press—to take this creature with his meager, modest demands, and turn him into a ravenous, disco-stomping, bank-card-punching, fast-car-driving, expensive-girl-letching, modern jerk. He'll sit there and say, "So where did you get this phobia about power boats? Why shouldn't you have what M. has?" Or he'll say "Aren't you as much of a man as W.?

Why, W. has a fast car." The psychiatrist is the guy who says, if you're getting laid all the time and that's all you do, "So what's so bad about that?" And then if you don't get laid for ten years, he says, "What about people in the army?" But of course maybe I've just encountered some of the lesser lights in the field.

If someone performs an *action*, and then you give me a description of that action, I can tell whether your description is true or not because I can tell whether it corresponds to the evidence. You say, "John walked out the door," and in actuality John did walk out the door, then that is true. If you say, "John jumped out the window," and he didn't, then that is false. But if you say "John walked out the door because he didn't want to deal with the work that he had to do," I have to say "Maybe." It sounds like nonsense to me, but I can't tell. Or if you say "John walked out the door because it was a sunny spring morning and he wanted to look at the girls," then I'll say, "Probably. Makes sense to me." A lot of psychiatry talks about motives. It talks about not just what there is or what happens, what I did or what you did, but why we did it. And that "why" is a very perplexing thing when it comes to true or false, because in a lot of cases you can never really tell, and in many cases it doesn't much matter anyway. There are a lot of discussions I engaged in when I was a patient that, although they might have been unnerving at the time or touched certain feelings, such that an onlooker would say, "That obviously means a lot to him, it disturbs him," in *fact*, outside of the artificial context of therapy, the subject might never even come up.

Therapists *must* impress. The explanations themselves are not powerful enough crutches to get somebody through life. So you have the whole business of transference, or the idealization of the therapist—though personally I never had the great good fortune to meet a therapist I respected as much as my friends. The saving grace of the whole proposition was the anonymity, the confessional aspect. There are certain tiresome details of our toilet and bed behavior that we suspect might try our friendships, so it's nice to have somebody to shit on who we don't know, and often don't like, and they don't mind taking it. As, I think, Henry Miller wrote, "Talk about whatever you want, as long as you want, and as long as you keep paying, he's got all the time in the world, he'll listen to anything. Whereas a priest is a busy man."

11

What Do
They Become?

It's a hard act to follow. They're
all bright, but offhand I can't think
of any analyst's son who's as good
as his father.

—AN ANALYST'S SON

I was struck early in my research by the types of professions into
which PsyKs go. Of those whom I interviewed, 32.4 percent were
artists, whether painters, sculptors, writers, musicians, photogra-
phers, performers, filmmakers, or designers; 31 percent had become
psychotherapists. Only 13.5 percent went into business of any kind,
and 12.2 percent were academics or educators, almost exclusively
involved in the humanities and social sciences rather than the hard
sciences or technical fields.*

The figures for psychotherapists may be slightly elevated: possibly
when people searched their minds for the names of PsyKs I could
interview, those who were themselves therapists came more readily
to mind. Conceivably, therapist PsyKs were also more eager to talk,
since their curiosity about the topic stemmed not only from being a
PsyK but also from being a therapist, and perhaps the parent of a
therapist's child. Nonetheless, the number is impressive and certainly more than coincidence. I am convinced that more PsyKs have
followed their parents' profession than have the children of lawyers,
dermatologists, or CPAs—it is almost a therapeutic tradition. A surprising number of the early group of psychoanalysts left children who

* Ralph Slovenko, a professor of law and psychiatry, has advanced the interesting argument
that psychiatrists' children have an affinity for the law. This has not been borne out by my
experience, though I can well imagine that PsyKs, exasperated with the arbitrary rules of
behavior with which they have grown up, might find the law's rigidity a welcome relief.
Conversely, their understanding of human motivation, their skill with dialectics, and their
relative views on right and wrong would make them very good at law.[1]

stayed in the field. One or more children of Sigmund Freud, Alfred Adler, Karen Horney, Melanie Klein, Wilhelm Reich, Ernst and Marianne Kris, Heinz Hartmann, Rudolph Loewenstein, Karl Abraham, Edward Hitschmann, and Oskar Pfister also became psychiatrists or psychoanalysts, and this is by no means an exhaustive list.

There are several obvious reasons why PsyKs should be tempted to become psychotherapists, and some more subtle, less conspicuous ones. Psychotherapy has always been made to seem fun and even relatively easy. All day long a succession of people who are sufficiently intellectual, sensitive, and psychologically enlightened to seek out psychotherapy parades through the office, talking to the therapist about their days and their difficulties, speaking of their jobs and accomplishments, being cheered or helped by the therapist's wise words. The therapist enjoys this living soap opera, and derives emotional satisfaction from the combination of such stimulating company and the gratification of helping people overcome their problems. Morever, the patients pay for the privilege of coming to be helped, they send little gifts, and they do little favors.

One man I interviewed said he had always found his mother's life as a therapist utterly delightful and fascinating, hardly a job at all. Her patients included lawyers, judges, university administrators, publishers, congressmen, academics, businessmen, scientists, and many others, all with great power and innumerable contacts, all very deeply in their therapist's debt. When, as a child or adolescent, he had questions on complex topics, one of his mother's patients could always find out the answer. Later, when he needed to know about college applications, had to find an apartment, or needed minor legal advice, one of her patients could help. Years afterward a doctor treated him for free because his mother had saved the doctor's marriage. He was given a substantial discount in an appliance store because the store owner, a former patient of his mother's, recognized the name on his credit card. He did not, ultimately, become a therapist himself. He started to do so, the idea seemed to fit him very comfortably, but finally he changed his mind. "It struck me in the end that the very fact that I had always known I would go into therapy was probably the best reason in the world not to do it. It would have been too easy, almost like never leaving home."

Because psychotherapy has such deep personal significance in the lives of so many psychotherapists, and they do not present it as being a chore with all the unpleasantness normally associated with jobs, it can be a surprise to the PsyK raised on this idyllic image to discover later that all work is not like this. The businesswoman daughter of a psychoanalyst says:

> The world of work is the hardest thing I have had to deal with. I think a lot of it is that I was never really exposed to what the working world was like. My father never talked about what he did for a living—not as though it was a job—it was always anecdotal: "A patient came in and told me this . . ." Most nights at dinner he related some story. He couldn't tell us who the patient was, but he could tell us the problem, especially if it was funny or unusual, or if somehow it involved a celebrity, and it would alway be interesting. He never came home and said "I had a hard day at the office today, and this bastard came in and did this . . ." Not once.
>
> There was no sense at all that my father had any kind of difficulty going off to work in the morning. On the contrary, he loved to go to work. He never missed a day of work, ever. He always got there on time, which was very important, and he always came home at the same time. He never had to work on weekends, he never had to work at night, he never brought the work home with him. When he left the office, that was it, the workday was over. Even now when I visit him, and I meet him at his office to get a ride home from the city, I'm waiting in the waiting room, the last patient leaves, and when that patient is five feet out the door my father is shutting off the light, picking up his paper, and is out the door and saying, "Hello, how're you doing? Let's go." It takes him five seconds to leave the office. It takes me about twenty minutes. I've got to think of what I did, and prepare my papers for the next day, and do my timesheet. I have to close shop. It isn't closing shop for him, it's just closing the door. The patient leaves, he leaves. That's it. It's all in his head. There's nothing to put away, nothing to file. He's happy-go-lucky and you'd never know that he worked. But he works hard. I'm sure he works hard for eight hours a day. So he must get a lot of gratification from it, though I don't know what it is. But I know it's there.
>
> I got a very clear message that going to work was a very satisfying thing. It was satisfying, it was fun, and it was important. There was never, somehow, any connection between work and making money. That was never discussed. You didn't work to make money, you worked because that was the thing you de-

rived your life satisfaction from. I never heard any negative aspects of the world of work. So I wasn't prepared. It's been a problem for me, because now I'm in a corporate setting, and I don't have the control that he's got. Growing up I felt that I was powerful and in control and relatively independent and autonomous. The high school I went to was small enough that I could do what I wanted, and my college was large enough that I could. And really, until I was about twenty-one, I kind of thought that when I knocked, doors were going to fly open. If I tried hard and was a good kid, then everything was going to be just fine. But the world of work doesn't operate that way. It was a real comeuppance for me to find that I would have to answer to somebody else, be responsible to somebody else, work on their schedule and with their set of expectations.

If I talk to my father about corporate settings or any work I do, I'm very resentful when he starts telling me, "Yes, this is how it's done, that's how it's done." I think: You don't know; you don't know anything about it. What do you do? You sit there in your chair all day and listen to people's problems. You don't have *any* idea what it's like to work for a major corporation. His response to that is: "I certainly do, because most of my patients work in major corporations, and most of the things they're complaining about are exactly what you're complaining about. So I have a very good idea." He's probably right. He probably does know a lot about it through secondhand experience. But it's not the same as firsthand, and I point that out to him, forcefully and resentfully. I really don't know what gives him satisfaction, but I do know that he's very satisfied, and he will never give up working, whereas I'm sure they won't have to drag me kicking and screaming away from my desk.

Since my father never had trouble working, and since he never had to answer to anyone, and since he had always treated me as special and led me to believe that I would find the same fulfillment in work as he had, it was a rude awakening to learn after I left home that I wasn't so special anymore, and that people weren't going to treat me special just because I was me. That didn't mean anything to them. I was like, "God, here I am, a secretary, and you're actually going to *treat* me like a secretary? Me? I mean, I guess this is my job, but this is *me*. Treat *me* like a secretary? How foolish of you!" I laugh about it now because I was an idiot: of course they were going to treat me like a secretary since that's what I was, but I was naïve enough to think that my aura was so powerful that everyone would know that I really wasn't a secretary, I really was just in a holding pattern while on my way to becoming president of this company or something, and they should treat me now the way they would treat me thirty years in the future. I can see that it would have been easier in some ways to go into psychotherapy, if I had been so inclined. I never would have had to face the reality; I could have kept assuring myself that I was just as wonderful as I wanted to be.

It is easy to succumb to the pleasant, familiar parental lifestyle not only because it has been portrayed in such a glowing way, but because PsyKs have the hunch that they will be very good at it. In this they very often are right, since they have acquired an early knack for therapeutic concepts and techniques. They have spoken about these concepts throughout their lives, whether couched in technical terms or not, and many PsyKs were always regarded as mini-therapists by friends and acquaintances and they cherished and cultivated that reputation. "The sickest minds have always sought me out," says one girl, rather proudly. "I have lots of friends who are friends because they need me. I'll come home and there's a message on my machine from one person who's about to throw herself off the Brooklyn Bridge. Would I give her a call? Another message from someone so depressed that he's about to quit school and move home. I'm always attracting flakes, probably because I know how to deal with them."

Another PsyK, the forty-year-old son of a psychologist and now a psychologist himself, after remarking that "instead of responding, my father would always analyze," said, "I'm not sure how useful that was for me, though ultimately, of course, it has become very useful for me to think in analytic terms. When I finally decided to become a therapist—I had several other aborted careers before this one—and when I finally decided to come back to this and recognized that this was really what I was good at and this was the thing that I really did enjoy, I found I was way ahead of all my peers, because I had started thinking analytically when I was about nine. I was used to doing it, and I had a facility for doing it that possibly someone who decides at age twenty-four to become a psychologist will never be able to acquire."

Going into the parent's mysterious profession is also a way of approaching the parent more intimately, of staying in the family, or of going back home. Just as PsyKs are said to want to grow up to be patients, as a way to get close to the parent who has neglected them in order to treat others, so, too, can they aspire to grow up to be therapists and to share with their parents this vitally important part of their practical and emotional lives. David Reiser remarks that even at times when he was having typically adolescent difficulties with his analyst father and looked down upon what he did, he nonetheless idolized Freud and dreamed of being a psychiatrist, a healthy sublimation of his need to identify with his father. Psychiatry was all the more appealing by being such a secret profession. There was added room to imagine the powers the parent might have and the satisfaction he might derive from it.

> I do believe that it might have been easier for me had the whole process not been so *mysterious*. For instance, had my father been an orthopedist, I think it really would have helped to go to his office with him or down to an emergency room to watch him set fractures. For the child of a psychiatrist, I believe the true nature of the parent's vocation remains enshrouded in mystery, a knowledge yearned for, yet inaccessible. It is, I am convinced, one compelling reason why I went into psychiatry myself. The fantasy went: Perhaps through training, even through analysis itself, I will at long last understand what my father does.[2]

A number of PsyKs who became psychotherapists described glowingly the transformation in their relationship with their therapist parent when they got their degrees and entered the profession. A parent and child who had been distant until then suddenly found they had something in common. Whereas there had never been time for playing games during childhood, no intimate talks at bedtime about the small things that matter to children, now they could sit down together and discuss clinical cases or recent professional papers or the latest gossip in the analytic society. Their work gave them, at last, something meaningful to share, even though each of them ultimately did it alone. The parent is delighted by the child's choice of profession and encourages it, not only out of the natural pleasure parents feel when their children wish to emulate them, but because this is a further validation of the life project the parent has carried out by going into psychotherapy.

Identification with the parental profession can also manifest a psychological defense mechanism in the child known as identification with the aggressor. The small child who is hurt and frightened by a doctor goes home and plays doctor with one of his friends, making himself feel a little bit better by commandeering the threatening position of power. The PsyK whose parent's uncompromised omnipotence and ability to manipulate leaves the child feeling victimized and defenseless, may see in the parent's extraordinary profession the key to gaining control at last. The child, too, will learn to understand, to harness emotions intellectually, to deflect the discomforts of certain human interactions by looking right through them at more profound and distant causes.

One woman whose psychoanalyst mother had always been poor at relating to her warmly, and whose intrusive, clinical manner of dealing with things had been felt as a threat to the daughter's identity, told me of her own first thoughts about becoming a psychotherapist, something she ultimately did:

> My mother was very smart, and she liked to let people know it. She loved to compete with us in various things, not in a harmful way, but she would outsmart us in puzzles, games that tested your wits. She took pleasure in being bright and in being regarded as very bright. She valued her abilities as a clinician, but it was more the insight aspect than the human piece of it. Her brightness seemed quite intimidating to me in some ways, and because of her profession I also saw her as holding a set of tools, and this had something to do with my initial interest in becoming a therapist.
>
> My first exposure to therapy was working as an aide one summer at a private psychiatric hospital. I thought, My God, what this opens up to me! To understand people seemed like an incredibly *powerful* position. It also seemed enormously exciting; nothing could be more exciting than to really understand what people were about. I think I really thought that you could sort of open up their heads and look inside. This was both exciting and it gave me the sense that I could be *master* of myself. If I could do this, then I would no longer be victim to unhappiness and problems. As a kid I had felt very vulnerable, because my mother had possessed an intrusive, dangerous power that had the potential to be quite harmful to me. And I thought that this was a power I could acquire, and then no one could be master of me, I could be master of myself.

Some PsyKs who become therapists, of course, examine themselves and come to grips with the problems of their childhood. They may become extraordinary therapists in consequence. Others, however, settle back just as their parents did, lured into carrying on the helping profession that has filled the emotional vacancy in their parents' lives, a vacancy that has often been passed on to the child. The narcissistically impaired breed the narcissistically impaired and, for scarcely coincidental reasons, psychotherapists often breed psychotherapists. The child who was treated intellectually and clinically by his parents, and who was so strongly if subtly encouraged during childhood to understand others, show compassion and empathy, is now in a position to do precisely the same thing. Not only do they find the means to protect themselves against further pain and violation, but they can reap the vicarious warmth and humanity of patients, carrying on the cycle of using intellectual tools to understand and master life rather than to live it.

Other PsyKs rebel against the lure of psychotherapy. Margot Adler, a reporter on National Public Radio, the daughter of a psychiatrist and the granddaughter of Alfred Adler, says:

> I remember deciding very early that I was going to have nothing to do with the profession. For about ten years the Alfred Adler Mental Hygiene Center was actually in the building where I lived, and a number of Adlerian therapists lived there, too, so there was a very direct and obvious presence. When I was about ten some woman who worked in the Clinic said to me, "Oh, isn't it sweet, you'll be a psychiatrist too, and all your children will be psychiatrists." I remember I was very struck by that comment, and I knew right then, even at ten, "Oh, no I won't."[3]

Oddly enough, she has felt a twinge of subsequent slight regret, and concedes that the work she does on the radio is not altogether removed from the fundamentals of therapy. Some friends consider the fact that she wrote a book on witchcraft as proof that she succumbed after all: "from witch-doctor to witch."[4]

Margot Adler is not alone in this somewhat ambivalent rejection of the field. Of those PsyKs I interviewed who had not become psychotherapists, fully 80 percent had at one point in college or afterward given it serious consideration and many continue to hold it in reserve somewhere in the back of their minds: if they don't succeed or are not happy in what they have set out to do, they suppose they could always go back to school and become a psychotherapist. They have no question at all that they could do it. It is a comforting presence, like a safety net.

Another PsyK, the son of a psychoanalyst and a social worker, said:

> Up until the middle of college I thought that psychiatry was the answer to my problems. I thought I could cure my own problems by being in therapy, and that I would cure other people's problems by becoming a doctor and an analyst like my father.

However, amidst college, I changed my mind. First away from psychiatry, then away from medicine, and then I got more involved in the arts, and found that I was much happier approaching the world as—not something that I would react to, and evaluate my response, but as something that I would *share* a *part* in, and influence by actively impinging upon it. Ever since then, I have felt that psychiatry has, in fact, been very detrimental to my development, and I believe that now, at this point, I am more interested in pursuing things that are more artistic and creative and spontaneous, that are physical as opposed to cerebral, and emotional rather than intellectual.

If PsyKs do not go into therapy, why should so many of them go into the arts? One suggested reason is that psychotherapists themselves are often artistically and certainly humanistically inclined.* Though family pressure or financial necessity prevented them from becoming artists, they chose the profession that they found closest to art, and in the case of psychiatrists, the medical specialty farthest from medicine. Now that they have arduously succeeded in life, they encourage their children to take the leisure to do something that they find worthwhile. One analyst's son quoted John Adams to me: "I must study politics and war, that my sons may have liberty to study mathematics and philosophy, geography, natural history and naval architecture, navigation, commerce, and agriculture, in order to give their children a right to study painting, poetry, music, architecture, statuary, tapestry, and porcelain."[5]

This benevolent wish to make a better world for one's children undoubtedly comes into play, though one might have supposed that people in certain other professions or medical specialties, who make more money than psychotherapists and are less devoted to their work, might be even more inclined to spare their children from the harsh demands life has made of them and subsidize their elevation to a higher and more beautiful plane. But psychotherapists, in addition, impart to their children a somewhat different concept of what is valuable in life.

One analyst's son made the interesting comment that when he was a child and spied on his parents' patients, what he saw was a lot of people who had good jobs and a lot of money, and who were re-

---

* When I asked PsyKs what their therapist parents would have done had they not gone into psychotherapy, a large number said "the arts." Most of them allegedly would have been writers, and a smaller number musicians—mostly concert violinists, interestingly enough. In contradistinction to their children, none was said to have been destined for painting or sculpture, though quite a few therapists do collect art.

spected or even famous. By all external standards they had succeeded in life. They had done just what one is supposed to. They were the people in his city who appeared in the newspapers, belonged to the right organizations, had the best houses, were greeted on all sides when they walked into a restaurant. Yet despite it all, there was something so fundamentally wrong with their lives that they were compelled to sneak anonymously into a room where, behind closed doors, they could pay someone to listen to their miseries. It struck him quite early that material, apparent success must be a poor measure of somebody's life, and he developed scorn for the notion of setting one's sights on such achievement alone while courting disaster in more intimate and critical areas of one's life. The more meaningful work, he concluded, was moral and aesthetic, learning about oneself and the world. This view led him to the arts. Art is worthwhile. Like religion, it permits one to approach life's large issues, on a scale larger even than psychotherapy. It enables one to create something new.

The art that PsyKs engage in tends to carry on the psychological work of their parents and of their own childhoods. When someone asked the psychoanalyst father of writer and filmmaker Nicholas Meyer why his son had not followed him into his profession, Dr. Meyer replied, "Oh, but he did."[6] The father approached human beings with science, while the son approached them through art. It is interesting to note that of all the painters and sculptors I have encountered, not one creates pure abstract or geometric art. All of their work involves people, situations, or histories. A sculptor who is the son of two psychiatrists says:

Introspection is absolutely the heart of who I am and of everything I do. All of my work is self-reflecting, or going beyond self and taking the personal or interpersonal and trying to make it more universal. I am analytic about everything—it tends to drive my kids crazy, because I'll see somebody on the street and start analyzing them from the little I know and can see of them: who they are, where they're from, what they do for a living, what their heritage is. It's absurd, but I do it as automatically as everything. I ask myself, "Why is this person interesting? They're not beautiful or good-looking, what is it that makes me want to look at them? Is it body language, demeanor, association, what?" In a funny way it is research for my work, and it carries on what I have always done. If it doesn't touch upon people in some way, then it doesn't really interest me at all.

Similarly, PsyK writers and poets do not write about things, they write character studies, novels about relationships, or nonfiction that examines the actions and motives of people. "I have always, from adolescence, been interested in being inside other people's minds," says one successful novelist. "There is some kind of coalescence of artistic and psychiatric requirements. I wanted to know what people were thinking, to be inside someone else, inside thought, and to know how other personalities are different from mine and how they are related to mine. As a writer I am top-heavily interested in characterization, so that my books tend to have events more than they have plots."

In addition to this pleasant interpretation of why PsyKs go into the arts, as a striving for understanding and for aesthetic creation that is condoned and encouraged by enlightened parents, there are other factors more closely related to the pathology in therapists' families. Psychiatrist Barry Schwartz made an interesting remark in the course of a conversation on therapists and their children. Some time ago, he said, someone wrote a paper on self-made millionaires. The author conducted extensive surveys and administered tests in an effort to find common denominators, and concluded that they had only one thing in common. "That one thing was that they all viewed their fathers as failures. Now turn that around, and ask yourself the question: if you see your father as a success, could this have a negative effect on you? I'm inclined to think that it could, because a father is a tough act to follow."[7]

Psychotherapists appear to be a particularly difficult act to follow. The trouble that many PsyKs have had in their attempts to break away from the parent and establish their own identities underlines the impossibility of cutting the therapist parent down to size. It is sad to hear how many PsyKs make comments to the effect that psychiatrists' kids aren't as good as their fathers or that they themselves could never live up to what their own parents had done. One man remarked that if one judges a man by the company he keeps, when he looks around at his own friends and compares them to his father's friends, he is embarrassed—this despite the fact that in the rest of his conversation he speaks deprecatingly of his father as a lonely and emotionally stunted man who had no life at all outside of his work. Even those PsyKs who have grown to dislike their fathers still speak of them with a degree of admiration and respect rather out of proportion with the father's real accomplishments, and tinged with an unfortunate feeling of hopelessness.

Freud's eldest son Martin, who had a varied and not especially successful career as publisher of the psychoanalytic press, then as a lawyer, finally as a tobacconist in Bloomsbury, rather pathetically wrote, on the very first page of a book about his father, significantly entitled *Glory Reflected*:[8]

> I have never had any ambition to rise to eminence, although, I must admit, I have been quite happy and content to bask in reflected glory. Nevertheless, I believe that if the son of a great and famous father wants to get anywhere in this world he must follow the advice given to Alice by the Red Queen—he will have to go twice as fast if he does not want to stop where he is. The son of a genius remains the son of a genius, and his chances of winning human approval of anything he may do hardly exist if he attempts to make any claim to a fame detached from that of his father.*

I suspect that an underlying belief in the parent's omnipotence and a sense of futility about attempting to compete may contribute to the fact that PsyKs do not go into business, or generally into the hard sciences, technical fields, or other sorts of areas where success and failure can be easily gauged. Since they feel that they cannot compete, they shun competitive fields, or those where one eventually completes a project, says it is the best he can do, and lets it stand on its own to be judged. Psychotherapy has the convenient attribute that success, failure, and termination are elusive and meaningless concepts in a never-ending process. One can, if so inclined, take credit for improvement that takes place spontaneously, and blame failures on the obduracy of the problem or the patient's lack of motivation. Thanks to the process of transference, patients tend to respect and admire even the most mediocre therapist. With the exception of supervised analyses during training, no one ever oversees or evaluates a therapist's work. In the arts, the question of how well one has done is also quite impossible to determine.

Art, in a very real sense, provides a way of emulating the parent without competing, since there are such strong similarities between

---

* Another of Freud's sons, Oliver, became a structural engineer for the Budd Company in the United States and lived in the East Falls section of Philadelphia. A psychoanalyst I interviewed once overheard Oliver Freud telling someone at a party that he lived in East Falls, "where Grace Kelly grew up." This analyst was astonished: "Here is a man who is the son of Sigmund Freud, and the most important association he could find in his life was that he lived near where a movie star had lived." Of course, it is clear that as far as this analyst was concerned Oliver Freud should have been content to be nothing but Sigmund Freud's son.

therapy and art. The therapist who relates a clinical vignette at the dinner table is a storyteller who has captured the extraordinary or bizarre and brought it back to explain it. Analytic understanding has an aura of mystical artistic creation—disparate elements are intuitively assembled into a harmonious whole. Like the writer or painter, the therapist derives his value from an ability to perceive things differently than other people do, to recognize the significance of shadow and detail, and the delicate, barely perceptible underpainting that give both life and art their richness and beauty. The artistic PsyK follows the parent without competing, and yet does successfully compete in a very real way, because unlike the therapist who helps others do things but does nothing himself, the artist child creates on his own. Many therapist parents of artist PsyKs are intensely jealous of their children.

For the PsyK whose childhood has left him narcissistically impaired, art is as natural a profession as psychotherapy. Narcissists need constant achievement, or at least the appearance of achievement, in order to buttress their fragile self-image. Painting, writing, acting, music, are all fields that solicit conspicuous and highly personal admiration and praise, unlike many other occupations where admiration may be wholly secret, based on one's own estimation of the worth of one's work, or where appreciation is reserved, diffuse, and postponed. The praise one receives is clearly for oneself, for one's vision and inspiration, not for the skillful use of tools or knowledge that someone else might also have acquired. One is not one's job: one is one's art.

Moreover, the arts are areas in which it is very easy to deceive oneself about the quality of one's work—even more so than for the psychotherapist who takes credit for his successes and blames the patients for his failures. The narcissistic PsyK who feels sublimely entitled to adoration all the while that he secretly doubts himself, can find in art a means of presenting what amounts to a physical manifestation of his supposed internal greatness and cleverness that others should praise and admire.[9] The inspiration alone should excite wonder. To a person uncomfortable with direct human contact on an equal footing, art, like therapy, offers a life of freedom and isolation from which one can communicate with others in a carefully controlled and awe-inspiring way, without interacting directly. One can influence people from afar, by using one's own perceptions to change other people's understanding. One is immune to criticism, because who can really judge the value of art? Much of the world's greatest art was misunderstood or derided in its time. For the same reason, one is immune from any accusation that one has failed in life: failure can be reinterpreted as an indication of success.

It is easy to entertain delusions of grandeur when working with aesthetic notions in solitude. It is also more terrifying to commit oneself to finishing a work and presenting it as complete to the public; what is judged, after all, is not only the quality of a product, but the validity of the artist's self-valuation. Too often, when narcissistic artists move farther into the business of art, they learn that inspiration alone is not enough, and that they must go on to finish the creation and deal with the pedestrian business and politics of life in this world. They are left disillusioned, with the bitter consolation that they are simply misunderstood. Kernberg comments that narcissists often appear to be quite successful, but careful observation over time may reveal evidence of superficiality, flightiness, and a void behind the glitter. "Quite frequently these are the 'promising' geniuses who then surprise other people by the banality of their development."[10]

While choosing the arts may be a result of narcissism and emotional scars in the therapist's child, it may also be a sign of striving for health. For the PsyK who has grown up in an intellectual household, where actions were interpreted and emotions discouraged, who has felt hemmed in by the rational consideration of his life, art provides a welcome release. Art is a way of quitting the bounds of reality and the intellect and of pushing emotions to their extremes. Through art the PsyK can rejoin life, and can do so in an indirect way. Art has the advantage that one can work at it alone and at a distance, and go through the tumult of emotions in privacy. The artist can in large part avoid the discomfort of emotional relations to others, and as the artist regresses in search of his emotional self he need not be embarrassed by his childish atavisms. Art is not judged by the standards of daily life. Paintings can be gone over, words can be edited. As one PsyK told me:

One of the few things that struck me early on as what I interpret as being an effect of growing up in the household I did, was that I tended to scrutinize my own emotions and to mistrust them and intellectualize everything. I had been brought up thinking that there was a cause for everything, and that somehow your emotions were never very honest because there was something else that caused them and you had to look and figure out exactly what it was. It made things very unpleasant in a way, because I envied the simple ability to feel that I believed other people, through their naïveté, possessed. I remember going out of my way to make myself much more emotional than I really was. I would have these dramatic scenes, even just with myself, showing off for my own benefit, where I would be terribly upset about something. I would try to work myself up, sort of put the hand to the brow and burst into tears, or sob, or choke manfully, or whatever, and I really didn't care. If the telephone rang and it was somebody else, then none of it really meant anything to me. But somehow it seemed like something to aspire toward, to have an emotion that was so big and overwhelming that you couldn't rationalize about it. But it was very hard to do, because I always was in control of things somehow. There was always this part of me that stood aside and said, "Well, really, it doesn't make a hell of a lot of difference in the great scheme of things, does it? A year from now you won't even remember that any of this happened."

This man subsequently went into acting, an interesting extension of what he describes. But rather than using acting solely to extend his ability to impersonate a person, he found that it provided a welcome excuse for behaving differently from what his normal, well-controlled personality would permit. He felt, in some sense, that he was treating himself through the theater, and that rather than mimicking emotion the way he had as a child, he was beginning to learn emotion from the outside in, by following scripts and molding himself. As elements of his characters lapsed into his personal life, people responded to him a bit differently and gave him the opportunity to move farther away from his constricted role.

Conclusion

> Fortunately analysis is not the only
> way to resolve inner conflicts. Life
> itself still remains a very effective
> therapist.
>
> —KAREN HORNEY

There is no easy or definitive conclusion to what began as a work of curiosity. Not all psychotherapists are conspicuously troubled: this work deals only with a significant, very interesting, rather sizable subpopulation. Therapists' children are not, by and large, crazy. PsyKs tend to be bright and articulate, and it is a pleasure to have the chance to talk with them. They are perceptive and creative people who were given many advantages and a great deal of freedom and responsibility as they grew up. What problems some of them may have are not necessarily obvious, they are not ubiquitous, and they are not limited to the children of therapists.

The problem with many therapists, as one PsyK put it, is not that psychotherapy made them the way they are, but that it did not make them any other way. The truth of the matter is that, though some people may go into psychotherapy for impersonal and objective reasons, as just a career choice and nothing more, for most therapists the field has some deeper significance. It is not a profession that one seeks out unless one has problems of one's own or a preoccupation with the workings of human behavior.

One can abuse one's position in any profession. Lawyers and doctors can turn into despots. Bureaucrats, teachers, auto mechanics, salesclerks—anyone who under some circumstance has somebody else at his mercy can use power immaturely, carelessly, or malevolently. The source of the psychotherapists' ostensible authority is, however, closer to home. They are supposed to know about people and human behavior.

The practical routine of a psychotherapist can be alienating in itself, even for the most psychologically equilibrated practitioner. To sit in an office motionless, day after day, and hear the confidences of a succession of strangers, to be swamped with powerful emotions and overwhelming problems and to train oneself to maintain poise and objectivity amidst this difficult onslaught, to suppress or modify one's natural response, is a trying task for anyone. It can be draining on one's emotions, and can leave one numbed and indifferent at the end of the day, so that the paltry domestic problems in one's family seem barely worthy of notice compared to the horror and disillusionment that drive patients into therapy.

What is worse, though, is the fact that the therapist who has urgent problems and questions about himself may find in his job a way to avoid looking for meaningful answers and even, paradoxically, apparent justification for doing so. The wounded healer who might have healed himself and become better as a result, may take the route of the encapsulated wound, where his ultimate aim is to protect himself, and where his wounds grow forever invulnerable to cure. Things are too easily reduced to dogmatic explanations. The gaining of insight comes to assume more importance than the behavior itself. Life turns into an enigma to be solved rather than something to live. The therapist who is ill at ease with himself, feeling lonely and lost and without power, finds an almost wholly satisfying refuge in the profession of psychotherapy, where he is admired and seemingly loved and can enjoy intimacy without the risks of involvement, where he learns techniques to deflect criticism and justify himself, and where he is engaged in an unquestionably valuable profession. Yet the fact that he has come to the job in search of fulfillment, rather than brought his personal fullness to the job and placed it at the service of others, leads to a fundamental perversion of the helping relationship. Often he can still do a great deal of good, but ultimately his aims are at variance with the purpose at hand.

At home, the dependence and artificial certainty of the therapist with the encapsulated wound make the give-and-take of family life much more difficult. Life is conducted intellectually, by systems. The therapist tries to help himself further through the agency of his children, and hopes to carry out some plan whereby his knowledge and techniques will spare them the suffering he himself has felt. There is nothing wrong with this within limits. Every parent has an investment in his child and feels good when he makes the child happy or proud, but there is a point at which the interests of parent and child diverge and at which the parent profits at the ultimate expense of the child. Childhood simply is a tough business at times, and the end result of this well-meaning meddling may be that the children are denied the robust impact of real life. They are subdued by the need to support the weak parent, at the same time as they are made unsure of themselves by the parent's seeming omniscient authority. All the while, there is the suspicion that something is not quite true.

Life may end up with a fragile, precious, and privileged quality that rushes the child into premature maturity and sensitivity. PsyKs seem wonderful to everyone else, and they genuinely are more perceptive than most of their peers or even, in many ways, than most of the adults around them. There are limits to how sensitive and empathic one can be, however. We grow from being selfish and belligerent creatures into disciplined ones. Our more primitive urges are subli- mated into higher ones. But these processes must take place at their own rate or else there is no power there to be harnessed, and the child has been denied that primordial, exuberant, megalomaniacal sense of self that, when tempered and domesticated, provides the solid foundation for a substantial sense of self. Without this founda- tion, life seems theoretical, intellectual, and arbitrary. One may be clever at living it, but one might ask whether this is really life.

The natural process of growth and individuation can be severely undercut by the parent who abdicates his parental role and authority in favor of being too close to his children. The wonderful closeness that typifies the relationships between many therapists and their children feeds the parent and supports the child, but finally makes it difficult for the child to break away. The child has no inner substance or values of his own, he has formed himself to fulfill an anticipation, and he is frightened of hurting his parent by signaling that he has outgrown him. This unhealthy psychological symbiosis can be found in many families, but therapists appear particularly prone to it, and through their interest in knowing about other people, their added understanding about the meanings of things, and their preemptive interpretation of the child's secret thoughts and developmental stages, they are capable of more insidious and better camouflaged penetration.

Children are a curious mixture of credulousness and perspicacity. They know very little, but by dint of their innocence and of constant exposure they are very adept at seeing through fraud. The parent's posture may have its effect, but in some way it will not quite ring true. In the end it is probably better to be an honestly bad parent than to try to be dishonestly good. The child will see, or feel that he sees, through the falsehood, yet, being a child, may not be able to maintain full confidence, in the face of fierce contradiction, that his judgment is valid. By inflicting artificial good at the expense of credibility, the parents will have undermined some of the child's sense of confidence in his own perceptions and ability to cope with reality. What he believes he sees, and which is really true, the parent skillfully and emphatically denies.

It is easier to find one's way in the world when one knows the real importance of things, has made mistakes and learned from experience, and had a normal dose of life's hard knocks. The child who is rushed into premature responsibility and forced to understand and manage his own behavior before he has developed a spontaneous self that can really call anything its own, is stunted and dissatisfied. He has grown up very fast, but he has left himself behind.

Notes

Introduction

1. David Reiser, interview, 26 March 1987.
2. Ross Wetzsteon, "Do Psychiatrists Drive Their Kids Crazy?" *Village Voice,* 14 February 1977, pp. 21–22, 24.
3. Lawrence Hartmann, interview, 11 April 1985.
4. Sigmund Freud, "New Introductory Lectures on Psycho-Analysis," in vol. 22 of *The Standard Edition of the Complete Psychological Works of Sigmund Freud,* edited by James Strachey (London: Hogarth Press, 1953–1974), p. 58.

Chapter 1

1. Bob Fisher and Arthur Marx, *The Impossible Years* (New York: Samuel French, 1964), p. 5.
2. J. Storer Clouston, *The Lunatic at Large* (Edinburgh and London: William Blackwood, 1903).
3. Frederick C. Redlich, "The Psychiatrist in Caricature: An Analysis of Unconscious Attitudes toward Psychiatry," *American Journal of Orthopsychiatry* (1950) 20:560–71.
4. Walter Freeman, *The Psychiatrist* (New York and London: Grune and Stratton, 1968), p. 160.
5. Alan F. Blum and Larry Rosenberg, "Some Problems Involved in Professionalizing Social Interaction: The Case of Psychotherapeutic Training," *Journal of Health and Social Behavior* 9 (1968):72–85.
6. Everett Dulit, interview, 8 April 1985.
7. Jay Rohrlich, interview, 26 June 1986.
8. Howard Page Wood, interview, 20 September 1984.
9. Robert R. Holt and Lester Luborsky, *Personality Patterns of Psychiatrists: A Study of Methods for Selecting Residents,* Menninger Clinic Monograph Series no. 13 (New York: Basic Books, 1958).
10. Ross Wetzsteon, "Do Psychiatrists Drive Their Kids Crazy?" *Village Voice,* 14 February 1977, pp. 21–22, 24.
11. Heinz Kohut, *The Restoration of the Self* (New York: International Universities Press, 1977).

12. Alice Miller, *The Drama of the Gifted Child* (New York: Basic Books, 1981).

13. Ibid., pp. 27–28.

Chapter 2

1. Thomas Monro, quoted in Kathleen Jones, *Lunacy, Law and Conscience, 1744–1845* (London: Routledge & Kegan Paul, 1955), pp. 15–16.

2. Albert Deutsch, *The Mentally Ill in America*, 2d ed. (New York: Columbia University Press, 1949), p. 52.

3. See, e.g., Henri F. Ellenberger, *The Discovery of the Unconscious* (New York: Basic Books, 1970).

4. Myles Johnson, telephone communication, 17 September 1986.

5. Bernard D. Beitman, "The Demographics of American Psychotherapists: A Pilot Study," *American Journal of Psychotherapy* 37 (1983): 37–48.

6. Lorrin M. Koran, ed., *The Nation's Psychiatrists* (Washington, D.C.: American Psychiatric Association, 1987).

7. Mary Ann Eiler, *Physician Characteristics and Distribution in the U.S.*, 1982 ed. (Chicago: American Medical Association, 1983).

8. David J. Knesper and Steven S. Sharfstein, "The Economics of Psychiatric Practice," in Koran, ed., *The Nation's Psychiatrists*, p. 157.

9. Koran, ed., *The Nation's Psychiatrists*, p. 21.

10. David J. Knesper and Steven S. Sharfstein, "The Economics of Psychiatric Practice," in Koran, ed., *The Nation's Psychiatrists*, p. 139.

11. Joint Information Service, *Psychiatrists and Their Patients* (Washington, D.C.: Joint Information Service of the American Psychiatric Association and the National Association for Mental Health, 1973); Marianne D. Mattera, "Why Psychiatrists Are Behind the Economic Eight Ball," *Medical Economics*, 5 February 1979, pp. 158–62; Carl A. Taube et al., "Patients of Psychiatrists and Psychologists in Office-based Practice, 1980," *American Psychologist* 39 (1984): 1435–47.

12. American Medical Association, *Socioeconomic Characteristics of Medical Practice 1983* (Chicago: American Medical Association, 1983), p. 116; David J. Knesper and Steven S. Sharfstein, "The Economics of Psychiatric Practice," in Koran, ed., *The Nation's Psychiatrists*, p. 119.

13. American Medical Association, *Socioeconomic Characteristics of Medical Practice 1983*, page 66.

14. Ibid., p. 80.

15. Robert Wood Johnson Foundation, *Medical Practice in the United States* (Princeton: Robert Wood Johnson Foundation, 1981), p. 35.

16. American Psychoanalytic Association, "Interpretative Commentary on Issues Raised by April 1976 Survey of Psychoanalytic Practice," Manuscript, 13 December 1979; membership of American Psychoanalytic Association from Helen Henry, telephone communication, 6 October 1987; average number of patients from American Psychoanalytic Association, "Interpretative Commentary," p. 27; Boston study from Lawrence E. Lifson,

"Analysis of a Psychoanalytic Society: Boston, 1984" *American Psychoanalytic Association Newsletter* 21, no. 3 (Fall 1987): 6–7.

17. Early estimates from Marquis Earl Wallace, "Private Practice: A Nationwide Study," *Social Work* 27 (1982): 262–67: estimate of social workers practicing psychotherapy from Myles Johnson, telephone communication, 15 September 1986.

18. "1985 Survey Report," *Psychotherapy Finances* 12, no. 9 (1985): 1–8.

19. American Psychological Association, Human Resources Research, "Preliminary Report: 1983 Doctorate Employment Survey" (Washington, D.C.: American Psychological Association, 1985), p. 6.

20. "1985 Survey Report."

21. William E. Henry, John H. Sims, and S. Lee Spray, *The Fifth Profession: Becoming a Psychiatrist* (San Francisco: Jossey-Bass, 1971).

22. William E. Henry, "Personal and Social Identities of Psychotherapists," in *Effective Psychotherapy: A Handbook of Research*, edited by Alan S. Gurman and Andrew M. Razin (Oxford: Pergamon Press, 1977), pp 47–62.

23. Henry, Sims, and Spray, *The Fifth Profession*, p. 181.

24. National Medical Care Utilization and Expenditure Survey, cited in Taube et al., "Patients of Psychiatrists," p. 1437; NIMH study cited in Myrna M. Weissman, "Psychiatric Diagnoses," *Science* 235 (1987): 522.

25. Lorrin M. Koran, Zebulon Taintor, and Mahmud Mirza, in Koran, ed., *The Nation's Psychiatrists*, p. 107.

26. Joint Information Service, *Psychiatrists and Their Patients*, p. 25–40.

27. Lawrence S. Kubie, *Practical and Theoretical Aspects of Psychoanalysis*, rev. ed. (New York: International Universities Press, 1975), p. 16; Sigmund Freud, "New Introductory Lectures on Psychoanalysis," in *The Standard Edition of the Complete Psychological Works of Sigmund Freud*, edited by James Strachey (London: Hogarth Press, 1953–1974), vol. 22, p. 80; Sigmund Freud, *Studies in Hysteria*, vol. 2 of *Standard Edition*.

28. Sigmund Freud, "The Dynamics of Transference," in *The Standard Edition*, vol. 12, p. 107.

29. Robert Fliess, "The Metapsychology of the Analyst," *Psychoanalytic Quarterly* 11 (1942): 214.

30. Sigmund Freud, "Recommendations to Physicians Practicing Psycho-Analysis," in *The Standard Edition*, vol. 12, p. 115.

31. See Seymour L. Halleck and Sherwyn M. Woods, "Emotional Problems of Psychiatric Residents," *Psychiatry* 25 (1962): 339–46; Robert O. Pasnau and Stephen J. Bayley, "Personality Changes in the First Year of Psychiatric Residency Training," *American Journal of Psychiatry* 128 (1971); 79–84; and Robert D. Mehlman, "Becoming and Being a Psychotherapist: The Problem of Narcissism," *International Journal of Psychoanalytic Psychotherapy* 3 (1974): 125–40.

32. Mehlman, "Becoming and Being a Psychotherapist," p. 126.

33. Paul H. Ornstein, "Selected Problems in Learning How to Analyze," *International Journal of Psychoanalysis* 48 (1967): 448–61.

34. Ellenberger, *Discovery of the Unconscious*, p. 737.

35. The studies are summarized in Edward Erwin, "Is Psychotherapy More Effective than a Placebo?" in *Does Psychotherapy Really Help People?* edited by Jusuf Hariman (Springfield, Ill.: Charles C Thomas, 1986).

36. Albert Moll is cited in Ellenberger, *Discovery of the Unconscious*, p. 825.

37. Daniel B. Hogan, *A Review of Malpractice Suits in the United States*, vol. 3 of *The Regulation of Psychotherapists* (Cambridge, Mass.: Ballinger, 1979), p. 27.

Chapter 3

1. Jon A. Shaw, "Children in the Military," *Psychiatric Annals* 17 (1987): 539–44.

2. David E. Reiser, "The Sorcerer and the Mirror: Psychiatrists and Their Children." Paper presented to the Colorado Child and Adolescent Society, 5 March 1980, pp. 10–11.

3. Edward Futterman, interview, 15 April 1985.

4. Margaret S. Mahler, "*Les enfants terribles*," in *The Selected Papers of Margaret S. Mahler* (New York: Jason Aronson, 1979), vol. 1, pp. 17–33.

5. Nicholas Meyer, interview, 24 February 1985.

Chapter 4

1. Kurt Adler, interview, 6 September 1984.

2. John Warkentin, "The Therapist's Significant Other," *Annals of Psychotherapy* 4 (1963):

3. Gordon E. Bermak, "Do Psychiatrists Have Special Emotional Problems?" *American Journal of Psychoanalysis* 37 (1977): 141–46.

4. J. Willi, "Higher Incidence of Physical and Mental Ailments in Future Psychiatrists as Compared with Future Surgeons and Internal Medical Specialists at Military Conscription," *Social Psychiatry* 18 (1983): 69–72.

5. Connie J. Deutsch, "A Survey of Therapists' Personal Problems and Treatment," *Professional Psychology* 16 (1985): 305–15.

6. The survey of nonmedical psychotherapists is reported in Cynthia D. Scott and Joann Hawk, *Heal Thyself: The Health of Health Care Professionals* (New York: Brunner-Mazel, 1986), passim. of physician members of A.A., in Elaine J. Knutsen, "On the Emotional Well-Being of Psychiatrists: Overview and Rationale," *American Journal of Psychoanalysis* 37 (1977): 123–39; other studies are reported in James D. Guy and Gary P. Liaboe, "Suicide among Psychotherapists: Review and Discussion," *Professional Psychology* 17 (1986): 111–14.

7. "Suicide Among Doctors," *British Medical Journal* 1 (1964): 789.

8. I. Safinofsky, "Suicide in Doctors and Wives of Doctors," *Canadian Family Physician* 26 (1980): 837–44; James L. Evans, "Psychiatric Illness in the Physician's Wife," *American Journal of Psychiatry* 122 (1965): 159–63;

J. Lewis, "The Doctor and His Marriage," *Texas State Journal of Medicine* 6 (1965): 615–19.

9. See Charles L. Rich and Ferris N. Pitts, Jr., "Suicide by Male Physicians during a 5-Year Period," *American Journal of Psychiatry* 136 (1979): 1089–90; and Alec Roy, "Suicide in Doctors," *Psychiatric Clinics of North America* 8 (1985): 377–98. The Task Force report is in Charles L. Rich and Ferris N. Pitts, Jr., "Suicide by Psychiatrists: A Study of Medical Specialists among 18,730 Consecutive Physician Deaths during a Five-Year Period, 1967–74," *Journal of Clinical Psychiatry* 41 (1980): 261–63; the quoted phrase is at p. 262.

10. Steven L. Wolfgang, "Physicians Who Commit Suicide: A Stacked Deck," *Psychiatric Opinion* 12 (April 1975): 26.

11. Judd Marmor, "Some Factors Involved in Occupation-Related Depression among Psychiatrists," *Psychiatric Annals* 12 (1982): 912–20.

12. Wittels is quoted in Walter Freeman, *The Psychiatrist* (New York & London: Grune & Stratton, 1968), p. 264.

13. William E. Henry, John H. Sims, and S. Lee Spray, *The Fifth Profession: Becoming a Psychotherapist* (San Francisco: Jossey-Bass, 1971), p. 113.

14. See, e.g., E. S. C. Ford, "Being and Becoming a Psychotherapist: The Search for Identity," *American Journal of Psychotherapy* 17 (1963): 472–82; and Arthur Burton and Associates, *Twelve Therapists* (San Francisco: Jossey-Bass, 1972). The quoted phrase is from Karl Menninger, "Psychological Factors in the Choice of Medicine as a Profession," *Bulletin of the Menninger Clinic* 21 (1957): 104.

15. Burton and Associates, *Twelve Therapists*, p. 17.

16. G. R. Racusin, S. I. Abramowitz, and W. D. Winter, "Becoming a Therapist: Family Dynamics and Career Choice," *Professional Psychology* 12 (1981): 271–79; William E. Henry, "Personal and Social Identities of Psychotherapists," in *Effective Psychotherapy: A Handbook of Research*, edited by Alan S. Gurman and Andrew M. Razin (Oxford: Pergamon Press, 1977).

17. C. Jess Groesbeck and Benjamin Taylor, "The Psychiatrist as Wounded Physician," *American Journal of Psychoanalysis* 37 (1977): 133.

18. See, e.g., Barbara Low, "The Psychological Compensations of the Analyst," *International Journal of Psychoanalysis* 16 (1935): 1–8; Ella Sharpe, "The Psycho-analyst," *International Journal of Psychoanalysis* 28 (1947): 1–6; Thomas S. Szasz, "On the Experience of the Analyst in the Psychoanalytic Situation," *Journal of the American Psychoanalytic Association* 4 (1956): 197–223; and Ralph R. Greenson, "That 'Impossible' Profession," *Journal of the American Psychoanalytic Association* 14 (1966): 9–27.

19. See C. W. Christensen, "The Occurrence of Mental Illness in the Ministry," *Journal of Pastoral Care* 13 (1959): 79–87; 14 (1960): 13–20; 17 (1963): 1–10; and 17 (1963): 125–35. See also J. Reid Meloy, "Narcissistic Psychopathology and the Clergy," *Pastoral Psychology* 35 (1986): 50–55.

20. Margaret C.-L. Gildea and Edwin F. Gildea, "Personalities of American Psychotherapists," *American Journal of Psychiatry* 101 (1945): 460–67.

21. Analogy courtesy of Joan Grant.

22. Alexander McCurdy, interview, 18 April 1984.

23. Cited by Robert Foulkes, interview, 23 October 1984.

24. William Dewart, interview, 9 July 1986.

25. See, e.g., Robert M. Dorn, "Psychoanalysis and Psychoanalytic Education: What Kind of 'Journey'?" *Psychoanalytic Forum* 3 (1969): 237–74.

26. Ernest Jones, "The God Complex," in idem, *Essays in Applied Psychoanalysis* (London: Hogarth Press, 1951), vol. 2, pp. 262–63.

27. Myron R. Sharaf and Daniel J. Levinson, "The Quest for Omnipotence in Professional Training," *Psychiatry* 27 (1964): 135–49; Donald Light, "Professional Superiority," paper presented at the annual meeting of the American Sociological Association, Montreal, August 1974; Judd Marmor, "The Feeling of Superiority: An Occupational Hazard in the Practice of Psychotherapy," *American Journal of Psychiatry* 110 (1953): 370–76.

28. Paul Roazen, *Freud and His Followers* (New York: Knopf, 1975), p. 10.

29. Ernest Jones, *Free Associations: Memories of a Psycho-Analyst* (New York: Basic Books, 1959), p. 14.

30. Ernest Jones, *The Life and Work of Sigmund Freud* (New York: Basic Books, 1953), vol. 1, p. 348.

31. From manuscript autobiography of Mervyn Jones.

32. Cf. Thomas Maeder, *Crime and Madness: The Origins and Evolution of the Insanity Defense* (New York: Harper & Row, 1985).

33. C. G. Jung, *Analytic Psychology: Its Theory and Practice* (New York: Pantheon, 1968), pp. 171–72.

34. See, e.g., American Psychiatric Association, *Diagnostic and Statistical Manual of Mental Disorders*, 3d ed. (Washington, D.C.: American Psychiatric Association, 1980); Gerald Adler, "Psychotherapy of the Narcissistic Personality Disorder Patient: Two Contrasting Approaches," *American Journal of Psychiatry* 143 (1986): 430–36; Otto F. Kernberg, "Factors in the Psychoanalytic Treatment of Narcissistic Personalities," *Journal of the American Psychoanalytic Association* 18 (1970): 51–85; and Heinz Kohut, *The Restoration of the Self* (New York: International Universities Press, 1977).

35. Dragan M. Švrakić, "On Narcissistic Ethics," *American Journal of Psychoanalysis* 46 (1986): 55–61.

36. Kohut, *Restoration of the Self*; Alice Miller, *The Drama of the Gifted Child* (New York: Basic Books, 1981).

37. Miller, ibid., pp. 8–9.

38. K. Daniel Rose and Irving Rosow, "Marital Stability among Physicians," *California Medicine* (1972): 95–99; William E. Henry, John H. Sims, and S. Lee Spray, *The Fifth Profession: Becoming a Psychotherapist* (San Francisco: Jossey-Bass, 1971).

39. Richard C. Robertiello, "The Occupational Disease of Psychotherapists," *Journal of Contemporary Psychotherapy* 9 (1978): 123–29.

40. Ibid., p. 127.

41. William E. Henry, "Some Observations on the Lives of Healers," *Human Development* 9 (1966): 47–56.

42. Willard Gaylin, personal communication, 16 April 1985.

43. Adolf Guggenbühl-Craig, *Power in the Helping Professions* (Dallas: Spring Publications, 1971), pp. 56–57.

44. Guggenbühl-Craig, *Power in the Helping Professions;* Phyllis Greenacre, "Problems of Overidealization . . . ," in *Emotional Growth,* edited by Phyllis Greenacre (New York: International Universities Press, 1971), vol. 2, pp. 743–61.

Chapter 5

1. Philippe Ariès, *Centuries of Childhood* (New York: Vintage Books, 1962).

2. Erik H. Erikson, *Childhood and Society* (New York: Norton, 1950), p. 12.

3. Quoted in Daniel Beekman, *The Mechanical Baby* (New York: New American Library, 1977), pp. 61–62.

4. Bruce H. Addington, "Masters of the Mind," *American Magazine,* November 1910, pp. 74–77.

5. Boris Sidis, *Philistine and Genius* (New York: Moffat, Yard, 1911).

6. William James Sidis, *The Animate and the Inanimate* (Boston: Richard C. Badger, 1925); William James Sidis, *Notes on the Collection of Transfers* (Philadelphia: Dorrance, 1926); James Thurber (as Jared L. Manley), "Where Are They Now?" *New Yorker,* 14 August 1937, pp. 22–26; *Sidis v. F. R. Publishing Corp.,* 311 U.S. 711 (1940). For further information on the life of William James Sidis, see Amy Wallace, *The Prodigy* (New York: Dutton, 1986).

7. John B. Watson, *Behaviorism* (New York: Norton, 1939), p. 104.

8. David Cohen, *J. B. Watson: The Founder of Behaviourism* (London: Routledge & Kegan Paul, 1979), chap. 8; Rosalie R. Watson, "I Am the Mother of the Behaviorist's Sons," *Parents' Magazine,* December 1930, pp. 16–18, 67.

9. Cohen, *J. B. Watson,* pp. 118–20.

10. John B. Watson, *Psychological Care of the Infant and Child,* quoted in Christina Hardyment, *Dream Babies* (New York: Harper & Row, 1983), p. 172.

11. Darrell Sifford, "Facing the Real Issues in Parent-Child Conflicts," *Philadelphia Inquirer,* 15 January 1985.

12. Richard C. Robertiello and Jonathan Goldman, "The 'Spock' Children," *Voices* 10 (1974): 71–75.

13. Sigmund Freud, "Explanations, Applications and Orientations," Lecture 24 of the "New Introductory Lectures on Psycho-Analysis," *The Standard Edition of the Complete Psychological Works of Sigmund Freud,* edited by James Strachey (London: Hogarth Press, 1953–1974), vol. 22, p. 150.

14. D. W. Winnicott, "Ego Distortion in Terms of True and False Self," in idem, *The Maturational Processes and the Facilitating Environment* (New York: International Universities Press, 1965), p. 145.

15. Heinz Kohut, *The Restoration of the Self* (New York: International Universities Press, 1977), p. 274.

16. Winnicott, "Ego Distortion," p. 145.

17. Alice Miller, *The Drama of the Gifted Child* (New York: Basic Books, 1981), p. 10.

18. David E. Reiser, "The Sorcerer and the Mirror: Psychiatrists and Their Children." Paper presented to the Colorado Child and Adolescent Society, 5 March 1980, pp. 22–23; idem, interview, 17 March 1987.

Chapter 6

1. Sigmund Freud, *The Origins of Psycho-analysis: Letters to Wilhelm Fliess* (New York: Basic Books, 1954), p. 192; Celia Bertin, *Marie Bonaparte: A Life* (New York: Harcourt Brace Jovanovich, 1982), p. 174; Paul Roazen, *Freud and His Followers* (New York: Knopf, 1975), p. 58. Mrs. Freud is quoted in Henri F. Ellenberger, *The Discovery of the Unconscious* (New York: Basic Books, 1970), p. 458.

2. Sigmund Freud, *Interpretation of Dreams*, vol. 4 of *The Standard Edition of the Complete Psychological Works of Sigmund Freud*, edited by James Strachey (London: Hogarth Press, 1953–74), pp. 127–29.

3. Sigmund Freud, *The Psychopathology of Everyday Life*, vol. 6 of *The Standard Edition*, p. 180.

4. Arthur Reik, interview, 6 September 1984.

5. Paul J. Stern, *C. G. Jung: The Haunted Prophet* (New York: Braziller, 1976), pp. 76–77.

6. Ernest Jones, *The Life and Work of Sigmund Freud* (New York: Basic Books, 1953–55), vol. 2, pp. 388–89; Roazen, *Freud and His Followers*, pp. 445–46.

7. Edward S. Levin, "The 'Doctor Game' Revisited: Doctors' Treatment of Their Own Children," *International Journal of Psychoanalytic Psychiatry* 10 (1984–85): 508 n.

8. Roazen, *Freud and His Followers*, pp. 438–42.

9. Edoardo Weiss, *Sigmund Freud as a Consultant: Recollections of a Pioneer in Psychoanalysis* (New York: Intercontinental Medical Book Corp., 1970), p. 81.

10. Sigmund Freud, "Analysis of a Phobia in a Five-Year-Old Boy," *The Standard Edition*, vol. 10, pp. 5–149.

11. Max Graf, "Reminiscences of Professor Sigmund Freud," *Psychoanalytic Quarterly* 11 (1942): 465–76.

12. Freud, "Analysis of a Phobia," pp. 15, 148.

13. Francis Rizzo, "Memoirs of an Invisible Man—I," *Opera News* 36 (5 February 1972): 25–26.

14. Hilda C. Abraham, *Karl Abraham: Biographie inachevée* (Paris: Presses Universitaires de France, 1976): "Some Illustrations on the Emotional Relationship of Little Girls towards Their Parents" (1917), in Karl Abraham, *Clinical Papers and Essays on Psycho-analysis*, vol. 2 of *The Selected Papers of Karl Abraham* (New York: Basic Books, 1955), pp. 52–54.

15. Dinora Pines, "*Note introductoire*," in Hilda Abraham, *Karl Abraham*.

16. Helene Deutsch, "A Two-Year-Old Boy's First Love Comes to Grief," in idem, *Neuroses and Character Types: Clinical Psychoanalytic Studies* (New York: International Universities Press, 1965), pp. 159–64.

17. Martin Deutsch, interview, 19 March 1987.

18. Ernst Simmel, "A Screen-memory in *Statu Nascendi*," *International Journal of Psychoanalysis* 6 (1925): 454–57.

19. Melanie Klein is quoted in Phyllis Grosskurth, *Melanie Klein: Her World and Her Work* (New York: Knopf, 1986), pp. 77–78.

20. Ibid., pp. 97–98, 99–100.

21. J. L. Moreno, Zerka Moreno, and Jonathan Moreno, *The First Psychodramatic Family* (Beacon, N.Y.: Beacon House, 1964); Jonathan Moreno, interview, 13 March 1987.

22. Jules Barron, "A Father-Son, Therapist-Patient Relationship," *Voices* 7, no. 4 (Winter 1971–72): 43–45.

23. Alexandra Adler, interview, 27 June 1984.

24. Levin, "The 'Doctor Game' Revisited," pp. 519–20.

25. Anna Freud, *Normality and Pathology in Childhood: Assessments of Development* (New York: International Universities Press, 1965), pp. 58–60.

26. Levin, "The 'Doctor Game' Revisited," pp. 519–20.

27. Ernst Simmel, "The 'Doctor-Game,' Illness and the Profession of Medicine," *International Journal of Psycho-Analysis*, pp. 470–483; Levin, "The 'Doctor Game' Revisited," p. 519.

28. Lawrence Hartmann, interview, 11 April 1985.

29. Herbert Strean, interview, 17 January 1985.

30. Ralph R. Greenson, *The Technique and Practice of Psychoanalysis* (New York: International Universities Press, 1967), vol. 1, p. 220.

Chapter 7

1. Martin Deutsch, interview, 11 June 1985.

2. Ralph R. Greenson and M. Wexler, "The Non-transference Relationship in the Psychoanalytic Situation," *International Journal of Psycho-Analysis* 50 (1969): 27–39.

3. Martin Deutsch, interview, 11 June 1985.

4. See, for example, Jules Glenn, "Freud's Advice to Hans's Father: The First Supervisory Sessions," in *Freud and His Patients*, edited by M. Kanzer and Jules Glenn (New York: Jason Aronson, 1980), pp. 121–27; and Jules Glenn, "Notes on the Causes and Effects of Therapy by Parents," *International Journal of Psychoanalytic Psychotherapy* 10 (1984–85): 525–31.

5. Sandor Ferenczi, "The Sons of the 'Tailor,' " in idem, *Further Contri-*

butions to the Theory and Technique of Psychoanalysis, edited by John Rickman (New York: Basic Books, 1926), pp. 418–19.

6. Glenn, "Freud's Advice," pp. 122–23.

7. Ibid.

8. Sigmund Freud, "Explanations, Applications and Orientations," Lecture 34 of *New Introductory Lectures on Psycho-Analysis,* in *Standard Edition,* vol. 22, p. 149.

9. Bruno Bettelheim, *The Uses of Enchantment* (New York: Knopf, 1976), pp. 18–19.

10. David Reiser, interview, 17 March 1987.

11. Ibid.

12. Jeffrey Moussaieff Masson, *The Assault on Truth: Freud's Suppression of the Seduction Theory* (New York: Farrar, Straus & Giroux, 1984).

Chapter 8

1. Sigmund Freud, *The Interpretation of Dreams,* vol. 5 of *The Standard Edition of the Complete Psychological Works of Sigmund Freud,* edited by James Strachey (London: Hogarth Press, 1953–74), p. 485.

2. Jules Romains, *Knock, ou le triomphe de la médecine* (Paris: Librairie Gallimard, 1924).

3. Allen Wheelis, "The Vocational Hazards of Psycho-Analysis," *International Journal of Psychoanalysis* 37 (1956): 176.

4. Stephen A. Appelbaum, "The Idealization of Insight," *International Journal of Psychoanalytic Psychotherapy* 4 (1975): p. 280.

5. See, for example, Brian Bird, "The Curse of Insight," *Bulletin of the Philadelphia Association for Psychoanalysis* 7 (1957): 101–104; and Appelbaum, "The Idealization of Insight."

6. Dragan M. Švrakić, "On Narcissistic Ethics," *American Journal of Psychoanalysis* 46 (1986): 55–61.

7. Alice Miller, *The Drama of the Gifted Child* (New York: Basic Books, 1981), pp. 40–41.

Chapter 9

1. Letters from A. Wilmot Jacobsen, 1 March and 23 March 1985.

2. Henriette Klein, interview, 21 February 1985.

3. Everett Dulit, interview, 8 April 1985.

4. Paul Roazen, *Freud and His Followers* (New York: Knopf, 1975), pp. 445–46, and p. 15.

5. Herbert Strean, interview, 21 February 1985. For further discussion of this issue, see idem, "Psychotherapy with Children of Psychotherapists," *Psychoanalytic Review* 56 (1964): 377–86.

6. Jules Glenn, interview, 10 January 1987.

7. Heinz Kohut, *The Restoration of Self* (New York: International Universities Press, 1977), pp. 274–75.

Chapter 10

1. Marianne von Eckardt, interview, 16 December 1986.
2. Jack L. Rubins, *Karen Horney: Gentle Rebel of Psychoanalysis* (New York: Dial, 1978), pp. 83–84; Susan Quinn, *A Mind of Her Own: The Life of Karen Horney* (New York: Summit Books, 1987), p. 183.
3. Mervyn Jones, "Autobiography," p. 11.
4. Letter of 22 September 1927, quoted in Vincent Brome, *Ernest Jones: Freud's Alter Ego* (New York: Norton, 1983), p. 156 n.
5. Sigmund Freud, "The Paths to Symptom Formation," Lecture 23 in *Introductory Lectures on Psycho-analysis*, vol. 16 of *The Standard Edition of the Complete Psychological Works of Sigmund Freud*, edited by James Strachey (London: Hogarth Press, 1953–74), p. 365.
6. Herbert S. Strean, "Psychotherapy with Children of Psychotherapists," *Psychoanalytic Review* 56 (1969), pp. 378–79.
7. Richard D. Chessick, "Intensive Psychotherapy for the Psychiatrist's Family," *American Journal of Psychotherapy* 31 (1977): 516–24.
8. Melitta Schmideberg, " 'After the Analysis . . . ,' " *Psychoanalytic Quarterly* 7 (1938): 126–27.
9. Jules Glenn, interview, 10 January 1987.

Chapter 11

1. Ralph Slovenko, "On the Metamorphosis of Psychiatrists, Their Spouses and Offspring into Lawyers," *Journal of Psychiatry and Law* 15 (1987): 325–66.
2. David E. Reiser, "The Sorcerer and the Mirror: Psychiatrists and Their Children," Paper presented to the Colorado Child and Adolescent Society, 5 March 1980.
3. Margot Adler, interview, 16 December 1986.
4. Margot Adler, *Drawing Down the Moon* (Boston: Beacon Press, 1981).
5. *Letters of John Adams Addressed to His Wife*, edited by Charles Francis Adams (Boston: Little, Brown, 1841), vol. 2, letter 78.
6. Nicholas Meyer, interview, 24 February 1985.
7. Barry Schwartz, interview, 11 April 1985.
8. Martin Freud, *Sigmund Freud: Man and Father* (New York: Vanguard Press, 1958; originally published as *Glory Reflected*, London: Angus & Robertson, 1957), p. 9.
9. William F. Murphy, "Narcissistic Problems in Patients and Therapists," *International Journal of Psychoanalytic Psychotherapy* 2 (1973): p. 115.
10. Otto F. Kernberg, "Factors in the Psychoanalytic Treatment of Narcissistic Personalities," *Journal of the American Psychoanalytic Association* 18 (1970): 54.

Bibliography

Aaron, Ruth. "The Analyst's Emotional Life During Work." *Journal of the American Psychoanalytic Association* 22 (1974):160–69.

Abraham, Hilda C. *Karl Abraham: Biographie inachevée.* Paris: Presses Universitaires de France, 1976.

Abraham, Karl. *Clinical Papers and Essays on Psycho-analysis,* vol. 2, of *The Selected Papers of Karl Abraham.* New York: Basic Books, 1955.

Adler, Gerald. "Helplessness in the Helpers." *British Journal of Medical Psychology* 45 (1972):315–26.

————. "Psychotherapy of the Narcissistic Personality Disorder Patient: Two Contrasting Approaches," *American Journal of Psychiatry* 143 (1986):430–36.

Adler, Margot. *Drawing Down the Moon.* Boston: Beacon Press, 1981.

Alexander, Franz, and Sheldon Selesnick. *The History of Psychiatry.* New York: Harper & Row, 1966.

American Medical Association. *Socioeconomic Characteristics of Medical Practice 1983,* Chicago, American Medical Association, 1983.

American Psychiatric Association. *Diagnostic and Statistical Manual of Mental Disorders,* 3d ed. Washington, D.C.: American Psychiatric Association, 1980.

American Psychoanalytic Association. "Interpretive Commentary on Issues Raised by April 1976 Survey of Psychoanalytic Practice." 13 December 1979. Typescript.

American Psychological Association. "Preliminary Report: 1983 Doctorate Employment Survey." Human Resources Research, Washington, D.C.: American Psychological Association, 1985.

Anderson, George Christian. "Emotional Health of the Clergy." *Christian Century* 70 (1953):1260–61.

Appelbaum, Stephen A. "The Idealization of Insight." *International Journal of Psychoanalytic Psychotherapy* 4 (1975):272–302.

Ariès, Philippe. *Centuries of Childhood*. New York: Vintage Books, 1962.

Avila, Donald L., Arthur W. Combs, and William W. Purkey. *The Helping Relationship Sourcebook*. Boston: Allyn & Bacon, 1971.

Barron, Jules. "A Father-Son, Therapist-Patient Relationship." *Voices* 7, no. 4 (winter 1971–72):43–45.

Beekman, Daniel. *The Mechanical Baby*. New York: New American Library, 1977.

Beitman, Bernard D. "The Demographics of American Psychotherapists: A Pilot Study." *American Journal of Psychotherapy* 37 (1983):37–48.

Benedek, Elissa P. "Training the Woman Resident to Be a Psychiatrist." *American Journal of Psychiatry* 130 (1973):1131–35.

Benedek, Therese. "Countertransference in the Training Analyst." *Bulletin of the Menninger Clinic* 18 (1954):12–16.

Bennet, Glin. *Patients and Their Doctors*. London: Baillière Tindall, 1979.

Bergman, Jerry. "The Rate of Suicide among Psychiatrists: Why Not Lower?" *Psychology: A Quarterly Review of Human Behavior* 16, no. 4 (winter 1979–80):7–19.

Bermak, Gordon E. "Do Psychiatrists Have Special Emotional Problems?" *American Journal of Psychoanalysis* 37 (1977):141–46.

Bertin, Celia. *Marie Bonaparte: A Life*. New York: Harcourt Brace Jovanovich, 1982.

Bettelheim, Bruno. *The Uses of Enchantment*. New York: Knopf, 1976.

———. "Punishment versus Discipline." *Atlantic Monthly*, November 1985, pp. 51–59.

Bird, Brian. "The Curse of Insight." *Bulletin of the Philadelphia Association for Psychoanalysis* 7 (1957):101–4.

Blos, Peter. *The Adolescent Personality*. New York and London. Appleton-Century, 1941.

———. *The Young Adolescent*. New York: Free Press, 1970.

Blum, Alan F., and Larry Rosenberg. "Some Problems Involved in Professionalizing Social Interaction: The Case of Psychotherapeutic Training." *Journal of Health and Social Behavior* 9 (1968):72–85.

Bromberg, Walter. *The Mind of Man*. New York: Harper & Row, 1959.

Brome, Vincent. *Ernest Jones: Freud's Alter Ego*. New York: Norton, 1983.

Bucher, Rue. "The Psychiatric Residency and Professional Socialization." *Journal of Health and Human Behavior* 6 (1965): 197–206.

Bugental, J. F. T. "The Person Who Is the Psychotherapist." *Journal of Consulting Psychology* 28 (1964):272–77.

Burton, Arthur, and Associates. *Twelve Therapists*. San Francisco: Jossey-Bass, 1972.

Cameron, P., and E. Persad. "Recruitment into Psychiatry: A Study of the Timing and Process of Choosing Psychiatry as a Career." *Canadian Journal of Psychiatry* 29 (1984):676–80.

Cath, Stanley H., Alan R. Gurwitt, and John Munder Ross, eds. *Father and Child*. Boston: Little, Brown, 1982.

Chessick, Richard D. *How Psychotherapy Heals*. New York: Science House, 1969.

———. "Intensive Psychotherapy for the Psychiatrist's Family." *American Journal of Psychotherapy* 31 (1977):516–24.

———. "The Sad Soul of the Psychiatrist." *Bulletin of the Menninger Clinic* 42 (1978):109.

Christensen, C. W., "The Occurrence of Mental Illness in the Ministry." *Journal of Pastoral Care* 13 (1959):79–87; 14 (1960):13–20; 17 (1963):1–10; and 17 (1963):125–35.

Cogan, Thomas P. "A Study of Friendship among Psychotherapists." *Dissertation Abstracts International* 38/09B (1978):4445.

Cohen, David. *J. B. Watson: The Founder of Behaviourism*. London: Routledge & Kegan Paul, 1979.

Coles, Jane H., and Robert Coles. "Our Work Our Children." *Parents*, February 1979, pp. 70–73.

Cooper, Arnold M. "Some Limitations on Therapeutic Effectiveness: the 'Burnout Syndrome' in Psychoanalysts." *Psychoanalytic Quarterly* 55 (1986):576–98.

Cronkite, Kathy. *On the Edge of the Spotlight*. New York: Morrow, 1981.

deMause, Lloyd, ed. *The History of Childhood*. New York: Harper Torchbooks, 1975.

Deutsch, Albert. *The Mentally Ill in America*. 2d ed. (New York: Columbia University Press, 1949).

Deutsch, Connie J. "Self-Reported Sources of Stress among Psychotherapists." *Professional Psychology* 15 (1984):833–45.

———. "A Survey of Therapists' Personal Problems and Treatment." *Professional Psychology* 16 (1985):305–15.

Deutsch, Helene. *Neuroses and Character Types: Clinical Psychoanalytic Studies*. New York: International Universities Press, 1965.

————. *Confrontations with Myself.* New York: Norton, 1973.

Dorn, Robert M. "Psychoanalysis and Psychoanalytic Education: What Kind of 'Journey'?" *Psychoanalytic Forum* 3 (1969): 239–74. Includes discussions by Henriette R. Klein, Edith Weigert, Seward Hiltner, Leon Grinberg, David Kairys, and William S. Horowitz.

Draper, Edgar. "An Illusion's Past." In *Healer of the Mind,* edited by Paul E. Johnson, pp. 110–19. Nashville and New York: Abingdon Press.

Eber, Milton, and Lyle B. Kunz. "The Desire to Help Others." *Bulletin of the Menninger Clinic* 48 (1984):125–40.

Eiler, Mary Ann. *Physician Characteristics and Distribution in the U.S.* 1982 ed. Chicago: American Medical Association, 1983.

Ekstein, Rudolf. "Omnipotence and Omni-Impotence: Phases of the Training Process." *International Journal of Psychoanalysis* 4 (1967):443–48.

Ellenberger, Henri F. *The Discovery of the Unconscious.* New York: Basic Books, 1970.

Erikson, Erik H. *Childhood and Society.* New York: Norton, 1950.

————. *Identity: Youth and Crisis.* New York: Norton, 1968.

Evans, James L. "Psychiatric Illness in the Physician's Wife." *American Journal of Psychiatry* 122 (1965):159–63.

Farber, Barry A. "The Effects of Psychotherapeutic Practice upon Psychotherapists." *Psychotherapy* 20 (1983):174–82.

Felton, Judith. "A Psychoanalyst's 'First Sample of the Technique' to Work Through Inhibitions." *Current Issues in Psychoanalytic Practice* 1 (1984):73–77.

Ferenczi, Sandor. "The Sons of the 'Tailor.' " In idem, *Further Contributions to the Theory and Technique of Psychoanalysis,* edited by John Rickman. New York: Basic Books, 1926, 1952, pp. 418–19.

Finell, Janet S. "Narcissistic Problems in Analysts." *International Journal of Psychoanalysis* 66 (1985):433–45.

Fisher, Bob, and Arthur Marx. *The Impossible Years.* New York: Samuel French, 1964.

Fliess, Robert. "The Metapsychology of the Analyst." *Psychoanalytic Quarterly* 11 (1942):211–27.

Ford, E. S. C., "Being and Becoming a Psychotherapist: The Search for Identity." *American Journal of Psychotherapy* 17 (1963):472–82.

Fox, Ron. "Lessons from a Therapist's Wife." *Voices* 7, no. 4 (winter 1971–72):36–37.

Freeman, Walter. "Psychiatrists Who Kill Themselves: A Study in Suicide." *American Journal of Psychiatry* 124 (1967):846–47.

————. *The Psychiatrist*. New York and London: Grune & Stratton, 1968.

Freidson, Eliot, and Judith Lorber, eds. *Medical Men and Their Work*. Chicago and New York: Aldine-Atherton, 1972.

Freud, Anna. *Introduction to the Technic of Child Analysis*. New York and Washington: Nervous and Mental Disease Publishing, 1928.

————. *The Ego and the Mechanisms of Defense*. New York: International Universities Press, 1946.

————. *Normality and Pathology in Childhood: Assessments of Development*. New York: International Universities Press, 1965.

Freud, Martin. *Sigmund Freud: Man and Father*. New York: Vanguard Press, 1958.

Freud, Sigmund. *The Origins of Psycho-analysis: Letters to Wilhelm Fliess*. New York: Basic Books, 1954.

————. *The Standard Edition of the Complete Psychological Works of Sigmund Freud*, edited by James Strachey. 24 vols. London: Hogarth Press, 1953–74.

Freudenberger, Herbert J., and Arthur Robbins. "The Hazards of Being a Psychoanalyst." *Psychoanalytic Review* 66 (1979):275–96.

Fried, Edrita. *The Courage to Change*. New York: Brunner-Mazel, 1980.

Fromm-Reichmann, Frieda. *Principles of Intensive Psychotherapy*. Chicago: University of Chicago Press, 1950.

Fuller, Robert E. "Headshrinker: The Psychiatrist in Cartoons." *Bulletin of the Menninger Clinic* 36 (1972):335–45.

Gartrell, Nanette, et al. "Psychiatrist-Patient Sexual Contact: Results of a National Survey, I: Prevalence." *American Journal of Psychiatry* 143 (1986):1126–31.

————. "Reporting Practices of Psychiatrists Who Knew of Sexual Misconduct by Colleagues." *American Journal of Orthopsychiatry* 57 (1987):287–95.

Garvey, Michael J. "Stability of Physicians' Marriages." *Medical Aspects of Human Sexuality* 14 (1980):34–40.

Garvey, Michael, and Vincente B. Tuason. "Physician Marriages." *Journal of Clinical Psychiatry* 40 (1979):129–31.

Gilberg, Arnold L. "Adaptation and the Psychiatrist in a World of Change." *Journal of the American Academy of Psychoanalysis* 2 (1974):55–61.

———. "The Psychoanalyst: An Agent of the Social Milieu." *American Journal of Psychoanalysis* 36 (1976):325–29.

Gildea, Margaret C.-L., and Edwin F. Gildea. "Personalities of American Psychotherapists." *American Journal of Psychiatry* 101 (1945):460–67.

Ginott, Haim. "How Psychotherapists Deal with Their Own Children." *Voices* 7, no. 4 (winter 1971–72):39–42.

Gitelson, Maxwell. "The Emotional Position of the Analyst in the Psycho-analytic Situation." *International Journal of Psycho-Analysis* 23 (1952):1–10.

Glenn, Jules. "Freud's Advice to Hans's Father: The First Supervisory Sessions." In *Freud and his Patients*, edited by Mark Kanzer and Jules Glenn, pp. 121–27. New York: Jason Aronson, 1980.

———. "Notes on the Causes and Effects of Therapy by Parents." *International Journal of Psychoanalytic Psychotherapy* 10 (1984–85):525–31.

Glover, Edward. "The Psychology of the Psychotherapist." *British Journal of Medical Psychology* 35 (1962):47–57.

Goldberg, Arnold L. "On the Prognosis and Treatment of Narcissism." *Journal of the American Psychoanalytic Association* 22 (1974):243–54.

Goldney, Robert, et al. "The Psychiatrist's Family: A Comparative Study." *Australian and New Zealand Journal of Psychiatry* 13 (1979):341–47.

Goode, William J. "Community Within a Community: The Professions." *American Sociological Review* 22 (1957):194–200.

Goz, Rebecca. "On Knowing the Therapist 'as a Person.' " *International Journal of Psychoanalytic Psychotherapy* 4 (1975):437–58.

Graf, Max. "Reminiscences of Professor Sigmund Freud." *Psychoanalytic Quarterly* 11 (1942):465–76.

Greben, Stanley E. "Some Difficulties and Satisfactions Inherent in the Practice of Psychoanalysis." *International Journal of Psychoanalysis* 56 (1975):427–34.

Greenacre, Phyllis. "Problems of Overidealization of the Analyst and of Analysis: Their Manifestations in the Transference and Countertransference Relationship." In idem, *Emotional Growth*, vol. 2, pp. 743–61. New York: International Universities Press, 1971.

Greenson, Ralph R. "That 'Impossible' Profession." *Journal of the American Psychoanalytic Association* 14 (1966):9–27.

———. *The Technique and Practice of Psychoanalysis*. New York: International Universities Press, 1967.

Greenson, Ralph R., and M. Wexler. "The Non-transference Relationship in the Psychoanalytic Situation." *International Journal of Psycho-Analysis* 50 (1969):27–39.

Groesbeck, C. Jess. "The Archetypal Image of the Wounded Healer." *Journal of Analytical Psychology* 20 (1975):122–45.

Groesbeck, C. Jess, and Benjamin Taylor. "The Psychiatrist as Wounded Physician." *American Journal of Psychoanalysis* 37 (1977):131–39.

Grosskurth, Phyllis. *Melanie Klein: Her World and Her Work.* New York: Knopf, 1986.

Guest, Lester. "The Public's Attitudes Toward Psychologists." *American Psychologist* 3 (1948):135–39.

Guggenbühl-Craig, Adolf. *Power in the Helping Professions.* Dallas: Spring Publications, 1971.

Guy, James D. *The Personal Life of the Psychotherapist.* New York: Wiley, 1987.

Guy, James D., and Gary P. Liaboe. "Suicide Among Psychotherapists: Review and Discussion." *Professional Psychology* 16 (1985):470–72.

———. "The Impact of Conducting Psychotherapy on Psychotherapists' Interpersonal Functioning." *Professional Psychology* 17 (1986):111–14.

Halleck, Seymour L., and Sherwyn M. Woods. "Emotional Problems of Psychiatric Residents." *Psychiatry* 25 (1962):339–46.

Halpern, Howard M., and Leona N. Lesser. "Empathy in Infants, Adults and Psychotherapists." *Psychoanalytic Review* 47 (1960):32–42.

Hardyment, Christina. *Dream Babies.* New York: Harper & Row, 1983.

Hariman, Jusuf, ed. *Does Psychotherapy Really Help People?* Springfield, Ill.: Charles C Thomas, 1984.

Henry, William E. "Some Observations on the Lives of Healers." *Human Development* 9 (1966):47–56.

———. "Personal and Social Identities of Psychotherapists." In *Effective Psychotherapy: A Handbook of Research*, edited by Alan S. Gurman and Andrew M. Razin. Oxford: Pergamon Press, 1977, pp. 47–62.

Henry, William E., John H. Sims, and S. Lee Spray. *The Fifth Profession: Becoming a Psychotherapist.* San Francisco: Jossey-Bass, 1971.

———. *Public and Private Lives of Psychotherapists.* San Francisco: Jossey-Bass, 1973.

Herron, William G., and Sheila Rouslin. *Issues in Psychotherapy.* Bowie, Md., Robert J. Brady, 1982.

Hersh, Stephen P. *The Executive Parent.* New York: Sovereign, 1979.

Hogan, Daniel B. *A Review of Malpractice Suits in the United States*. vol. 3 of *The Regulation of Psychotherapists*. Cambridge, Mass.: Ballinger, 1979.

Hollingshead, August B., and Frederick C. Redlich. *Social Class and Mental Illness: A Community Study*. New York: Wiley, 1958.

Holt, Robert R., and Lester Luborsky. *Personality Patterns of Psychiatrists: A Study of Methods for Selecting Residents*. Menninger Clinic Monograph Series no. 13. New York: Basic Books, 1958.

Humphrey, Frederick G. "Therapists' Own Marriages." *Family Therapy Newsletter*, May–June 1984, p. 6.

Hunt, David. *Parents and Children in History*. New York: Basic Books, 1970.

Jackson, Michael R. *Self-Esteem and Meaning: A Life Historical Investigation*. Albany: State University of New York Press, 1984.

Janowitz, Tama. *American Dad*. New York: Putnam, 1981.

Jensen, Peter S., Ronel L. Lewis, and Stephen N. Xenakis. "The Military Family in Review: Context, Risk, and Prevention." *Journal of the American Academy of Child Psychiatry* 25 (1986):225–34.

Joint Information Service. *Psychiatrists and Their Patients*. Washington, D.C.: Joint Information Service of the American Psychiatric Association and the National Association for Mental Health, 1973.

Jones, Ernest. "The God Complex." In idem, *Essays in Applied Psychoanalysis*, vol. 2, pp. 244–65. London: Hogarth Press, 1951.

———. *The Life and Work of Sigmund Freud*. 3 vols. New York: Basic Books, 1953–55.

———. *Free Associations: Memories of a Psycho-Analyst*. New York: Basic Books, 1959.

Jones, Kathleen. *Lunacy, Law and Conscience, 1744–1845*. London: Routledge & Kegan Paul, 1955.

Jung, C. G., *Analytical Psychology: Its Theory and Practice*. New York: Pantheon, 1968.

Kakar, Sudhir. *Shamans, Mystics, and Doctors*. New York: Knopf, 1982.

Kales, Joyce D., Enos D. Martin, and Constantin R. Soldatos. "Emotional Problems of Physicians and Their Families." *Pennsylvania Medicine* 81, no. 12 (December 1976):14.

Kanzer, Mark, and Jules Glenn. *Freud and His Patients*. New York: Jason Aronson, 1980.

Kaplan, Louise J. *Adolescence: The Farewell to Childhood*. New York: Simon & Schuster, 1984.

Kardener, Sheldon H., and Marielle Fuller. "The Firstborn Phenomenon Among Psychiatric Residents." *American Journal of Psychiatry* 129 (1972):350–52.

Kerényi, Carl. *Asklepios: Archetypal Image of the Physician's Existence.* New York: Bollingen–Pantheon, 1959.

Kernberg, Otto F. "Factors in the Psychoanalytic Treatment of Narcissistic Personalities." *Journal of the American Psychoanalytic Association* 18 (1970):51–85.

————. "Contrasting Viewpoints Regarding the Nature and Psychoanalytic Treatment of Narcissistic Personalities: A Preliminary Communication." *Journal of the American Psychoanalytic Association* 22 (1974):255–67.

Khan, M. Masud R. *Hidden Selves*. New York: International Universities Press, 1983.

Kiev, Ari. "Primitive Therapy: A Cross-Cultural Study of the Relationship between Child Training and Therapeutic Practices Related to Illness." *Psychoanalytic Study of Society* 1 (1960):185–217.

Kirschenbaum, Howard. *On Becoming Carl Rogers*. New York: Delta, 1979.

Klein, Henriette. "Myths of Psychiatric Training." *International Journal of Psychoanalysis.* 4 (1967):448–50.

Klein, Melanie. *Narrative of a Child Analysis*. New York: Delta Books reprint, 1975.

Knutsen, Elaine J. "On the Emotional Well-Being of Psychiatrists: Overview and Rationale," *American Journal of Psychoanalysis* 37 (1977):123–29.

Kohut, Heinz. *The Restoration of the Self*. New York: International Universities Press, 1977.

————. *The Search for the Self*. 2 vols. New York: International Universities Press, 1978.

————. *How Does Analysis Cure?* Chicago and London: University of Chicago Press, 1984.

Koran, Lorrin M., ed. *The Nation's Psychiatrists*. Washington, D.C.: American Psychiatric Association, 1987.

Kottler, Jeffrey A., *On Being a Therapist*. San Francisco: Jossey-Bass, 1986.

Kreitman, Norman. "Psychiatric Training: A Transatlantic Viewpoint." *International Journal of Psychoanalysis* 4 (1967):451–52.

Kubie, Lawrence S. *Practical and Theoretical Aspects of Psychoanalysis*. Rev. ed. New York: International Universities Press, 1975.

Landis, Bernard, and Edward S. Tauber. *In the Name of Life*. New York: Holt, Rinehart & Winston, 1971.

Langs, Robert. *Madness and Cure*. Emerson, N.J.: Newconcept Press, 1985.

Levin, Edward S. "The 'Doctor Game' Revisited: Doctors' Treatment of Their Own Children." *International Journal of Psychoanalytic Psychotherapy* 10 (1984–85):505–25.

Levinson, Daniel J., et al. *The Seasons of a Man's Life*. New York: Knopf, 1978.

LeVine, Robert A. *Culture, Behavior, and Personality*. Chicago: Aldine, 1973.

Lewis J. "The Doctor and His Marriage," *Texas State Journal of Medicine* 6 (1965):615–19.

Lewis, Jerry M. *To Be a Therapist*. New York: Brunner/Mazel, 1978.

Lifson, Lawrence E. "Analysis of a Psychoanalytic Society: Boston 1984." *American Psychoanalytic Association Newsletter* 21, no. 3 (Fall 1987):6–7, 10–11.

Light, Donald. "Professional Superiority." Paper presented at the annual meeting of the American Sociological Association, Montreal, August 1974.

———. *Becoming Psychiatrists*. New York: Norton, 1980.

Low, Barbara. "The Psychological Compensations of the Analyst." *International Journal of Psycho-Analysis* 16 (1935):1–8.

McDonald, Marjorie. "The Psychoanalytic Concept of the Self." *Psychiatric Clinics of North America*, 4 (1981):429–34.

Mackie, R. E. "Family Problems in Medical and Nursing Families." *British Journal of Medical Psychology* 40 (1967):333–40.

Maeder, Alphonse. *Ways to Psychic Health*. New York: Scribner's, 1953.

Maeder, Thomas. *Crime and Madness: The Origins and Evolution of the Insanity Defense*. New York: Harper & Row, 1985.

Mahler, Margaret S. "*Les enfants terribles*." In *The Selected Papers of Margaret S. Mahler*, vol. 1, pp. 17–33. New York: Jason Aronson, 1979.

Marmor, Judd. "The Feeling of Superiority: An Occupational Hazard in the Practice of Psychotherapy." *American Journal of Psychiatry* 110 (1953):370–76.

———. "The Psychoanalyst as a Person." *American Journal of Psychoanalysis* 37 (1977):275–84.

———. "Some Factors Involved in Occupation-Related Depression Among Psychiatrists." *Psychiatric Annals* 12 (1982):913–20.

Masson, Jeffrey Moussaieff. *The Assault on Truth: Freud's Suppression of the Seduction Theory*. New York: Farrar, Straus & Giroux, 1984.

Mattera, Marianne D. "Why Psychiatrists Are Behind the Economic Eight Ball." *Medical Economics*, 5 February 1979, pp. 158–62, 167.

Mehlman, Robert D. "Becoming and Being a Psychotherapist: The Problem of Narcissism." *International Journal of Psychoanalytic Psychotherapy*, 3 (1974):125–40.

Menninger, Karl. "What Are the Goals of Psychiatric Education?" *Bulletin of the Menninger Clinic* 16 (1952):153–58.

———. "Psychological Factors in the Choice of Medicine as a Profession." *Bulletin of the Menninger Clinic* 21 (1957):51–58, 99–106.

Meloy, J. Reid. "Narcissistic Psychopathology and the Clergy." *Pastoral Psychology* 35 (1986):50–55.

Miller, Alice. *The Drama of the Gifted Child*. New York: Basic Books, 1981.

———. *For Your Own Good*. New York: Farrar, Straus & Giroux, 1983.

———. *Thou Shalt Not Be Aware*. New York: Farrar, Straus & Giroux, 1984.

Moreno, J. L., Zerka Moreno, and Jonathan Moreno. *The First Psychodramatic Family*. Beacon, N.Y.: Beacon House, 1964.

Morgan, David W. "A Note on Analytic Group Psychotherapy for Therapists and Their Wives." *International Journal of Group Psychotherapy* 21 (1971):244–47.

Murphy, William F. "Narcissistic Problems in Patients and Therapists." *International Journal of Psychoanalytic Psychotherapy* 2 (1973):113–24.

National Institute of Mental Health. *The Nation's Psychiatrists*. Public Health Service Publication no. 1885. Chevy Chase, Md., 1969.

Neill, John R., and Arnold M. Ludwig. "Psychiatry and Psychotherapy: Past and Future." *American Journal of Psychotherapy* 34 (1980):39–50.

Nelson, Sarah B. "Some Dynamics of Medical Marriages." *Journal of the Royal College of General Practitioners* 28 (1978):585–86.

———. "Is There a Doctor in the House?" *Journal of the Royal College of General Practitioners* 31 (1981):715–22.

Nieporent, James. Letter to the editor. *Village Voice*, 28 February 1977.

Olch, Gerald B. "Technical Problems in the Analysis of the Preoedipal and Preschool Child." *Journal of the American Psychoanalytic Association* 19 (1971):543–51.

Olden, Christine. "On Adult Empathy with Children." *Psychoanalytic Study of the Child* 8 (1953):111–26.

Olinick, Stanley L. "The Analytic Paradox." *Psychiatry* 22 (1959):333–39.

Ornstein, Anna. "Self-Pathology in Childhood: Developmental and Clinical Considerations." *Psychiatric Clinics of North America,* 4 (1981):444–53.

Ornstein, Paul H. "Selected Problems in Learning How to Analyze." *International Journal of Psychoanalysis* 48 (1967):448–61.

Pasnau, Robert O., and Stephen J. Bayley. "Personality Changes in the First Year of Psychiatric Residency Training." *American Journal of Psychiatry.* 128 (1971):79–84.

Payne, George Henry. *The Child in Human Progress.* New York and London: Putnam's, 1916.

Paul, Louis, "A Note on the Private Aspect and Professional Aspect of the Psychoanalyst." *Bulletin of the Philadelphia Association for Psychoanalysis* 9 (1959):96–101.

Peters, Uwe Henrik. *Anna Freud: A Life Dedicated to Children.* New York: Schocken Books, 1984.

Psychotherapy Finances. "1985 Survey Report." *Psychotherapy Finances,* 12, no. 9 (1985):1–8.

Pumpian-Mindlin, Eugene. "Problems of Professional Identity in Training Psychiatrists." *Journal of Nervous and Mental Disease* 144 (1967):535–38.

Quinn, Susan. *A Mind of Her Own: The Life of Karen Horney.* New York: Summit Books, 1987.

Racusin, G. R., S. I. Abramowitz, and W. D. Winter. "Becoming a Therapist: Family Dynamics and Career Choice." *Professional Psychology* 12 (1981):271–79.

Rank, Otto. *The Myth of the Birth of the Hero.* New York: Basic Books, 1952.

Redlich, Frederick C. "The Psychiatrist in Caricature: An Analysis of Unconscious Attitudes toward Psychiatry." *American Journal of Orthopsychiatry* 20 (1950):560–71.

Reich, Peter. *A Book of Dreams.* New York: Harper & Row, 1973.

Reik, Theodor. *Listening with the Third Ear.* New York: Farrar, Straus, 1948.

———. *Curiosities of the Self.* New York: Farrar, Straus & Giroux, 1965.

———. *The Search Within* (1956). New York: Jason Aronson, reprint, 1974.

Reiser, David E., "The Sorcerer and the Mirror: Psychiatrists and Their Children." Paper presented to the Colorado Child and Adolescent Society, 5 March 1980.

Reynolds, Roger A., and Jonathan B. Abram, eds. *Socioeconomic Characteristics of Medical Practice, 1983*. Chicago: American Medical Association, 1983.

Rich, Charles L., and Ferris N. Pitts, Jr. "Suicide by Male Physicians during a 5-Year Period." *American Journal of Psychiatry* 136 (1979):1089–90.

————. "Suicide by Psychiatrists: A Study of Medical Specialists Among 18,730 Consecutive Physician Deaths During a Five-Year Period, 1967–72," *Journal of Clinical Psychiatry* 41 (1980):261–63.

Rieman, Fritz. "The Personality Structure of the Analyst and Its Influence on the Course of Treatment." *American Journal of Psychoanalysis* 28 (1968):69–79.

Rizzo, Francis. "Memoirs of an Invisible Man—I," *Opera News* 36 (5 February 1972):25–28.

Roazen, Paul. *Freud and His Followers*. New York: Knopf, 1975.

————. *Helene Deutsch: A Psychoanalyst's Life*. New York: Anchor-Doubleday, 1985.

Robert Wood Johnson Foundation. *Medical Practice in the United States*. Princeton: Robert Wood Johnson Foundation, 1981.

Robertiello, Richard C. "The Occupational Disease of Psychotherapists." *Journal of Contemporary Psychotherapy* 9 (1978):123–29.

————. *A Man in the Making: Grandfathers, Fathers, Sons*. New York: Richard Marek, 1979.

————. *A Psychoanalyst's Quest*. New York: St. Martin's-Marek, 1986.

Robertiello, Richard C., and Jonathan Goldman. "The 'Spock' Children." *Voices* 10 (1974):71–75.

Roberts, Caton. "In Retrospect: Son of a Shrink," *Voices* 12, no. 4 (winter 1976–77):11–15.

Robinson, David Owen. "The Medical-Student Spouse Syndrome: Grief Reactions to the Clinical Years." *American Journal of Psychiatry* 135 (1978):972–74.

Roeske, Nancy A. "Women in Psychiatry: Past and Present Areas of Concern." *American Journal of Psychiatry* 130 (1973):1127–31.

————. "Women in Psychiatry: A Review." *American Journal of Psychiatry* 133 (1976):365–72.

————. "Life Stories as Careers: Careers as Life Stories." *Perspectives in Biology and Medicine* 28 (1985):229–42.

Rogers, Carl. *On Becoming a Person*. Boston: Houghton Mifflin, 1961.

Rogow, Arnold A. *The Psychiatrists*. New York: Putnam, 1970.

Rohrlich, Jay B. *Work and Love: The Crucial Balance*. New York: Harmony Books, 1980.

Rose, K. Daniel, and Irving Rosow. "Marital Stability among Physicians." *California Medicine* 116 (1972):95–99.

Rosen, Winifred. *Cruisin for a Bruisin*. New York: Dell, 1977.

Rossner, Judith. *August*. Boston: Houghton Mifflin, 1983.

Roy, Alec. "Suicide in Doctors." *Psychiatric Clinics of North America* 8 (1985):377–87.

Rubins, Jack L. *Karen Horney: Gentle Rebel of Psychoanalysis*. New York: Dial Press, 1978.

Russell, Andrew T., Robert O. Pasnau, and Zebulon C. Taintor. "Emotional Problems of Residents in Psychiatry." *American Journal of Psychiatry* 132 (1975):263–67.

Safinofsky, I. "Suicide in Doctors and Wives of Doctors." *Canadian Family Physician* 26 (1980):837–44.

Salk, Lee. *My Father, My Son*. New York: Putnam, 1982.

Saul, Leon J. *The Childhood Emotional Pattern and Corey Jones*. New York: Van Nostrand Reinhold, 1977.

Schafer, Roy. *A New Language for Psychoanalysis*. New Haven and London: Yale University Press, 1976.

———. *The Analytic Attitude*. New York: Basic Books, 1983.

Schatzman, Leonard, and Anselm Strauss. "A Sociology of Psychiatry: A Perspective and Some Organizing Foci." In *Medical Men and Their Work*, edited by Eliot Friedson and Judith Lorber (Chicago and New York: Aldine-Atherton, 1972), pp. 128–44.

Scher, Maryonda. "Women Psychiatrists in the United States." *American Journal of Psychiatry* 130 (1973):1118–22.

Scher, Maryonda, et al. "Psychiatrist-Wife-Mother: Some Aspects of Role Integration." *American Journal of Psychiatry* 133 (1976):830–34.

Schmideberg, Melitta, " 'After the Analysis. . . .' " *Psychoanalytic Quarterly* 7 (1938):122–42.

———. "Iatrogenic Disturbance." Correspondence. *American Journal of Psychiatry* 119 (1963):899.

Schwartz, Lynne S. *Acquainted with the Night*. New York: Harper & Row, 1984.

Scott, Cynthia D., and Joann Hawk. *Heal Thyself: The Health of Health Care Professionals*. New York: Brunner/Mazel, 1986.

Searles, Harold F. "Feelings of Guilt in the Psychoanalyst." *Psychiatry* 29 (1966):319–23.

————. "The Patient as Therapist to His Analyst." In *Countertransference*, vol. 2 of *Tactics and Techniques in Psychoanalytic Therapy*, edited by Peter L. Giovacchini, pp. 95–195. New York: Jason Aronson, 1975.

Sedgwick, John: *Rich Kids*. New York: Morrow, 1985.

Sharaf, Myron. *Fury on Earth: A Biography of Wilhelm Reich*. New York: St. Martin's Press-Marek, 1983.

Sharaf, Myron R., and Daniel J. Levinson. "The Quest for Omnipotence in Professional Training." *Psychiatry* 27 (1964):135–49.

Sharaf, Myron R., Patricia Scheider, and David Kantor. "Psychiatric Interest and Its Correlates among Medical Students." *Psychiatry* 31 (1968): 150–60.

Sharpe, Ella, "The Psycho-analyst." *International Journal of Psychoanalysis* 28 (1947):1–6.

Shaw, Jon A. "Children in the Military." *Psychiatric Annals* 17 (1987):539–44.

Shem, Samuel. *Fine*. New York: Dell, 1985.

Shepherd, Michael. "A Failure of Omnipotent Strivings." *International Journal of Psychoanalysis* 4 (1967):453–54.

Sherman, Murray H. "Theodor Reik: The Man." Introduction to *The Search Within*, by Theodor Reik. New York: Jason Aronson, 1974.

Sidis, Boris. *Philistine and Genius*. New York: Moffat, Yard, 1911.

Sidis, Wiliam James. *The Animate and the Inanimate*. Boston: Richard G. Badger, 1925.

————[Frank Folupa, pseud.]. *Notes on the Collection of Transfers*. Philadelphia: Dorrance, 1926.

Sifford, Darrell. "Facing the Real Issues in Parent-Child Conflicts." *Philadelphia Inquirer*, 15 January 1985.

Silverberg, W. "Acting Out versus Insight: A Problem in Psychoanalytic Technique." *Psychoanalytic Quarterly* 24 (1955):527–44.

Silverman, M. A. "A Fresh Look at the Case of Little Hans." In *Freud and His Patients*, edited by Mark Kanzer and Jules Glenn, pp. 96–120. New York: Jason Aronson, 1980.

Simmel, Ernst. "A Screen-memory in *Statu Nascendi*." *International Journal of Psycho-Analysis* 6 (1925):454–57.

————. "The 'Doctor-Game,' Illness and the Profession of Medicine." *International Journal of Psycho-Analysis* 7 (1926):470–83.

Skinner, B. F. *The Shaping of a Behaviorist*. New York: Knopf, 1979.

Slovenko, Ralph. "On the Metamorphosis of Psychiatrists, Their Spouses and Offspring into Lawyers." *Journal of Law and Psychiatry* 15 (1987): 325–66.

Snyder, Susan, and C. R. Snyder. "The Therapist at Home: Her Side and His." *Voices* 7, no. 4 (winter 1971–72):23–25.

Stern, Paul J. *C. G. Jung: The Haunted Prophet*. New York: Braziller, 1976.

Strean, Herbert S. "Psychotherapy with Children of Psychotherapists." *Psychoanalytic Review* 56 (1969):377–86.

———. *Controversy in Psychotherapy*. Metuchen, N.J., and London: Scarecrow Press, 1982.

"Suicide Among Doctors." *British Medical Journal* 1 (1964):789.

Sulman, A. Michael. *The Freudianization of the American Child: The Impact of Psychoanalysis in Popular Periodical Literature in the United States, 1919–1939*. Ann Arbor, Mich.: University Microfilms, 1973.

Švrakić, Dragan M. "On Narcissistic Ethics." *American Journal of Psychoanalysis* 46 (1986):55–61.

Szasz, Thomas S. "On the Experiences of the Analyst in the Psychoanalytic Situation." *Journal of the American Psychoanalytic Association* 4 (1956): 197–223.

Tartakoff, Helen H. "The Normal Personality in Our Culture and the Nobel Prize Complex." In *Psychoanalysis: A General Psychology*, edited by Rudolph Loewenstein et al., pp. 222–52. New York: International Universities Press, 1966.

Taube, Carl A., et al. "Patients of Psychiatrists and Psychologists in Office-based Practice, 1980." *American Psychologist* 39 (1984):1435–47.

Taylor, Gordon Rattray. *The Angel Makers*. London: Heinemann, 1958.

Thoreson, Richard W., Frank C. Budd, and Charles J. Krauskopf. "Perceptions of Alcohol Misuse and Work Behavior among Professionals: Identification and Intervention." *Professional Psychology* 17 (1986):210–16.

Thurber, James. "Where Are They Now?" *The New Yorker*, 14 August 1937, pp. 22–26.

Torrey, E. Fuller. *The Mind Game*. New York: Bantam, 1973.

Tournier, Paul. *Secrets*, translated by Joe Embry. Richmond, Va.: John Knox Press, 1963.

Van der Waals, H. G. "Problems of Narcissism." *Bulletin of the Menninger Clinic* 29 (1965):293–311.

Vincent, M. O. "Doctor and Mrs.: Their Mental Health." *Canadian Psychiatric Association Journal* 14 (1969):509–15.

Viscott, David S. *The Making of a Psychiatrist*. Greenwich, Conn.: Fawcett, 1972.

Waelder, Robert. *Basic Theory of Psychoanalysis*. New York: International Universities Press, 1960.

Wallace, Amy. *The Prodigy*. New York: Dutton, 1986.

Wallace, Marquis Earl. "Private Practice: A Nationwide Study." *Social Work* 27 (1982):262–67.

Wallerstein, Robert S. *Becoming a Psychoanalyst*. New York: International Universities Press, 1981.

Walton, H. J. "Personality Correlates of a Career Interest in Psychiatry." *British Journal of Psychiatry* 115 (1969):211–19.

Warkentin, John. "The Therapist's Significant Other." *Annals of Psychotherapy* 4 (1963):54–59.

Warner, Silas L. "What Is a Headshrinker?" *American Journal of Psychotherapy* 36 (1982):256–63.

Watson, John B. *Behaviorism*. New York: Norton, 1930.

Watson, Rosalie R. "I Am the Mother of a Behaviorist's Sons." *Parents' Magazine*, December 1930, pp. 16–18, 67.

Wechsler, Henry. *Handbook of Medical Specialties*. New York: Human Sciences Press, 1976.

Weiss, Edoardo. *Sigmund Freud as a Consultant: Recollections of a Pioneer in Psychoanalysis*. New York: Intercontinental Medical Book Corp., 1970.

Weissman, Myrna M. "Psychiatric Diagnoses." *Science* 235 (1987):522.

Welwood, John, ed. *Awakening the Heart*. Boulder, Colo.: New Science Library, 1983.

Wetzsteon, Ross. "Do Psychiatrists Drive Their Kids Crazy?" *Village Voice*, 14 February 1977, pp. 21–22, 24.

Wheelis, Allen. "The Vocational Hazards of Psycho-analysis." *International Journal of Psychoanalysis* 37 (1956):171–84.

———. *The Quest for Identity*. New York: Norton, 1958.

———. *The Illusionless Man*. New York: Harper Torchbooks reprint, 1971.

———. *How People Change*. New York: Harper Colophon, 1975.

Will, Otto A., Jr. "The Patient and the Psychotherapist: Comments on the 'Uniqueness' of Their Relationship." In *In the Name of Life*, edited by

Bernard Landis and Edward S. Tauber, pp. 15–43 (New York: Holt, Rinehart & Winston, 1971).

Willi, J. "Higher Incidence of Physical and Mental Ailments in Future Psychiatrists as Compared with Future Surgeons and Internal Medical Specialists at Military Conscription." *Social Psychiatry* 18 (1983):69–72.

Winnicott, D. W. "Ego Distortion in Terms of True and False Self" (1960). In *The Maturational Processes and the Facilitating Environment*, edited by idem. New York: International Universities Press, 1965, pp. 140–52.

Wishy, Bernard. *The Child and the Republic*. Philadelphia: University of Pennsylvania Press, 1968.

Wittenberg, Clarissa K. "Psychiatrists Discuss Their Parenting Skills." *Psychiatric News* 16, no. 15 (3 August 1979): 21.

Wolff, Werner. *Contemporary Psychotherapists Examine Themselves*. Springfield, Ill.: Charles C Thomas, 1956.

Wolfgang, Steven L. "Physicians Who Commit Suicide: A Stacked Deck." *Psychiatric Opinion* 12 (April 1975): 26.

Zilbergeld, Bernie. *The Shrinking of America*. Boston: Little, Brown, 1983.

Index

abandonment and betrayal feelings, 213–15

Abraham, Karl, 126–27, 127n, 242

accusatory nature of interpretations, 166–67

Adler, Alexandra, 129–30

Adler, Alfred, 69, 129–30, 242, 248

Adler, Margot, 248

alcohol abuse, 71–72, 163, 179, 180, 181, 201n, 205–6, 238

American Academy of Psychotherapists, 70

American Medical Association, 32–33

American Psychiatric Association, 4–5, 32, 40n, 42, 63, 72

American Psychoanalytic Association, 34, 35

amorality, 41, 149n, 229

appearances, 185–88, 193–94

Appelbaum, Stephen, 181

Ariès, Philippe, 94–95

army brats, 49n

arts, 237, 249–55

Asklepios, 76

asylums, 25–27

authority: and career choice, 80–81; and interpretations, 148–50, 161; and parenting, 98, 109, 115–16, 118, 141–42, 258; and private practice, 80–81; and responsibility, 204–5, 213; source of therapist's, 256. *See also* God complex

Beers, Clifford, 30

behaviorism, 98–99, 177

Bettelheim, Bruno, 156–57

blame, 160, 166–67, 227–30, 252, 253

Bloomingdale Asylum [New York], 28

Boston Psychoanalytic Society and Institute, 35

bribery, 210

camp environment, 112, 135

capitulation, 172–73

capriciousness, 178–80, 258

career choice: and alcohol abuse, 71–72; and authority, 80–81; and avoidance of dealing with problems, 77, 257; and childhood of therapists, 75–76, 79–80, 92; and clinical social workers, 74; and craziness of therapists, 70–71; and emotional problems of

career choice (*cont.*)

parent-therapist, 71–72, 74–75, 76–77, 159, 181, 256, 257; and God complex, 80–84; and insight, 181; and intellectualization, 77–78; and less-than-selfless motives, 76–77; and narcissism, 22–23, 84–86, 92, 108–9; and personal analysis, 76–78; and personality of psychotherapists, 17–18; and psychiatrists, 74; and psychoanalysts, 74; and psychologists, 74; and psychopathology, 69–70; reasons for, 69–70, 74, 256; and relationships with others, 71, 86–93; role of family in, 73–75; and self-assurance, 82–83; and therapeutic attitude, 44–45; and therapist's need for parenting, 204–5; and voyeurism, 92. *See also* professions of PsyKs

castration complex, 81n, 150n, 199

cause and effect, 179

causes and effects, 179, 183–84

Charcot, Jean Martin, 29–30

child analysis: beginnings of, 125–26; consequences of, 130–35; and emotional problems of parent-therapist, 142–45; and family life, 137; and family lore, 136–37; Freud's views about, 103–4, 121–23; and grandiosity, 132–33; and interpretations, 216–17; and personality of psychotherapist, 129–30; preventive, 198; and professions of PsyKs, 245; and proof of success, 217; and spontaneity, 129; subtle nature of, 129–30; as a taboo, 128–29; and therapeutic attitude, 132–45; and the training process, 129–30. *See also name of specific child or parent*

childhood experiences and professions of PsyKs, 247–48

childhood of therapists: and career choice, 74–75, 79–80, 92; and narcissism, 85–86; and parenting, 103, 107–8, 116–17; and permissiveness, 201, 203

child rearing. *See* parenting

children: historical views of, 94–96

children of God, 189–94

children of psychotherapists. *See* PsyKs; *name of specific topic*